SOCIAL WORK PRACTICE

WITH THE ELDERLY

SOCIAL WORK PRACTICE WITH THE ELDERLY

Third Edition

Edited by
Michael J. Holosko
and
Marvin D. Feit

Canadian Scholars' Press Inc.
Toronto

Social Work Practice with the Elderly, Third Edition
Edited by Michael J. Holosko and Marvin D. Feit

First published in 2004 by
Canadian Scholars' Press Inc.
180 Bloor Street West, Suite 801
Toronto, Ontario
M5S 2V6

www.cspi.org

Canadian Scholars' Press gratefully acknowledges financial support for our publishing activities from the Government of Canada through the Book Publishing Industry Development Program (BPIDP).

Library and Archives Canada Cataloguing in Publication

Social work practice with the elderly / edited by Michael J. Holosko and Marvin D. Feit. -- 3rd ed.

Includes bibliographical references.
ISBN 1-55130-233-0

1. Social work with older people. I. Holosko, Michael J. II. Feit, Marvin D. (Marvin David), 1942-

HV1451.S62 2004   362.6   C2004-904425-7

Cover design by Aldo Fierro
Page design and layout by Brad Horning
Cover photographs: Health Canada, © Minister of PWGSC, 2001

04 05 06 07 08   5 4 3 2 1

Printed and bound in Canada by AGMV Marquis Imprimeur Inc.

Canada

FOR OUR PARENTS,

Joseph John Holosko, Maria Mary Klochko,
and Abraham Feit and Sara Gleicher.

We thank you for not only dispelling but
shattering the societal myths associated with old age.

TABLE OF CONTENTS

Section I: Direct Practice Elements

Section II: Selected Practice Settings

Section III: Future Considerations

PREFACE

Canadian Scholars' Press and the co-editors are pleased to present the 3rd edition of *Social Work Practice with the Elderly*. The question—so what's new?—seems relevant here. This text includes: an update of all the older chapters, including a complete rewrite of some, a deletion of a few chapters, and the addition of seven new chapters on issues that students and professionals told us need to be included. Each chapter also includes a minimum of three to five Internet references as well as three to five related readings that students may find helpful for finding additional information about the subject matter in each chapter. Experienced practitioners and academics working in the field of gerontology in North America wrote this text. It is intended for use by undergraduate or graduate social work students and other helping professionals who work with the elderly.

In the past 30 years or so, we have been deluged with demographic trends and statistics that clearly project the rapid growth of the elderly population and the inability of existing health and human service agencies to adequately serve their immediate or future needs. Indeed, health and social service institutions have currently been extending their mandates and organizational parameters to serve this population. The long-standing North American tendency toward reactive (rather than proactive) policy making, and a symptom-disease orientation to helping the elderly is slowly changing. Social workers have responded by developing creative approaches to caring for the elderly, by initiating and using more holistic interventions in treatment, by injecting liberal doses of humanism into the overall care process, and being flexible in working within the contradictions of these agencies and their existing policies and procedures. The profession of social work has once again shown that its malleability and adaptation is its greatest single asset, and in this evolution it has never lost sight of its mission—to help serve the needs of its clients. Certainly, all of the chapters in this text serve as testimony to this legacy.

The revised text is organized in two main sections: Direct Practice Elements and Selected Practice Settings. The former provides the context for understanding generic practice issues that typically transcend all practice settings. The latter provide setting-specific content and case examples about working with clients in a range of different institutional, daycare, and community-based settings. These are our organizations practice domains.

In Section I, Feit and Cuevas-Feit set the stage in the first chapter for understanding both the dynamics of working with the elderly and also the multifaceted aspects of such work. They provide an overview of nine salient trends confronting workers in this field. Holosko and Holosko then attempt to distill elements about the uniqueness of social work practice with the elderly by "seeking the difference that makes the difference." In Chapter 3, Watt and Soifer present in detail both the rationale for conducting psychosocial assessments with the elderly and a protocol for how to conduct them. Birnie-Marino (in Chapter 4) diligently articulates five generic cornerstone practice issues that social workers need to address if they are to be successful in counselling the elderly. Further, Giannetti, in Chapter 5, clearly describes an important yet neglected practice issue confronting gerontological social workers—medication utilization problems and their implications. In Chapter 6 Leslie and Holosko present a case for social workers becoming more actively involved in policies that influence practice with the elderly. They outline and analyze all the social policies affecting the elderly in North America today. Holosko and Gallant identify a unique niche for gerontological social work practice—identifying the elderly alcoholic. Austin and McClelland then present a comprehensive overview of the emerging field of case management practice with the elderly. Leslie and Leslie (in Chapter 9) articulate the importance of sensory impairment losses in hearing, taste, touch, smell, and vision. Chapter 10, by Bobyk-Krumins and Holosko, presents an overview of the growing phenomenon of elder abuse. St. John and Holosko (in Chapter 11) address yet another neglected area of study with this population—social work practice with clients who have HIV/AIDS. MacKenzie presents her insightful first-hand practice accounts of working with the rural elderly in Saskatchewan in Chapter 12. Taylor and Holosko (in Chapter 13) then provide an overview of the issues regarding retirement. In Chapter 14, Wheeler presents a comprehensive analysis of volunteerism and the elderly in the final chapter of Section I.

Section II presents 10 chapters formatted in the same way: The Clientele, Practice Roles and Responsibilities, Potential for Role Development, Concluding Remarks, and Case Examples. Indeed, these chapters reflect the diverse practice settings in which gerontological social work is practised. These range from urban to rural, institutional to community-based care, acute to chronic, and wellness to disease orientations. They are all written by (and for) front-line practitioners, and are all reminders of the integral role that social work plays in serving the elderly in a variety of health and human service settings. In each of these, social workers have carved out unique niches in caring for the elderly, and have demonstrated considerable leadership, creativity, collaboration, initiative, and ability to be effective in these respective settings. The case examples in each chapter convey this message.

In Chapter 15, Martyn and Fabiano present the full range of practice issues that confront social workers practising with the growing numbers of frail elderly in North America. Patchner and Patchner then enlighten us about the realities and conduct of social work practice in nursing homes. In Chapter 17, MacKenzie focuses on practice in specialized geriatric assessment units prevalent in hospitals in both Canada and the U.S. Kleiner, Kopstein, Lagunoff, and Urman (in Chapter 18) describe the realities of practice in an integrated adult daycare program at a well-regarded, Toronto-based facility, the Baycrest Centre for Geriatric Care. Toseland, Smith, and Zinoman then provide an insightful overview of issues related to practice with the important cohort of family caregivers of frail older persons. Dicks and Venturini then describe the nuts and bolts of rural practice with mentally challenged elderly in Mississippi. Fitch, Slivinske, and Nichols (in Chapter 21) describe and analyze practice roles and responsibilities in a unique private retirement community in Ohio. Subsequently, Fitch, Slivinske, Green, and Hinkson describe practice issues affecting geriatric patients in a U.S. midwest rehabilitation hospital. Jurkowski, Kemp, and Patterson describe a current community trend of assisted living and the unique social work practice roles in such settings. Section II concludes with Kindiak, Grieve, Randall, and Madsen presenting an overview of practice in community psychogeriatric programs.

Finally, Section III, written by Holosko, White, and Feit, projects the realities of practice with the elderly in the future, pointing to the new challenges and exciting frontiers for the profession. They conclude, as do many chapters in this text, by pointing out that the future is now for gerontological social work and the profession has an important role to play in the future of service delivery for the elderly.

All of the chapters in this revised text are both descriptive and analytic and are intended to enhance an understanding of the realities of front-line social work practice with the elderly. We have learned much about practising with the elderly and it is only by sharing our knowledge that we can learn more.

Upon completion of this text, it became apparent that we still have new or budding areas of practice that social workers are currently involved in. These include: sexuality and intimacy; grandparents raising grandchildren; English as a second language (ESL) classes as an entry point for practice; elderly offenders in correctional facilities; and gay, lesbian, and transgender (GLTG) issues. Hopefully, the next edition of this text will include these and other emerging domains of social work practice. Our profession's hallmark characteristic of "starting where the client is at" is indeed an ever-evolving testimony to its mission-driven commitment to the needs of its clients and their day-to-day concerns.

Finally, it is apparent in these chapters that our education and training have lagged far behind our practice initiatives, and the profession has much work to do in this regard. Another is that much more research of a clinical, theoretical, empirical, and evidence-based nature is needed to discover, refine, test, or verify some of our cherished practice wisdom.

This is not a book about what is wrong with social work practice (which may feed the fragile insecurity of some social workers), but about what is right! We would like readers to be the judge of that.

M.J.H.

ACKNOWLEDGEMENTS

A cast of many directly and indirectly supports a work of this undertaking. Susan Silva-Wayne of Canadian Scholars' Press believed in this project and its relevance to practitioners from its inception to printing. She worked tirelessly in supporting and bringing it to fruition. Her guidance, gentle persuasion, and constructive comments greatly shaped this work. My son Joel Holosko did the important initial editing and worked diligently for long hours to move this project along with much research assistance. Cecil Houston, the dean of the Faculty of Arts and Social Science at the University of Windsor, provided much needed support in various phases of this endeavour. Donald R. Leslie provided a sounding board for the numerous iterations of this text. Katilyn Lauzon and Adrienne Holosko provided ideas for the cover concept. Finally, we acknowledge those numerous faculty, social work practitioners, researchers, and academics who used the earlier editions of this text and encouraged us to update our work. To all of them we offer sincere thanks.

M.J.H. and M.D.F.

SECTION I

DIRECT PRACTICE
ELEMENTS

CHAPTER 1

AN OVERVIEW OF SOCIAL WORK PRACTICE WITH THE ELDERLY

MARVIN D. FEIT AND

NURIA M. CUEVAS-FEIT

This chapter assesses social work practice with the elderly by identifying nine trends useful for practitioners and social work students. These are: (1) more people are getting older, particularly in the over-85 age group, and they are likely to be more active politically, economically capable, independent, and mobile; (2) older people will both need and demand more social, health, and medical services; (3) they will be hit hardest by chronic illnesses and diseases; (4) many unique situations will arise requiring attention; (5) despite possessing more resources than their predecessors, a greater share of the economic pie will be consumed by costly medical and health care; (6) benefits will continue to be provided unevenly; (7) for many people, old age will be the first time they have had any contact with health, social, and/or medical services; (8) responding to death and dying issues; and (9) the impact of technology on practice. The effects that these trends are likely to have on social work practice with the elderly are discussed.

I.   Introduction

The focus of this introductory chapter is on identifying emerging trends to better understand social work practice with the elderly. One must be able to look beyond numbers and statistics and react to the present or immediate needs of the elderly in providing meaningful services. Thus, in order to prepare practitioners for work with this clientele, one must start with the present and offer suggestions about the future direction of practice.

Two fundamental premises of this overall text have long been accepted by our society. One is that there will be more elderly people in the United States and Canada during the next 20 to 30 years than ever before. Indeed, no one doubts this reality and its importance. Kaihla (2003) noted that during the next 20 years or through the year 2023 the baby boom generation will retire, and cites Anthony Carnevale's model which "shows that within 7 years 30 million people now in the North American workforce will be older then 55, that's not a guess. It is virtually a certainty" (p. 99).

Less clear is the precise impact that this population will have on the social, economic, and political structures of the respective societies of each country. An impending impact the aging population is expected to have on society is a large skilled labour shortage. This labour shortage added to the number of unskilled workers is anticipated to reach 21 million in year 2020 (Kaihla, 2003). The problem appears to be the result of the current workforce aging and retiring and the numbers in the younger workforce just not being there.

The second premise is that as people age they require and use more health and social welfare services. It should, therefore, be of no surprise to learn of the continuous increases in Medicaid and Medicare costs resulting from increased provider costs, the increase in the number of senior citizen programs, and the increased costs of basic goods and services to this population.

Based on these factors, one is able to provide an overview of the salient issues, problems, and concerns likely to be faced by social workers as they engage in practice with the elderly during the next 20 to 30 years. The purpose of this chapter, then, is to identify these particular trends and discuss ways that they may influence gerontological social work practice. Certainly one must start with the present, and in many chapters of this text practitioners provide, in exceptional detail, their current practice realities in various social work settings. Thus, these chapters, taken as a whole, provide quite a picture of the landscape and offer a better understanding of the range of agencies and services provided to the elderly. They also reveal some interesting gaps in services and disparities among programs while offering insights about very important practice and policy issues.

However, as social workers continue to practise in this emerging field, it is likely that changes will occur as a result of, or in response to, several factors. For instance, current programs are likely to be modified or changed, new or different programs are likely to be developed (as well as specialized services), the political infrastructures and resulting policies most certainly will be different, and the character of social work practice with the elderly is likely to be profoundly affected.

Nine significant trends identified in this regard are as follows:

- While many people are getting older, they are likely to be more politically sophisticated and active, more economically capable, more mobile and independent than ever before.
- Older people will need and demand significantly more social, health, and medical services, and these services will have to be integrated in order to be most effective.
- Older people will continue to be hit hardest by illnesses and diseases that require chronic care, in addition to periodic acute medical and psychosocial problems.
- Many unique subpopulation situations and their problems will emerge and require attention, such as minority elderly not living to age 65, the "sandwich" or "squeezed" generation, etc.
- While the elderly as a group may possess more resources than their predecessors, a greater share of the economic budget is likely to be consumed by costly medical and health care.
- Benefits will continue to be provided unevenly to the elderly, i.e., those with money and/or insurance will have better health care than those without money or insurance. In turn, many elderly are likely to receive no care or inadequate care.
- For many people, old age will be the first time in their lives that they or their families have had to formally access and engage health, social, and medical programs and their services on a regular and continuing basis. These people, predominantly from the private sector, will inevitably find these programs not what they expected.
- There will be an increased need to respond to death and dying issues, particularly with the inclusion of the client and/or family members in decisions.
- There is increasingly an impact of technology on practice, and as this aspect of practice grows rapidly, it increases independence and enhances communication, albeit with caution.

A. The Politics of Aging in North America

While many persons are getting older, the largest increases among the elderly are projected to be in the 75-and-over age group. Specifically, the population of adults aged 65 and older has increased by 24 percent, while the population under age 65 has increased by only six percent in the past 20 years. Further indications are that this population will more than double in North America by 2020, and by the year 2030, 21 percent of the elderly population will be 65 years of age or older.

However, the largest relative proportionate growth of the elderly population is projected to be in the 85-and-older group in the next 20 years. This age category is estimated to grow three to four times faster than the population aged 65 to 84. The primary reason given for this is the high birth rates prior to 1920 and during the post-World War II period between 1945–1959. A number of other factors such as improved diets and better nutrition, better personal health care, better health care services, advances in medical technology, etc., have also contributed to these longevity patterns (Fitch and Slivinske, 1989).

There appears to be some disagreement in the literature regarding when actual aging begins. The definition ranges from those aged 65 years of age and older, as defined by government agencies such as Medicare or the Canadian Pension Plan, to those 50 years of age and older as defined by the American Association of Retired Persons (AARP). The most widely used definition associated with the development and implementation of age-specific programs for older adults appears to be 65 years of age or older, which is the retirement age established in the original U.S. Social Security legislation of 1935. [This is the same age for receipt of benefits in Canada.]

It is our contention, consistent with many authors in this field, that the elderly will be more politically active, more mobile, and more independent than ever before. One reason for their being more politically active is the decline in the number of labour force workers supporting persons receiving Social Security retirement benefits. For example in the U.S.A. in 1960, 20 workers supported one retired person. Currently in the U.S.A., three workers support one retiree (Dobelstein and Johnson, 1985). Thus, the growing political significance of older persons is likely to focus on the Social Security debate even more so in the future. Preferences for the living styles of older adults and their ability to maintain the standards of living for which they worked all of their lives, when contrasted with the uncertainty of future Social Security retirement benefits, will likely trigger sharp debate in America.

Future elderly will also be more economically viable and have more financial security than the elderly of today. Pension plans, stocks and bonds, and other non-wage-related income serve as the cornerstone of the various pre-retirement plans of today's 30- to 60-year-old group. For example, Feit and Tate (1986) reported that in one company the financial aspect of one pre-retirement program accounted for 75 percent of its content and emphasis.

At the same time, this population will also be more mobile. First, with "aged" starting at 50 years of age for membership in the AARP, and one of their services being discounts at many service establishments (e.g., hotels, restaurants, car rental agencies, etc.) throughout the country, significantly greater numbers of these "elderly" will be mobile and able to travel. Programs that define elderly at younger ages such as 50 generally attract persons who are in the prime of their lives and are physically and mentally healthy. Also, in North America, many elderly live independently until age 75 to 80 before requiring assistance. Should the current emphasis on illness and health continue, it is conceivable that considerably more elderly will live independently and perhaps extend their independence to 90 years of age.

B. Service Demands

Older people need more social, health, and medical services. The vulnerability of this population includes issues related to a series of life-cycle processes and adjustments identified by a number of authors in this text. These adjustments include:

- Educational and cognitive issues, e.g., quality of life, the ability to remain active and to maintain personal interests, and mental and intellectual functioning;
- Emotional and psychological issues, e.g., isolation, depression, anxiety, loss of friends and spouses, unfulfilled expectations, and communication abilities;
- Physical health concerns, e.g., how vision, illness, mobility, etc., affect social and financial resources;
- Family dynamics, e.g., is the family helpful or do they exacerbate problems;
- Financial realities, e.g., a high percentage of their income, about 20–25 percent is out-of-pocket expenses and go to health care and long-term care in the U.S.A.;
- Leisure and recreational outlets;

- Domestic life and home maintenance issues, e.g., shopping, household chores, preparing meals, managing money, etc.; and,
- Personal care, e.g., walking, going outside, bathing, dressing, using the toilet, getting in and out of bed or a chair, eating, etc.

As individuals age, they undergo gradual changes in most of their psychological and physical areas of functioning. Most of these are hardly noticeable except when greater than average exertion is required. For example, one may need more time to complete tasks or to remember things, or be unable to move as quickly as before. Cognitive changes reflect an actual slowing down of functioning rather than a loss of functioning. For instance, new learning can occur; however, one must allow adequate time to learn various tasks, information, and/or skills. Further, in this regard, sexual functioning may reflect the same slowing of response mechanisms rather than the actual loss of functioning, libido, or physiologic response (Edinberg, 1985).

While medical and health services play a prominent role in the lives of many elderly, the need for social services will be enormous. Although case management may be the most utilized service, there will be need for services such as home-based care, family treatment, substance abuse counseling and mental health counseling (with an emphasis on depression and suicide). Such services will inevitably require a base line knowledge in other health- and medical-related disciplines, such as pharmacology, medicine, dentistry, and so forth, for effective social work practice [see Giannetti, Chapter 5, for a good example for this].

Finally, in this regard, increased age brings on increased susceptibility to illness and disease. Most older adults have at least one chronic impairment in their lives, yet it is remarkable that most can manage on their own with appropriate supports. Many problems are often overlooked because medical symptoms are similar to one another, complaints can be incorrectly recognized as signs of aging and, also, older persons may be reticent about discussing their actual problems for a variety of reasons.

C. The Impact of Chronic Illness

The elderly suffer more from illnesses and diseases, and a substantial number are chronic in nature. While the perceived self-reported health status of the elderly is generally "excellent" or "good" for most, 20 percent of older adults report their health status to be only "fair" or "poor." By contrast, older adults make up 12 percent of the general population yet use 40 percent of all prescription drugs in the U.S.A. Further, they account for approximately 31 percent of the total health care expenditures nationally in America (Myers, 1989).

About 80 percent of older persons can carry out and manage their daily lives without assistance despite chronic problems. In North America, they can generally live independently and in good health until at least age 75, although by age 85 most need some form of assisted living. As indicated previously, most can cope with physical limitations and chronic illnesses and maintain independence despite chronic conditions, which are usually debilitating in nature, such as arthritis, hypertension, hearing and vision impairment, heart disease, diabetes, etc. However, blanket assumptions about chronic health care needs can be misleading as such needs include the categories of acute, transitional, and long-term care. For instance, acute care involves a hospital stay, which is needed when an episodic flare-up occurs or when certain health and medical problems don't respond to treatment. Transitional care usually involves a period of 90 days or fewer, which follows a hospital stay, and is necessary before an elderly person can return to regular community living. Long-term care involves continuous care in a facility in which the elderly person resides. Thus, while chronic health care needs imply symptomatic treatment of a condition that remains with people for a long time, other types of continuing care will be needed from time to time in the life course.

Arthritis, gout, gastritis, gall bladder disease, hiatus hernia, Alzheimer's disease, nutritional and vitamin problems, hypertension, coronary artery disease, diabetes, prostatitis, and certain cancers (e.g., stomach, testicular, cervix, uterine) are just a few of the frequent and major medical problems among the elderly. Generally, those elderly with money and insurance receive care and those without either go without attention or seek service at emergency facilities.

However, there are many problems that reimbursement usually doesn't cover or doesn't cover fully. For example, Medicare in the U.S.A. doesn't cover the cost of sensory-correcting devices such as glasses, hearing aids, or corrective shoes. Similarly, American medical insurance coverage for eye care is limited; however, vision problems among the aged are common and may be severe. For example, 50 percent of the population of blind Americans is over 65 years of age, 55 percent of the new cases of blindness each year occur among older people, and 25 percent may be using incorrect lens prescriptions (American

Association of Retired Persons, 1990). Similarly, foot and dental care needs are often neglected and/or not addressed at all.

With regard to functional disorders, depression seems to be the most common. As well, alcoholism affects ten to 15 percent of the elderly, suicide is three times more likely to occur among the elderly, and elder abuse is increasing rapidly in every urban centre in North America. The exacerbating realities of isolation and loneliness contribute greatly to these frequently occurring disorders (Edinberg, 1985). Finally, in this regard, older adults use more than twice as much medication as younger people, and 75 percent of the American elderly regularly use both prescribed and over-the-counter medications.

In summary, the future health picture of the elderly may seem cloudy. Ironically, at the same time that many elderly need more services to address the increase in their health and medical problems and they consume a larger portion of national health care costs, many are better able to function independently for many years despite having one or more chronic illnesses. The realities of the impact of such illnesses on care providers and programs has profound implications for social and health care institutions in general, and social work practitioners in particular.

D. Emerging Unique Situations

Many unique population situations and their problems will inevitably emerge and require attention in the future. In one such situation many minority people do not live to age 65. For example, in an American study by McGhee et al. (1986–1987), approximately 90 percent of persons aged 65 and over were white, 8 percent were black, and 2 percent were categorized as "other." In the same vein, the life expectancy of Native Americans is approximately 63 years of age (Gelfand, 1982), and the life expectancy for black men in 2000 was 64.8 years down from 65.4 years in 1995, about 8 years lower than the life expectancy of white men (and this has been steadily declining) (National Center for Policy Analysis, 2001).

Similarly, in Canada the total visible minority population over 65 years is 7.2 percent. Blacks make up 12.5 percent, Chinese make up 38.98 percent, South Asians make up 21.3 percent. These are the three highest non-white populations over 65 years (Statistics Canada, 2001).

Another interesting observation about our contemporary society is that more couples have elected to remain childless. Specifically, almost

5 percent of older American adults are married and have remained childless, and 5 percent are single and childless. With lower fertility rates, and an increased possibility for outliving their children, it seems that 10 percent of future older U.S. adults will have no children to help with their needs and/or to support them (Myers, 1989).

One spin-off effect of this is that new roles emerge for both older adults and their children. For instance, children may provide assistance to older adults in housework, financial assistance, transportation, and caring for them in their homes. Older adults may, in turn, help with children, financial assistance, advice on business or other matters, running errands, and taking in grandchildren or other relatives to live with them.

These new roles certainly assume a different character when the older adult requires extensive care, attention, and, in some cases, financial help. Some children may then become part of the "squeezed" or "sandwich" generation, in that they must choose between financial help for their parent(s) or support for their nuclear family or between spending considerable time being a caregiver to their parent(s) or spending time with their own family. Being part of the squeezed generation is becoming much more common in our society and will emerge as a major problem in the near future.

Further, family and in-home caregivers and services will continue to grow in number and importance as elderly persons live longer and suffer more debilitating illnesses and diseases that require round-the-clock care, e.g., Alzheimer's disease, chronic depression, stroke, etc. As a result, these caregivers will also demand help and support services as they try to regain some control over their own lives. Part of this effort is very likely to entail an increase in many social, health, and some medical support services provided in the home.

E. The Costs of Care

The future population of the elderly may have more money than their previous counterparts, yet a greater share of the overall economic pie will be taken by increasing health and medical care costs. Currently, retirement benefits, including Social Security benefits, and public and private pensions make up almost half of the income for older adults in the U.S.A. Further, one-third of their income comes from employment earnings and the remainder comes from savings, investments, and gifts. Presently, the overall income of older adults may be greater than at any time before; however, poverty rates remain high among subgroups of the elderly, in particular Native and black men and women, and white women.

In addition, living on a fixed income poses serious problems for a number of elderly. In general, any increases or adjustments in their fixed incomes fall far below the national increases in the cost of living and/or inflation. Moreover, expenditures change dramatically for many older adults. Specifically, older adults comprise 11 percent of the total U.S. population, but account for over 30 percent of public health expenditures (American Association of Retired Persons, 1989). Further, older adults tend to spend more of their household incomes on food and medical care, less on shelter and recreation, and more on household assistance and maintenance, which they usually cannot do for themselves (Dobelstein and Johnson, 1985).

When their incomes do not allow for paying for household assistance and maintenance, many elderly simply do without, and their domiciles often go unattended and/or fall into disrepair. Most older adults are forced to lower their accustomed standards of living when they retire (Dobelstein and Johnson, 1985). They also tend to be squeezed out of the workforce due to failing health, biases against older people, public policies and practices, and retirement incentives such as income support plans. In general, most experience as much as a one-half drop in annual income upon retirement (Dobelstein and Johnson, 1985). Since health and medical costs have continued to increase each year, minimally at a two-digit rate, the pressure involved in maintaining themselves in their homes while continuing to pay for escalating costs for such care will become tremendous. At some point in the not-too-distant future, this situation will become intolerable for many elderly and changes in the system will be necessitated. Unfortunately, many elderly are likely to get caught in this dilemma and will suffer needlessly.

F.   Discrepant Benefits

Benefits received by the elderly in North America tend to be uneven. Poverty proportions among various subgroups are unequal, e.g., American blacks were 1.5 times as likely as whites to be included among the older adult poor in 1990. Similarly, American Hispanics represented 5 percent and blacks represented 20 percent of the elderly poor in 1980, despite accounting for 3 percent and 5 percent, respectively, of the over-65 population. As one might assume, older blacks and other minorities are among the least able to afford private health insurance

(McGhee et al., 1986–1987). These authors also noted that as a result of past and recent discrimination practices in hiring, promotions, firing, and underemployment, it is expected that older blacks will also have lower rates of Social Security benefits, few if any union pensions, and will be more dependent on Supplemental Social Insurance, Medicare, and Medicaid than their older adult white counterparts in the U.S.A. Furthermore, we concur that much is yet to be learned from future research about the ways to defray out-of-pocket health care costs, the effects of Diagnostic Review Groups (DRGs) on social class and ethnicity and other problems faced by the elderly, in particular the minority aged, in either financing their health care and/or living on an annual fixed amount.

In Canada, according to the 1996 Census, 43.4 percent of Aboriginal people, 35.9 percent of visible minorities, and 30.8 percent of persons with disabilities were poor in 1995. These rates were significantly higher than the national average (Canadian Council of Social Development, 2000).

Further complicating the disproportionate benefits received by many elderly subgroups will be their place of residence. Specifically, the American black elderly population is projected to migrate and have high concentrations living in central U.S. cities while the white elderly are likely to remain in the suburbs with only a very slight increase migrating to less costly central corridor cities. Thus, some projections estimate that elderly blacks may come to constitute one-fourth of the population living in central cities in the 2000s (American Association of Retired Persons, 1995; McGhee et al., 1986–1987).

The picture is essentially not different when gender is considered in this formula. For instance, Hispanic elderly females in the U.S. were twice as likely as elderly white females to live in poverty. And black females were almost three times as likely as white women to be considered impoverished (Stone, 1985). The median income of black older persons is lower than that of white elderly: about $7,328 for black men, $5,239 for black women, compared to $14,775 for white men, and $8,297 for white women (American Association of Retired Persons, 1995).

Elderly persons with incomes between the poverty line and 12.5 percent above the poverty line (the "near poor") are the most vulnerable because they most often run the risk of not qualifying for public support programs (e.g., Supplemental Security Income, Medicaid, Food Stamps, etc.), but they do not have enough income to provide for their basic needs.

Another significant change lies in the sociodemographic characteristics of the ethnic aged. Specifically, there has been a decline in the number of European-born American older adults, an increase in American-born ethnic older adults, and also ethnic older adults immigrating from Indo-China, Asia, and Latin America. The educational level attained by the older adult is increasing. Between 1970 and 2000, the number of older adults who had completed high school increased from 28 percent to 70 percent. Approximately 16 percent of older adults hold a bachelor's degree or higher (American Association of Retired Persons, 1995). The education level for blacks and Hispanics is likely to remain almost five years below that of whites in the U.S. While the overall economic situation of older adults has improved since 1970 (over the past 30–35 years), the median income of older adult whites continues to be twice that of black and Hispanic older adults (Gelfand, 1982).

In the U.S.A., slower advancement of blacks, other minorities, and ethnic populations due to inadequate education, difficulties with English, unfamiliarity with American culture, and discrimination generally restrict their economic opportunities, advancement, and social mobility. As a result, there is a large discrepancy between white and black older adults in the availability of unearned income. For example, Gelfand (1982) noted that in 1976 two-thirds of white older adults had incomes from dividends, pensions, and/or investment interest. This source of income was found among one-sixth of all older adult black families. Black older adults, therefore, were more likely than whites to depend on Social Security, current earnings, and SSI for their incomes. Today's findings from the "Minorities Face Retirement: Worklife Disparities Repeated?" study indicate that Social Security benefits account for more than a half (54 percent) of black and two-thirds (66 percent) of Hispanic median household retirement wealth. They account for slightly more than a third (39 percent) of median white household retirement wealth (International Longevity Center, 2002). Finally, in this context, other minority older adults share the lower incomes and educational backgrounds of older American adult blacks. Lower educational levels and relegation to poor-paying positions have prevented many minority elderly from obtaining either the maximum benefits available from Social Security, pensions, and unearned income, or the quality services expected by high-income older adults.

G. The First Contact with Services

For many people, old age is the first time that either they or their families will have to contact and engage social, health, and/or medical services on a regular and/or continuing basis. These families are likely to need help to understand and sort through the various programs and services that may be required. As one might assume, they usually do not understand the social, health, and medical systems, how they function, the roles of various personnel, how to obtain services, and/or the extent of care needed. Specific information on what to expect from such agencies as Social Security, home health care, public welfare, Medicaid and Medicare, rehabilitation facilities, community mental health facilities, and others will be needed as well as basic information about accessing and using such services. Case management, a relatively new service covered by financial reimbursement, is the most likely form of service the elderly and their families are most likely to use in America. A case manager works to see that needed services are provided and coordinated on behalf of elderly clients and their families in their respective communities. However, case management is limited by the extent of available community services. For instance, discouragement and frustration are two common outcomes many families realize when needed community services do not exist, are inadequate in number, have waiting lists, or are poorly funded or staffed, etc. In other words, the public policies of the 1980s, which were usually supported by these baby boomers, will make for frustrating encounters with the service providers. Our contention is that many elderly will conclude that these policies and services are inadequate and not quite what they expected.

H. The Increased Importance of Responding to Death and Dying Issues

It seems clear that with the huge increase in people living longer, the concerns of death and dying will increase in importance (Chinchin, Ferster, & Gordon, 1994). There are many issues that surface during this phase of working with the elderly, none more important than an orientation to assisting older people in reviewing their personal histories (Horejsi et al., 2000). As one reviews his or her life, a sense of where a person sees himself or herself in the life cycle emerges, particularly as one reviews accomplishments and addresses remaining tasks.

A second critical issue is planning for continuity with regard to friends and family so that the elderly person may have greater control over the many life issues facing him or her. The work at this stage can be quite difficult and emotionally draining, such as assisting with wills, assisting with audio-visual tapes, planning funerals, and other activities that may leave a legacy to all. A continuous focus on addressing these issues can be emotionally draining for workers who may not have their own sense of personal struggle about the issue. It is critical for workers to reconcile their own feelings about death and dying in order to keep their own emotional balance and to be capable of listening to their client's concerns (Lowy, 1979). Finally, no matter the amount of planning and discussion, the finality of dying and its impact is often overwhelming and emotionally charged. It is, after all, for most family members a catastrophic event that no amount of planning and discussion seems to adequately address.

The emphasis of work needed by the family is also stressful (Cochran, 1999). Workers must recognize the tremendous stress on family caregivers who must often balance providing care and tending to their own needs and responsibilities. They must also address the end-of-life concerns and discuss how family members would be addressing support for death, such as grief and loneliness. As with caring for the elderly, workers should be sensitive to such problems as alcoholism and elder abuse, which have both shown significant increase during this time.

Workers must be cautious about giving legal advice since they do not usually have a legal background. It is advisable to refer the family to an attorney to handle such issues as power of attorney and wills, even though a worker may have some experience in such matters. In the context of fiscal matters, social workers may likely be called upon to assist with a host of budgetary concerns from determining discretionary funds to investments and annuities, to fixed costs, to reverse mortgages, and so forth. There is no question that social workers will need to better understand the economic and investing fields to be effective.

A spouse may often experience a sense of isolation when everyone leaves after the funeral. It is often better that the spouse remain in the community and among friends and other family members than to move to a new community where social support would be needed and basic services and acquiring friendships is likely to be problematic for a long time.

For many gerontological workers, who are usually younger than the people with whom they are working, many intergenerational issues may arise in an indirect manner. A central theme from a client's perspective would be that since workers are so young, they are likely to know about little about the problems of growing old, dying, and death. Clients are searching for a sense of how helpful a worker may be to their concerns, and also to develop a sense of credibility from the worker.

In summary, the trend of increased importance and responding to death and dying issues is critical. Workers will need to understand many aspects of law and economics. They must be able to recognize and deal with their own feelings about death and dying to be able to listen carefully and help the client and family during the phases of life. Shaefor, Horejsi, and Horejsi (2000) noted that social workers need to become administrators so as to help establish and implement policies and practices directed toward the elderly.

I.   The Impact of Technology on Practice

There is no doubt that technology has become a cornerstone of society, yet its total impact on every facet of our lives has not yet been fully realized. In working with the elderly, technology plays a significant role in medical, health, personal, and home improvements. In the medical field, technology is the norm for assisting with diagnosis and monitoring one's health. Significant advances of looking inside the body and performing surgery on an out-patient basis have become a normal occurrence for many elderly. Today, technology has made it possible to obtain immediate feedback, and/or monitoring of chronic illnesses such as diabetes and hypertension.

The Internet provides a sense of new independence to the elderly, particularly for those who are homebound. Improvements needed in the home can often be installed because technology allows one to control the device via portable handsets.

It has been pointed out that becoming old increases our sense of physical imbalance and chronic illness with the likelihood of loss of esteem, isolation, loss of transportation, and possibly loss of mobility and memory (Morales and Shaefor, 1995). Technology can play a rather significant role in increasing the connection to others in any locale. For example, the Internet places one in another world, connects us to others via chat rooms, and some may even get in touch with various self-help or treatment groups. In effect, the Internet has opened up a whole new world of communication.

The fascinating aspect of technology is that it provides an incredible array of possibilities, of which many are likely to emerge in the future. However, one must learn how to use the different components of technology so as to obtain its benefits. For example, the elderly can make extensive use of e-mail (Ellis, 1999), can play many games, and can place orders for clothing, food, and other items on-line. This is a tremendous advantage for people becoming increasingly less mobile and for those interested in bringing the external environment closer to their home.

There is an increasing set of problems that are also likely to emerge. For instance, one can receive much useless information. There is likely to be an increase in scams and con games directed at the elderly, such as participating in financial opportunities where they may lose a lot of money (Gordon, 2003). There is likely to be an increase in identity theft when clients place confidential information on the Internet. A worker must be aware of these possibilities and learn how to help older people protect themselves with issues such as identifying theft, reporting scams to the appropriate authorities, and helping clients contact the appropriate agencies in order to resolve their problems.

It has been noted that as one ages, the response time in learning new materials also lengthens. Yet, the speed of the Internet is breathtaking and thus it is likely to take older persons much more time and patience in order for them to feel comfortable using the Internet. Also, since workers tend to be much younger than the elderly, they are more likely to grow up in a technological world where the use of technology and the Internet is second nature. They may not be likely to understand the difficulty an older person may have or understand an older person's reluctance to use the Internet. Patience and understanding are needed by workers in dealing with such generational and technological gaps.

It is important to remember that dignity, self-determinism, and the ability to be involved in making decisions are often central when working with the elderly. Often the elderly may not respond quickly, nor move as fast as one might like, and cannot often interject a response before an individual forms his or her thoughts. Often, such behaviour may violate dignity or result in treating the older person as a child. At times, a worker may even have a tendency to talk about the older person as if the person were not present. A worker may also intervene by indicating that he or she has the clients' best interest at heart without talking with the clients, learning about their thoughts, or including them in discussing or completing treatment plans, discharge plans, or end-of-life decisions. Workers must ever be mindful that a client may be responsive as ever, may understand what's happening in his or her environment, and be fully capable of participating in decisions about his or her life (Moody, 1998).

II.   What Do the Trends Mean?

These trends provide a backdrop for understanding the certain challenges for social workers as they confront gerontological social work practice in the next generation. The major question for the field is, of course, what these trends are likely to mean and what impact they are likely to have in the preparation and practice of its professionals.

One way to initially grasp the meaning of these trends is by categorizing their effects or outcomes in two aspects: (1) those that have a direct effect on social work practice; and (2) those that have to do with the environments in which the practice occurs. In other words, we should think of how these trends are likely to change or alter social work practice and also how they are likely to shape the political climate and human service organizations in which social workers are employed.

As indicated, social work practice with older adults is very likely to be quite different. As it evolves over time, these changes may seem modest; however, when examined from one time period to another, these changes may become dramatic. For example, it is obvious that there will be a need for more social workers in this field and employment opportunities will be plentiful. However, social work practice with older adults will also become more highly specialized. In turn, the education and training of personnel will be dramatically altered due to the specialized knowledge requirements and requisite skills needed to be effective with this population.

Foremost, the concept of the older adult will be expanded to include several subgroups. The age range of older adults is likely to be from 50 to 90 years of age, and workers will be called upon to understand the lifespan needs and unique characteristics of the "young" older adults as being distinct from "old" older adults. Thus, the universality of the aged concept will give way to a body of unique knowledge; that is, the identification of needs translated into client services that reflect these age-specific subgroups. At the same time, a greater knowledge of the social, emotional, and physical problems of these subgroups is also likely to be required. Such knowledge is likely to occur in at least such areas as: pharmacology (drug interaction and substance abuse); chronic and debilitating illnesses and the problems they cause for an individual, family, and society; mental health (depression and isolation); domestic relations (older adult abuse); family interaction and caregiving; and developing community resources.

A critical component of social work practice will inevitably involve the interweaving of social services with medical care and health services. To be effective in this regard, a social worker must be able to move fluidly from one system to the other in an integrated community-based service network. Thus, as the chapters in Section II of this text exemplify, social work practice with older adults will include being able to work effectively in health and mental health care; being a hospital social worker; being skilled in individual, group, family, and community practice; being a substance abuse worker; being knowledgeable about legal and economic issues; understanding the impact of technology on communication and practical applications within the home; and so forth. This type of worker is very different from today's generic social worker.

The case management approach to service delivery will continue its prominence and become even more important in serving elderly clients [see Chapter 8]. Case management, with its emphasis on connecting clients with community resources, will probably be the major conduit for identifying gaps in service and, at times, bring public attention to many issues for resolution (e.g., advocacy in action). Such community resources as hospices, long-term care facilities, and home care services are a few of the services likely to be brought to public attention in this regard. Some issues likely to be highlighted are the need to deplete economic resources before obtaining public services, the high costs of insurance despite the availability of Medicare, and the lack of public support (in both Canada and the U.S.) for needed programs.

It seems clear that the nature of social work practice, i.e., what we do, will be affected greatly by the seven trends previously identified. However, another variable influencing social work practice is the agencies themselves, and authors in Section II of this text project how their social work roles may potentially develop over the years from their own organizational setting and perspective.

Probably one of the more obvious and important reasons why social work practice will be different with this clientele has to do with the clients themselves. They will be very different indeed. The population we are talking about is today in the age range of 35 to 65 and increasing to 85 and over. As a group, they are likely to have more education, more resources, increased mobility, live longer, and have the characteristics previously mentioned. As equally important, they are likely to have been part of the 1960s generation, with its social consciousness, be more technically and technologically competent, and may have been part of the individual human growth and development effort. They will have been a part of the computer age, an age where rapid technologic advances replaced the factories and foundries of the Industrial Revolution hangover. In short, many more will be used to working with their minds rather than their hands, have more resources then previous aged populations, and be politically active.

This scenario suggests that much of today's social work practice and the activities of the organizations in which they work *must* change if they expect to meaningfully serve tomorrow's clients. Future activities must be challenging, have relevancy to their clients' lifestyles, be needs appropriate to a computer-age population and reflect the age-specific and unique needs of these different older adults. It seems safe to assume that senior citizen daycare centres, with such activities as ceramics, quilting, knitting, arts and crafts, and the like, will have to change more than they imagine if they expect to attract and serve future clients.

III. The Environmental Context

The environmental context shaped by these trends is likely to produce at least four powerful outcomes: (1) political clashes between older and younger adults; (2) increased hostility among the served population and their families; (3) problems associated with accessing medical and health technology; and (4) complex ethical decision making.

Future older adults will inevitably become more politically active, in part to protect their economic resources as well as to lobby for equitable public policies and much needed services. Their competition is likely to come from fewer younger workers supporting Social Security, for example, with the majority of these younger workers expected to be minorities. A sizeable portion of the older adults will also have private pensions, Individual Retirement Accounts (IRAs), etc., which they will fight to protect through changes in public policies. It is quite possible that medical, health, and social services for chronic illness will be financially underwritten by insurers in the U.S.A. due to shifts in public attitudes and policies.

Increased hostility may be one consequence of future older adults who require service but find these services inadequate. In this regard, they may not connect the current national fiscal policies, which they supported, with the inadequate provision of services. In addition, they may be forced to participate in an unfamiliar system of care on a long-term basis for the first time in their lives. While one cannot predict with certainty how each client will respond, there is much evidence to support that these future clients will behave much differently than their predecessors.

North American society is already witnessing a raft of complex ethical decisions that are coming to the public's attention. Such decisions are likely to continue and will be difficult to make and/or understand. For instance, euthanasia, cryogenics, genetic splicing, and transplants are just some of the issues that society in general will face and for which decisions regarding the allocation of resources will be difficult.

Likewise, it is our contention that the accessibility of available technology will continue to plague public policy and negatively affect care of many elderly. Unless major changes are made, the financial means to pay or live close to major medical and health centres will determine who receives the benefits of a highly technological and exclusive system. People lacking these resources may find themselves receiving a poorer quality of services or no services at all.

This scenario regarding the environmental context of social work practice largely depends on the current situation continuing to endure without major changes. The whole picture would change radically in America should universal health insurance become public policy, as it is in Canada. In that case, social work practice would adjust accordingly in order to be an integral part of a comprehensive service system. While difficult to accurately predict each situation, it is important to remember the fundamental point made in this chapter and throughout this text—*social work practice with the older adults will be very different in the future as a result of current trends and public policies.*

IV. Concluding Remarks

The future practice of social work with older adults will change significantly as a result of the interaction of the nine trends previously described. These trends will directly affect the actual practice of social work by making it more specialized, requiring greater knowledge and improved training, by understanding and being sensitive to the various age-specific subgroups and their unique characteristics and needs, by identifying and developing needed services, and by emphasizing case management as a major service component.

These trends will significantly alter the environmental context within which social work is practised. Public policy will be affected dramatically as a result of legislative clashes between numerous future older adults and fewer, mostly minority, younger working persons. Many more people and their families are likely to enter the care system with and on behalf of older adults for the first time and remain in it due to chronic illness or loss of economic resources. The far-reaching effect of technology and the Internet will dramatically alter the nature of the nature of services provided and services utilized.

Most important, social work practice will change because the client population it is likely to serve will be quite different. A rule of thumb would be to project that the characteristics of future clients are likely to reflect today's 35- to 60-year-old group, for these will be tomorrow's older adult clients. Of central concern to this issue is whether social work will react to these trends, as it has done too often in previous situations, or will it respond proactively and be ready for these future challenges? We hope the latter.

References

American Association of Retired Persons. (1989). *Perspectives in health promotion and aging,* 4(3), Washington, DC.

American Association of Retired Persons. (1990). *Perspectives in health promotion and aging,* 5(2), Washington, DC.

American Association of Retired Persons. (1995). A portrait of older minorities. Retrieved from http://research.aarp.org/general/portmino.html.

Bloom, M. (1985). *Life span development,* 2nd ed. New York: Macmillan.

Canadian Council of Social Development. (2000). Highlights: The Canadian fact book on poverty 2000. Retrieved from http://www.ccsd.ca/pubs/2000/fbpov00/hl.htm.

Chichin, E., Ferster, L., & Gordon, N. (1994). Planning for the end of life with the home care client. *Journal of Gerontological Social Work,* 22(½), 147–158.

Cochran, D. (1999). Advanced elder care decision-making: A model of family planning. *Journal of Gerontological Social Work,* 32(12), 53–63.

Dobelstein, A.W. & Johnson, A.B. (1985). *Serving older adults: Policy, programs and professional activities.* Englewood Cliffs: Prentice-Hall.

Edinberg, M.A. (1985). *Mental health practice with the elderly.* Englewood Cliffs: Prentice-Hall.

Ellis, R. (1999). Patterns of e-mail requests by users of an Internet-based aging services information system. *Family Relations*, 48(1), 17–21.

Feit, M.D. & Tate, N.P. (1986). Health and mental health issues in preretirement programs. *Employee Assistance Quarterly*, 1(3), 49–56.

Fitch, V.L. & Slivinske, L.R. (1989). *Situational perceptions of control in the aged.* In P.S. Fry (ed.), *Psychological perspectives of helplessness and control in the elderly*, Chapter 6. North-Holland: Elsevier Science.

Gelfand, D.E. (1982). *Aging: The ethnic factor*. Boston: Little, Brown and Company.

Gordon, M. (2003). Investment schemes often target the elderly. *Journal of Gerontological Social Work*, 29(2/3), 13–17.

Horejsi, C.R., Horejsi, G.A., & Shaefor, B.W. (2000) *Techniques and guidelines for social work practice*, 5th ed. Boston: Allyn & Bacon.

Kaihla, P. (2003). The coming job boom. *Business 2.0*, 4(8), 96–105.

Lowy, L. (1979). *Social work with the aging*. New York: Longman.

McGhee, Jr., N., Reed, W., & Watson, W.H. (1986–1987). Health policy and the black aged. *The Urban League Review*, 10(2), 63–71.

Moody, H.R. (1998).Why dignity in old age matters. *Journal of Gerontological Social Work*, 29(2/3), 13–17.

Morales, A.T. & Shaefor, B.W. (1995). *Social Work: A profession of many faces*, 7th ed. Toronto: Allyn & Bacon.

Myers, J.E. (1989). *Adult children and aging parents*. Dubuque: Kendall/Hunt Publishing Company.

National Center for Policy Analysis. (2001). Social security issues—current problems. Retrieved from http://www.ncpa.org/pi/congress/socsec/socsec2.html.

Shaefor, Bradford W., Horejsi, Charles R., & Horejsi, Gloria A. (2000). *Techniques and guidelines for social work practice*, 5th ed. Boston: Allyn & Bacon.

Statistics Canada. (2001). Canadian census. Retrieved from http://www.statcan.ca/english/Pgdb/demo41.htm.

Stone, R. (1985). *The feminization of poverty among the elderly*. Washington: U.S. Department of Health and Human Services.

Internet Resources

American Association of Retired Persons
    A nonprofit membership organization dedicated to addressing the needs and interests of persons 50 and older.
    http://www.aarp.org

National Health Expenditures in Canada by Age and Sex, 1980–1981 to
2000–2001
http://www.hc-sc.gc.ca/english/care/expenditures/exp_age_sex.html
U.S. Bureau of the Census
http://www.census.gov

Additional Readings

American Association of Retired Persons. (1998). *Global aging report: Aging everywhere*. Washington: AARP.

Atchley, R.H. (1998). *The social forces of aging: An introduction to social gerontology*. Belmont: Wadsworth.

Hooyman, N. & Kiyak, M.A. (1999). *Social gerontology: A multi-disciplinary approach*. Boston: Allyn & Bacon.

CHAPTER 2

WHAT IS UNIQUE ABOUT SOCIAL WORK PRACTICE WITH THE ELDERLY?[1]

D. ANN HOLOSKO AND

MICHAEL J. HOLOSKO

This chapter attempts to answer the question—what is unique about social work practice with the elderly? The answer is based on examining gerontological social work practice trends with this diverse population group. The chapter contains three interrelated subsections: (1) attitudes about the elderly; (2) practice modifications with the elderly; and (3) educational issues. The main contention put forward is that the profession has made great strides in this area, but continues to have formidable challenges. These challenges are not only in meeting their unique needs, but also in defining an evolving social work practice role with this population.

I. Introduction

Any attempt to answer the question posed in the title is by its very nature limited because foremost, it is impossible to delineate all of the unique attributes involved in such social work practice and/or the elderly as a group. The chapters in this text serve as testimony to the fact that social work practice with the elderly is decidedly unique and the revisions of these chapters with each edition of this text have indicated that our knowledge and practice with the elderly is not static. What we have learned from the literature on gerontological social work practice is that the profession has accepted the position that practice with the elderly is indeed a unique sub-specialty. Specifically, while the principles of general social work practice guide our actions, there is recognition that the body of knowledge required to do the work must include specific gerontological knowledge (Kosberg & Kaufman, 2002). Such knowledge is required for gerontological social workers to effect competent practice at micro or macro levels with elderly and their families and to effect change with this population at all levels of the direct and indirect practice continuum.

Since the inception of social work practice (generally thought to be around the 16th century with the advent of the Elizabethan Poor Laws in England), the profession has generally taken its lead from society at large in terms of how to care for the elderly. Historically, the socio-political structures of the Western world have assumed that the elderly were "taken care of" through the major institutions and mechanisms of social welfare, e.g., the church, state, health care system, social and family agencies, social policies and programs, etc. Indeed, one may assume that they have had equal footing with other vulnerable populations such as children, families, the sick, and the poor.

Unfortunately, a closer examination of the evolution of services indicates that North American society has failed in providing minimally adequate care for the elderly, and social work has been slow to act on this injustice. For the most part, there appears to be a prevalent attitude that in the later years of life, the obligation of society and social work with the elderly is at best a maintenance function. Practice with the elderly often focuses on the management of increasing dependency of this group (Lentzner et al., 1992). Confirmation of this viewpoint can be found in the frequently posed question—how are we to manage the rising costs of supporting an aging population (Galambos & Rosen, 1999)?

The prevalence of such a question is best understood with a historical look at the development of aging policies and services. Hardina and Holosko (1990) indicated that with the exceptions of old age security benefits for the elderly (in North America), which arose after they served their country in at least one world war, the elderly have not been deemed as a distinct group for social policy consideration until about 1955. Interestingly, this was about the same time that their visibility in numbers became more viable to both politicians and policy-makers. Since then, a proliferation of social policies emerged to provide programs and services to this group in North American society supposedly to help with their quality of life on financial, health, and/or social dimensions (Graham et al., 2003).

Such responses typically categorized the elderly into two distinct groups—those needing to adjust socially and financially to retirement [the young/old] and those in declining health requiring increasing assistance [the old/old]. Both groups have contributed to the societal concern of supporting an elderly population and both have had different reactionary responses. The concern with the younger healthy elderly is usually that they can they afford retirement, particularly since the realities of pensions, better health, nutrition, and lifestyle coupled with no wars (in the Western world) have meant a longer retirement period [in some cases longer than 35 years]. As a "healthy group," this subgroup has wielded its political power, making "grey power" a political force to which some politicians have responded. Some of the more positive social work interventions with the elderly can been seen here. At present, the viewpoint advocated here is "productive aging" and subsequent interventions can be found at all levels of social work practice. Some of the more recent themes of this movement to harness seniors' productive value include: helping them stay in the workforce, connecting them to volunteer initiatives, promoting their abilities to care for their grandchildren, and involving them in community development activities.

The fastest-growing age group in society is not the baby boomers entering retirement as many think, but the over-85 age group [see Chapter 1]. Unfortunately, both society's and social work's response/ reaction to this cohort has not been as positive. This is the group that continues to have the historical definition and stigma of being "old"— those still viewed as dependent and needing caregiving. There are those who are active well past 85, but for many, this is when the issues of physical and mentally frailty begin to surface. Both on an individual and societal level the concerns are: Who will assist with any actual care? Who will assist financially? And who will make the care decisions?

Unfortunately, the responses to assist this particular subgroup remain based almost exclusively on the medical model with its orientation on symptomology of acute illness and recovery. This model, however, flies in the face of the traditional client-focused and holistic model of social work and does not provide easy practice answers to the challenging issues typically facing gerontological social workers, e.g., ethical dilemmas and/or ways to evaluate practice effectiveness, helping people to successfully "age in place" when they do not wish to.

The fortunate fallout from this concern [that is financing our aging population] is that as a whole, society is more willing to both acknowledge the elderly as a complex and diverse group and, to a lesser degree, as a group with potential and strengths. Indeed, over time in North America we are beginning to see a genuine interest addressing the needs of this group. It is not coincidental that as North American society ages, issues related to the elderly surface with greater frequency. The extent to which such issues, e.g., the health, education, and social welfare of the elderly evolve from "social conditions" of society to "social problems" and become identified as such by the politically powerful and economically privileged remains to be seen. But if our practice efficacy with the elderly is to develop, their concerns need to become labelled as social problems that have a more likely chance of making it to the agenda of government (Jurkowski & Tracey, 2000). This, in turn, encourages the profession to "practise outside the box" and direct practice energy toward issues of advocacy, social justice, redistributive justice, community development, and political lobbying for the elderly. The profession's track record in these areas historically has not been good. However, our knowledge, values, and skills are far ahead of other helping professions in this area and we are certainly positioned to assume a leadership role in these new practice domains (Jansson, 2003). The extent to which the profession picks up the gauntlet and assumes a leadership role in this regard remains to be seen.

II. Attitudes toward the Elderly

Attitudes toward the elderly can be viewed from at least three perspectives: (1) attitudes of the elderly toward themselves; (2) attitudes of social workers; and (3) attitudes of society at large. It is well documented that how a problem or situation is viewed will affect not only how the problem is perceived, but eventually defined and treated. The importance here is to acknowledge that each perspective addressed has a unique viewpoint that impacts on social work practice. With an emphasis on strengths-based and client-focused practice, it is particularly important to first emphasize and consider the elderly's attitude toward themselves.

A. Attitudes of the Elderly toward Themselves

Membership in a particular subgroup of society entitles a person to express an opinion about his or her status, which is often entrenched in how the person behaves. For the elderly, there are at least two predominant attitudes they have toward themselves. First, there is a sense of personal pride presented about surviving their life to date. Those who reach an older age all have unique stories with a common resiliency thread—basically they were able to live through whatever life threw at them. Associated with this is a licence to tell their stories, to provide wisdom and insight to others, and to reap the benefits of their earlier contributions to society via pensions, social security, and social/health programs. Such attitudes have been identified in the literature as resources or strengths with which social workers have drawn upon in their gerontological practice which promotes productive aging (Chappell et al., 2003).

Second, a common saying by older individuals is, "It's no fun to get old," or "Yes, retirement was great until ... [a stroke, heart attack, arthritis, macular degeneration, compromised finances, etc.]." An underlying message here is that the elderly hold, unconsciously or not, a dislike toward a part of their present reality and/or accepting who they are. Ironically, no longer is dying the predominant fear for many elderly, it is the dread of the coming years! In the extreme, the elderly may express a profound fear of losing abilities, competency, a particular lifestyle, and a sense of purpose that is outside of their control. The attitude reflected here is one of "getting old" as opposed to "growing old" as the latter entails an obvious sense of purpose through continued growth and development.

B. Attitudes of Social Workers

Social work practice has changed significantly with regard to its attitude toward vulnerable populations. Specifically, over the past decade there has been a decided shift toward identifying and building on existing strengths and resources of vulnerable populations in general rather than their problems (Chaplin & Cox, 2001; Silverstone, 2000). Practice with the elderly has attempted to follow suit. It can be argued that past practice attitudes about aging have restricted such a move (Chappell et al., 2003). For example, a classic task of old age has been coming to grips with the past and the reconciling of past conflicts. However, with many living 20 to 40 years in this life stage, the profession has finally come to realize that an equally relevant task for successful aging may be to focus on the present situation—"What should the elderly person be doing now and in the future? and How can it be a positive and meaningful experience?" (Katzko et al., 1998).

It is the "how" that is the real challenge for social workers as resources of the elderly are often viewed as limited (Chappel et al., 2003; Greene, 2000). Such attitudes emerge as social workers attempt to practice in the face of difficult realities such as health care and welfare reforms [including limited access to rehabilitation/home care/ appropriate housing, etc.]. These limitations are also reinforced at a personal level when elderly individuals are perceived to have a limited informal support network or limited physical or cognitive capacity. The issues of limited resources can often be a source of a disempowering attitude for social workers who find themselves caught in the middle of a resource tug of war. Politicians, policies, and agencies are demanding a conservation of funds and elderly clients are requiring more than is being offered (Galambos, 1997).

C. Attitudes of Society

The issue of scarce resources becomes increasingly damaging to the elderly as society often views their potential as non-productive members of society, thus providing the rationale to spend more of the already limited health and social programming dollars on them becomes difficult to reconcile. As with other vulnerable populations, social workers view the elderly as victims of certain discrimination or ageism and in need of redistributive justice. Within this context, the profession must actively work at dispelling societal myths about the elderly, which have trickled down to frustrate and challenge front-line practitioners as well as their families, friends, and the elderly themselves.

Whether we wish to admit it or not, North American society has generally promoted a negative attitude toward the elderly, which has permeated caregivers for centuries. Such stereotypes are largely perpetuated by: (1) social institutions, which are usually age-segregated, e.g., schools, hospitals, mental health centres, alcohol treatment centres, social/health welfare systems, etc.; (2) political-legal structures, which formulate laws that preclude the elderly from participation in avenues of society, e.g., mandatory retirement laws; and (3) economic institutions, which promote youthful employees, e.g., commercial and financial institutions, the service, fashion, and entertainment industries, etc. All of these stereotypes have been fuelled by a sometimes merciless media industry. Although society should become kinder to those who grow old, the best that can be said here is that "old age" has now been pushed to a later starting age. Once at "old age," however, these stereotypes prevail.

The extent to which such stereotypes have affected practitioners may be understood by exploring a series of myths articulated some 30 years ago that have contributed to such "ageism," or the prejudices and stereotypes that are applied to older people solely on the basis of their age (Butler, 1969). The sad fact is that they are still relevant. Greene (1986) listed some of these major myths and facts as follows. We [the chapter authors] have also added to this now growing list:

Myth: Being "old" is merely a matter of chronological age.

Fact: Aging refers to the processes of change in individuals that occur after maturity. Not all aspects of the human organism show the same age-related changes as a person advances in chronological age. Therefore, it is well to distinguish three aspects of aging: biological age, referring to organic changes and life expectancy; psychological age, referring to adaptive capacities; and sociocultural age, referring to social roles and expectations of the group. These are interrelated and together comprise an individual's functional age (Birren & Sloane, 1980; Haber 2003).

Myth: Older people talk about the good old days because they are garrulous or "senile."

Fact: The introspective qualities of older people are a result of a naturally occurring return to past experiences, reassessing them in an attempt to resolve and integrate them. This provides the opportunity for the ego to reorganize these events and come to terms with past conflicts and relationships. The process of reminiscing can occur at any age, particularly at times of transition. However, this takes place more frequently in some elderly who are not as actively involved in the present and may not be able to draw upon interesting current experiences. The tendency to reminisce also increases as the older person begins to deal with his or her own mortality. This process can be tapped as a therapeutic tool in life review (Butler, 1963). It can also be a tool to gain insight into the past as it relates to present coping and growth. Developing ego strength and self-concept is essential for coping and further growth and as well as being a specific purpose in itself.

Myth: Older people do not develop or grow [cannot change].

Fact: Lifespan theorists reject the view that growth ends with adulthood. They point out that while there may be growth limits for attributes such as height, other qualities such as creativity and abstract reasoning do not fit this model. In this context, growth refers to differentiation, increased complexity, and greater organization, and can occur at every age (Schell & Hall, 1979). The number of adaptations an elderly person eventually must make negates any statement about the lack of potential for development and growth. The statement and attitude seem to persist, however, as a coping mechanism for both elderly individuals and others who wish to resist or deny the need to adapt to their changing situation.

Myth: Older people cannot learn new roles, skills, or competencies.

Fact: Unfortunately, mature individuals are usually thought of as having reached a stage when no further socialization takes place. However, research on aging and the life cycle indicates that as people mature, they must "continually learn to play new or altered roles and to relinquish old ones" (Riley et al., 1969). It is now understood that at every stage of life the individual must master certain developmental tasks requiring new skills and competencies. Some of the skills to learn and practise can include: practising healthy lifestyle options, making and maintaining social contacts after retirement, finding volunteer activities, and learning how to collaborate and network on difficult situations (Chappell et al., 2003).

Myth: Older people are not suitable candidates for insight therapy.

Fact: Because of their introspective qualities, capacity for growth, and lifelong coping styles, many elderly clients have exceptional adaptation skills to draw upon in a crisis (Devries, 1996; Scogin & McElreath, 1994).

Myth: Older people are alienated from their families.

Fact: The family continues to be the primary source of social support in old age. While most Americans do not live in three- or four-generation households, the family continues to be the primary caregiver for the frail and impaired elderly. Research affirms that there is frequent contact between the elderly and their families, particularly at times of illness. Exchange of services and regular visits are common among old people and their children whether or not they live under a single roof (Shanas, 1979). Indeed, research has found that children get satisfaction from being able to give to their parents (Haber, 2003).

Myth: Older people are cared for by their families, but do not give anything in return.

Fact: Survey data suggest there is a high degree of interdependence between generations in today's families. There is generally ongoing contact between adult children and their parents in the form of shared social activities and the mutual exchange of material and emotional support (Bengston & Treas, 1980). Issues of reciprocal family relationships are frequently highlighted in the literature as the elderly have become a resource for childcare (Greenwell & Bengston, 1997). The phenomenon of grandparents raising grandchildren is a unique practice and study area (Cooney & Smith, 1996; Tucker, 2002).

Myth: When older people experience a biopsychosocial crisis, they are best helped without the involvement of the family.

Fact: A family system is composed of interrelated members who constitute a group. A change in the life of one of the members brings about change throughout the system. Therefore, a biopsychosocial crisis in one of the members can be expected to result in change affecting everyone in the family system. An awareness of this phenomenon can enhance casework services to the aged and their families (Greene, 1986). Presently, family involvement is actively sought and supported [in some cases mandated] as a potential and viable resource in helping their loved one. Unfortunately, professionals socialized in a medical model may experience difficulty transitioning to client and family focused intervention. Advocacy is often necessary to ensure inclusion.

Myth: The family usually knows how to make good decisions for their elderly members.

Fact: Family members, even those with good intentions, can unconsciously put their needs before that of their loved one. Information and decisions are often kept from the elderly family member—"for their own good"—when, in reality, it is often the other family members who wish to avoid an uncomfortable issue. Even when the elderly person does participate, there can be pressure to make decisions to please the family rather than the individual's desires. Overall, most families do assist effectively with decision making; however, a careful assessment of the dynamics and advocacy on the part of the elderly client may have to be addressed.

Myth: Incompetent individuals can't participate in decision making.

Fact: Except in the case of extreme dementia, individuals are usually capable of expressing need, which is the basis for a communication entry point. With an understanding of an individual's stage-specific dementia, skilled workers are able to present choices and pose questions in a way that allows participation in decision making and problem solving. As well, workers in the area of gerontology must be able to pick up on the subtle and numerous non-verbal cues of persons with diminished capacity.

Confronting the above myths [perceived as barriers to service delivery] through advocacy and addressing them are the primary roles for some social workers; however, all social workers should be able to incorporate such elements into any practice position. For example, the literature points out that social workers have: (1) worked creatively within existing institutions and structures of care (sometimes stretching their mandates) to provide for the differential needs of the elderly; (2) consistently promoted the uniqueness of the elderly in both assessment and interventions; and (3) attempted to maintain clients' rights for self-determinism and decision making in the face of complex capacity issues. Such initiatives have taken time, but all of them have been driven by a pervasive positive attitude toward the elderly on behalf of the profession. As one might assume, all of these types of activities have assisted in socializing not just social work but other helping professions and the general public toward creating more favourable attitudes toward caring and helping the elderly.

III.   Practice Modifications

Social workers have had a half century to refine practice ideologies, assumptions, and frameworks to fit the unique needs of the elderly.

From a strengths-based framework, the uniqueness of practice with the elderly is to promote factors of successful aging. These include the avoidance of disease and disability, involvement in society, continued high cognitive and physical functioning, and a maintained or acquired sense of purpose (Rowe & Kahn, 1997). Presently, a simplified view of how to do this in terms of social work practice is to ensure that there is just distribution or redistribution of resources to age successfully (Wiener et al., 1994). The question then is how to identify and define these resources (Wakefield, 2001).

Changes in practice did not occur overnight, but clearly gerontological social work has been a front runner in recognizing and responding to the practice and political realities of the elderly today. As mentioned in the previous subsection, social workers' practice with vulnerable populations has perhaps made them more prepared and clearer about how to effectively approach practice in a time of rationed health and social services. Clearly, there is a more support for a client-centred focus with the elderly than ever before, as society attempts to place responsibility for care back to communities and individuals. The elderly person, despite capacity, physical abilities, and financial resources, is to be considered as *the person with the resources to make changes in his/her situation in order to be more functional.* For example, what service eligibility does his/her situation offer? What support systems does he or she have in place? What creative support systems can he or she develop? And what coping skills is he or she using? These are the types of important questions and issues that fit our professional social work domain as they speak to self-determinism, autonomy, individuation, personal strengths, and tangible resource networking — all of which are imbedded in our professional code of ethics.

Common themes of practice with the elderly are still present: finding meaningful activities, dealing with loss, transitioning out of the labour force, offsetting the impact of ageism, and living with multiple disabilities. However, as well as growing in sheer numbers, the elderly are also expanding in terms of their diversity, e.g., ethnicity, family composition, and lifestyle choices. Thus, while these common themes still exist, their accompanying responses and interventions must also evolve. Many of the chapters in this text speak to various settings and populations that are included in practice with the elderly, therefore making a detailed list of specific practice modifications seems redundant here. However, we will present a general overview of how present ideologies and interventions have impacted on practice modifications in one area, the assessment process. Assessment is selected here for a few reasons: it set ups the intervention or practice process, it is within our practice repertoire, it is done well by our practitioners, and it is interdisciplinarily accountable.

Most of the helping professions, including social work, have realized the importance of modifying their practice assumptions regarding how to assess the elderly and have adapted their protocols and technologies accordingly [see Chapter 3]. Specifically, social workers are very aware that a comprehensive assessment requires a complex look at a number of systems of the elderly person in his/her environment. They also acknowledge that assessment outcome must determine functional status, quality of life, and health status as the process goal (Rubenstien, 1989). To accomplish this, the specific techniques advocated for here include: (1) accepting the principle of multiple symptomology in the analyses, e.g., one symptom interacts with a subsystem, which in turn influences another symptom and subsystem; (2) using a comprehensive assessment framework that includes individual capacity assessments (finances, housing, mental status, etc.), personality assessments, medication appraisals, family and/or social support network assessments, biographical or ecological considerations; (3) using significant others directly in the assessment process, e.g., family, friends, physicians, etc., to obtain a more complete and accurate appraisal; (4) finding ways to reiterate the importance of social work principles such as self-determinism and client autonomy in the assessment process particularly when capacity is compromised; (5) developing a personal assessment style conducive to elderly clients, e.g., using two to three sessions rather than one for conducting an assessment; using engagement techniques specific to the elderly; and (6) assessing health risks.

Active engagement to demonstrate empathy and building trust/confidence are keys to an accurate assessment. In this regard, Tobin and Gustafson (1987) posed the question: "What do social workers do differently with elderly clients?" Five unique intervention activities reported were: (1) touching to provide a more active approach to the elderly's needs; (2) activities such as concrete assistance, outreach, and talking by the social worker in sessions to assist with problems; (3) reminiscing to develop ego strength (by noting past coping) and adaptation capabilities, as well as helping to recapture and reaffirm the current self; (4) transference as a means to examine the meaning, wishes, and thoughts of the client; and (5) counter-transference to clarify or specify concerns by the worker to the client of dependency, helplessness, death.

When an elderly person's point of entry for help is a health service, many countries [including Canada and the U.S.] use or are considering a type of MDS (Minimum Data Set) or RAI (Resident Assessment Instrument) tool for standardizing assessments (Kikuta et al., 2002). While no judgment is being made on its utility here, such tools provide insights into the comprehensiveness required in conducting a thorough assessment. While there are variations of the tools in general, the areas of an MDS assessment typically include: finances, legal status, present lifestyle and abilities around activities of daily living, amount of physical assistance required, cognitive abilities, communication abilities, mood and behavioural issues, psychosocial strengths/problems, support networks, medical diagnoses, medication, signs of delirium or acute illness, required or ongoing medical treatments, sensory impairments, mobility, nutrition, and diet (www.cms.hhs.gov).

An MDS tool compiles assessment information and then flags areas of potential risk and strengths. Areas of intervention are assigned by the tool and in some cases prioritized. At this time, such tools are often mandated by health policies and are used to assess health risks, determine care levels, and assess environmental needs. A challenge here often can be to maintain a client focus as any assessment tool is only as good as the practitioner using it. In this regard, personal biases (attitudes toward the elderly) and professional orientation (client-focused versus problem/medical-focused) seriously impact on the validity of the data collected using such protocols.

Although the above discussion focuses only on gerontological practice modifications in conducting assessments, there are other practice areas that social workers in this field need to similarly modify. These are presented in Figure 2.1.

IV.   Educational Issues

Although the institutions of social welfare and health care are slow to change, educational institutions are slower. The training and education for social work practitioners offered on-site in gerontological settings has generally been more significant than that offered in traditional educational institutions. When one considers the extensive knowledge expectations of social workers practising in this field (e.g., biological,

Figure 2.1: What Do Gerontologists Do?

1. Direct Service
    *   Assesses clients needs
    *   Provides services directly to the older client and family
    *   Coordinates services with other agencies and institutions
    *   Works to ensure that the older client and family receive appropriate services that are of a high quality
    *   Evaluates and modifies the services needed
    *   Conducts outreach to expand and enhance client base
    *   Carries out advocacy on behalf of older persons
2. Program Planning and Evaluation
    *   Identifies the needs of the community
    *   Plans the programs and facilities
    *   Determines the level and timing of funds required
    *   Develops the staffing and management plans
    *   Determines the evaluation plan for the program
    *   Consults and coordinates with other agencies and programs
3. Education and Training
    *   Plans and conducts educational programs for older persons, their caregivers, and families
    *   Plans and conducts continuing education programs for paraprofessional and professionals interested in serving older people
    *   Instructs pre-professionals
    *   Intergenerational programs
4. Administration and Policy
    *   Designs the structure, motivates and supervises the activities of staff members
    *   Determines, monitors, and modifies organizational expenditures
    *   Coordinates activities within the organization and with outside organizations
    *   Conducts analyses of current and proposed programs
    *   Increases public awareness of needs and services
5. Research
    *   Designs and carries out evaluations and academic studies to clarify aspects of aging and program interventions

Source: Hooyman & Kiyak (1999, p. 519)

physiological, psychological, ethical, legal, familial, social supports, resources, sociological, life cycle, etc.), this is not surprising. As well, when considering the overall objectives of accredited BSW and MSW programs, the issue of how to successfully integrate gerontological content into the curriculae without overwhelming it is indeed a critical question (Holosko, 1995).

Since about 1980 onward, university-based social work degree-granting programs have taken the initiative in attempting to infuse gerontological content into their curriculae. Generally, such efforts have been more successful at the graduate level than undergraduate level, and have taken one of two avenues, either by developing speciality concentrations or by promoting such content in a more broad-based fashion across the entire curriculum. The use of speciality field practica, research projects, multidisciplinary training, case vignettes, and certificates have been instrumental in helping to educate and train professional social workers (MSWs or BSWs) in these settings (Schneider et al., 1984; Rathbone-McCuan and Hurwitz, 1988; Schneider and Nelson, 1984). To date, however, there is still no consensus on how to include gerontological content into BSW or MSW curricula (Holosko, 1995; O'Neill, 1999).

Areas where social work educators have not progressed in this regard have been in research, publication, and speciality teaching. As one administrator of a Canadian school of social work once remarked, however: "As a faculty begins to age or experience aging as an issue in their lives, more attention may be given [in the curriculum] to aging ... when it takes on a less abstract dimension" (Rathbone-McCuan & Hurwitz, 1988, p. 32). In an effort to bolster geriatric education programs, Macfadyen (1989), who conducted an international study on the subject for the World Health Organization, offered the following suggestions:

1. Identification and training of key faculty to act as institutional stimuli for curriculum development
2. Development of regional and/or national resource centres to strengthen multidisciplinary training, faculty development, continuing education, and mid-career retraining
3. Development of clearing houses on curricula and resources
4. Stimulation of research efforts in the field of aging both to strengthen the knowledge base and increase the level of faculty awareness and interest. One approach is the provision of traineeships and fellowships for research
5. Development of links between teaching institutions and community care facilities (p. 6)

He goes on to state that to fulfil the teaching and learning objectives that have been identified for care of the elderly, schools must develop teaching networks beyond the traditional institutions and teaching hospitals, which have conducted the bulk of clinical teaching so far. The processes of teaching must also allow maximum opportunity for active involvement and personal interaction of students with elderly people (pp. 7–8). Although these were offered some 15 years ago, they still hold current relevance today (Council on Social Work Education, 2001).

Despite the numerous global warnings about increased populations of elderly persons, this demographic imperative has not translated into: greater numbers of professionally trained social workers, increased educational and training initiatives for BSW or MSW students, increased numbers of BSW or MSW students preparing for the field, increased salaries for gerontological social workers, or greater numbers of teaching faculty (Holosko, 1995; Kosberg & Kaufman, 2002; O'Neill, 1999). Kosberg and Kaufman (2002) describe this curious irony the following way: "there has been a plethora of material warning about the growing elderly population, the lack of social workers prepared for such growth, and the need for the profession to do something about this discrepancy" (p. 3). The extent to which the profession can continue to exercise "conscious avoidance behaviour" about these concerns remains to be seen.

Of all the careers in gerontology, social work provides the greatest variety of employment opportunities for working with the elderly. The profession, by its very nature, has an ethical responsibility to promote the dignity of all human beings, elderly or otherwise. As indicated previously, we have made considerable strides in educating professionally trained BSWs and MSWs to work in this unique field. We still have, however, a long way to go in helping professionals in "seeking the difference that makes the difference." The future in this regard is nothing less than promising.

V.   Concluding Remarks

In summary, with the unfolding of a new millennium, it is safe to say that social work has made significant practice changes to work in an era when a growing population of elderly must contend with a rationing of social and health resources. Current definitions of practice are presently focused around social justice and the redistribution of resources. As well, the definitions of resources have been profoundly affected by strengths-based practices. Resources go beyond the tangible items of finances, health status, and support systems to now include the social capital currencies of community support systems, individual capacity, growing successfully while aging, automony, coping, and adaptation abilities. The goal is not on wellness and perfection but functional ability to live a meaningful quality of life until death. Perhaps the most positive impact for the elderly with these changes is the position of empowerment afforded the elderly in this model of practice. To ensure this requires social workers to modify their practice, maximizing client involvement and decision making in all interventions.

This chapter attempted to answer the question—What is unique about social work practice with the elderly?—by examining general practice issues related to: (1) attitudes toward the elderly; (2) practice modifications; and (3) educational issues. The main contention put forward was that the profession is rapidly evolving in "seeking the difference that makes the difference" in working in this field; however, it still has a long way to go. The demographic reality that the elderly will constitute the largest minority group in North American society by the year 2050 has resounding implications for social work and other professions. To attempt to meet the challenges of caring for this group in society, we believe that the profession has to continue to be creative, take initiative, advocate for change, and adapt its attitudes, assumptions, and interventions accordingly as the unique needs of this group warrant such modification. Certainly, the time is now for social work to take proactive measures in enhancing its knowledge, values, and skills related to care for the elderly.

Note

1.   Social work has had a long history of identity anxiety about its
     uniqueness (Lubove, 1973). William James's (1906) classic essay on
     pragmatism makes the point more succinctly as "seeking the difference
     that makes the difference." Since Section II of this text describes specific
     practice issues about the elderly in numerous and diverse settings (in
     attempting to "seek the difference"), this chapter will present some
     of the general social work practice issues that transcend these various
     settings.

References

Bengston, V. & Treas, J. (1980). The changing family context of mental health and aging. In J.E. Birren & R.B. Sloane (eds.), *Handbook of mental health and aging*, pp. 400–428. Englewood Cliffs: Prentice-Hall.

Birren, J.E. & Sloane, R.B. (eds.). (1980). *Handbook of mental health and aging.* Englewood Cliffs: Prentice-Hall.

Butler, R.N. (1963). The life review: An interpretation of reminiscence in the aged. *Psychiatry, 26,* 65–76.

Butler, R.N. (1969). Directions in psychiatric treatment of the elderly: Role of perspectives in the life cycle. *Gerontologist, 9*(2), 134–138.

Centers for Medicare and Medicaid Services. (2003). U.S. Government Department of Health and Human Services, Washington, www.cms.hhs. gov.

Chaplin, R. & Cox, E. (2001). Changing the paradigm: Strengths-based and empowerment-oriented social work with frail elders. *Gerontological social work practice: Issues, challenges and potential,* pp. 165–179. New York: Haworth.

Chappell, N., Gee, E., MacDonald, L., & Stores, M. (2003). *Aging in contemporary Canada.* Toronto: Prentice-Hall.

Cooney, T.M. & Smith, L. (1996). Young adult's relationship with grandparents following recent parental divorce. *Journal of Gerontology, 51*(B), 591–595.

Council on Social Work Education. (2001). *A blueprint for the new millennium.* Washington: Council on Social Work Education.

Devries, H.M. (1996). Cognitive-behavioral interventions. In J.E. Birren (ed.), *Encyclopedia of gerontology.* San Diego: Academic Press.

Galambos, C.M. (1997). Resolving ethical conflicts in providing case management services to the elderly. *Journal of Gerontologial Social Work, 27*(4), 57–67.

Galambos, C.M. & Rosen, A. (1999). The elderly are coming and they are us. *Health and Social Work, 24*(1), 73–77.

Graham, J., Swift, K., & Delaney, R. (2003). *Canadian social policy: An introduction,* 2nd ed. Toronto: Pearson Education Canada.

Greene, R. (1986). *Social work with the aged and their families.* New York: Hawthorne, Aldine de Gruyter.

Greene, R. (2000). Serving the aged and their families in the 21st century using a revised practice model. *Journal of Gerontological Social Work, 34*(1), 43–62.

Greenwell, L. & Bengston, V. (1997). Geographic distance and contact between middle-aged children and their parents: The effect of social class over 20 years. *Journal of Gerontology, 51*(B), 513–526.

Haber, D. (2003). *Health promotion and aging: Practical application for health professionals*, 3ʳᵈ ed. New York: Springer.

Hardina, D. & Holosko, M. (1990). Social policies which influence practice with the elderly. In M. Holosko & M. Feit (eds.), *Social work practice with the elderly*, pp. 103–131. Toronto: Canadian Scholars' Press.

Holosko, M.J. (1995). The inclusion of gerontology content into undergraduate social work curricula in Australia and New Zealand. *Gerontology and Geriatrics Education*, 15(4), 5–20.

Hooyman, N. & Kiyak, H.A. (1999). *Social gerontology: A multi-disciplinary perspective*, 5ᵗʰ ed. Boston: Allyn & Bacon.

James, W. (1906). What pragmatism means. *Pragmatism and other essays*, pp. 22–28. New York: Washington Square Press.

Jansson, B. (2003). *Becoming an effective policy advocate: From policy practice to social justice*, 4ᵗʰ ed. Pacific Grove: Thomson Brooks/Cole.

Jurkowski, E.T. & Tracey, M. (2000). Social policy and the aged: Implications for health planning, health education, and health promotion. *The Health Education Monograph Series 2000*, (18)2, 20–26.

Katzko, M., Steverink, N., Dittmann-Kohli, F., & Herrera, R. (1998). The self-concept of the elderly: A cross-cultural comparison. *International Journal of Aging and Human Development*, 46, 171–187.

Kikuta, S.C., Petch, C., & Dupuis, M. (2002, May/July). Supporting the use of MDS in everyday work. *Stride Magazine*, 1–22.

Kosberg, J. & Kaufman, A. (2002). Gerontological social work: Issues and imperatives in education. *Electronic Journal of Social Work*, 1(1), 1–15.

Lentzner, H.R., Pamuk, E.R., Rhodenhiser, E.P., Rothberg, R., & Powell-Given, E. (1992). Quality of life in the year before death. *American Journal of Public Health*, 82, 1093–1098.

Lubove, R. (1973). *The professional altruist*. New York: Harvard University Press.

Macfadyen, D. (1989, March). *Training professionals in health care of the elderly*. Hamilton: McMaster University Faculty Health Sciences.

O'Neill, J.V. (1999, February). Aging express: Can social work keep up? Washington: NASW News.

Rathbone-McCuan, E. & Hurwitz, E. (1988). *Crossroads: A report on Canadian gerontological social work education trends*. Burlington: University of Vermont, Canadian Studies Program.

Riley, M., Foner, B., Hess, B., & Toby, M. (1969). Socialization for the middle and later years. In D.A. Goslin (ed.), *Handbook of socialization, theory and research*. Chicago: Rand McNally College Publishing Co.

Rowe, J.W. & Kahn, R.L. (1998). *Successful aging*. New York: Pantheon Books.

Rubenstein, L.V., Calkins, D., Greenfield, S., & Jette, A. (1989, June). Health status assessment for elderly patients: Report of the society of general internal medicine task force on health assessment. *Journal of the American Geriatrics Society*, 37(6), 562–569.

Schell, R. & Hall, E. (1979). *Developmental psychology today*. New York: Random House.

Schneider, R., Decker, T., Freeman, J., & Syran, C. (1984). *The integration of gerontology with social work educational curriculum*. CSWE Series in Gerontology. Washington: Council on Social Work Education.

Schneider, R. & Nelson, G.M. (1984). *The current status of gerontology in graduate social work education*. CSWE Series in Gerontology. Washington: Council on Social Work Education.

Scogin, F. & McElreath, L. (1994). Efficacy of psychosocial treatments for geriatric depression: A quantitative review. *Journal of Consulting and Clinical Psychology*, 62, 69–74

Shanas, E. (1979). The family as a social support system in old age. *The Gerontologist*, 19, 169–174.

Silverstone, B. (2000). The old and the new in aging: Implications for social work practice. *Journal of Gerontological Social Work*, 33(4), 35–50.

Tobin, S. & Gustafson, J. (1987). What do we do differently with elderly clients? *Journal of Gerontological Social Work*, 10(3–4), 107–120.

Tucker, C. (2002). Grandparents raising grandchildren. The childcare solution? *Social Work Today*, 2(25), 12–15.

Volans, P. & Levy, R. (1982, June). A re-evaluation of an automated tailored test of concept learning with elderly psychiatric patients. *British Journal of Clinical Psychology*, 21(2), 93–101.

Wakefield, J. (2001). Social work as the pursuit of minimal distributive justice. Invited paper presented at the Kentucky conference "Re-Working the Working Definition," Lexington.

Wiener, J., Illston, L., & Manley, R. (1994). *Sharing the burdens: Strategies for public and private long term care insurance*. Washington: The Bookings Institute.

Internet Resources

Advocacy Centre for the Elderly (Canada)
> A community-based legal clinic for low-income senior citizens.
> http://www.advocacycentreelderly.org/

Benefits Check-up
> Eligibility for government programs for seniors in the U.S. Sponsored by the National Council of the Aging.

http://www.benefitscheckup.org/
http://www.ncoa.org
The care guide: "Everything under the sun for seniors" housing and care.
http://www.thecareguide.com
Centres for Medicare and Medicaid Services
Quantitative information on programs, from estimates of future
Medicare and Medicaid spending to enrolment, spending, and claims
data.
http://www.cms.hhs.gov/
Citizenship and Immigration Canada (2002).
Language Instruction for Newcomers to Canada (LINC). Guide for
Application.
http://www.cic.gc.ca/english/newcomer/linc-2e.html
Division of Aging and Seniors (Canada)
Provides federal leadership in areas pertaining to aging and seniors.
http://www.hc-sc.gc.ca/seniors-aines/
Dr. Weil.com
A unique medical and non-traditional orientation to illness and
wellness.
http://www/drweil.com
Health Finder
Health and information site through the government for seniors.
http://www.healthfinder.gov/
U.S. Administration on Aging
The advocate agency for older persons and their concerns. Works to
heighten awareness about older Americans and alerts the public to the
needs of vulnerable older people.
http://www.aoa.dhhs.gov/

Additional Readings

American Association of Retired Persons. (1998). *Global aging report: Aging everywhere*. Washington: AARP.
Beers, M. & Berkow, R. (2000). *The Merck manual of geriatrics*, 3rd ed. Whitehouse Station: Merck Research Laboratories.
Duffy, M. (ed.). (1999). *Handbook of counselling and psychotherapy with older adults*. New York: John Wiley & Sons Inc.
National Association of Social Workers. (2001). *Social work with other people: Understanding diversity*. Washington: NASW Press.

Saleebey, D. (1997). *The strengths perspective in social work practice*. New York: Longman.

Thorson, J. (2000). *Aging in a changing society*. New York: Taylor & Francis.

CHAPTER 3

CONDUCTING PSYCHOSOCIAL ASSESSMENTS WITH THE ELDERLY

SUSAN WATT AND

AHUVA SOIFER

Psychosocial assessments of elderly persons by social workers require the full range of knowledge and skills used in the assessment of any adult, coupled with particular sensitivities to the biological, cultural, social, and psychological factors that shape the lives of the elderly. Particularly, social workers must recognize the purposes to which the assessment may be used, which may lead to major life changes for elderly persons. The importance of history, obtained from the elderly person and collateral sources, is discussed. Two case examples illustrate some of the challenges of obtaining and interpreting information for such psychosocial assessments.

In our changing Canadian demography, social workers are increasingly being called upon to assess the ability of elderly persons to function in their environments. There are several aspects of psychosocial assessments of elderly persons that distinguish them from other types of assessments (Gold, 1999).

It should be noted that the elderly are not a homogeneous group. Some are physically well, some are frail, some are competent in all spheres, and some cannot remember the names of their children. Each has an individual history of life experiences and relationships with a unique meaning and importance to him or her.

We [the authors] reject the notion of "cookbook assessments," which are popular in many disciplines. We believe that social work brings to human caring the unique perspective of individuals in their social environments. Unlike a researcher who seeks to discover the commonality among disparate individuals, patterns of behaviour, common perceptions, shared difficulties, etc., a social worker focuses on the individual's strengths, deficits, and coping strategies in the unique environment. Thus, we depend upon the patterns established through the insights of practice wisdom and research to evaluate and predict both patterned and unique outcomes in individual cases (Kazi & Wilson, 1996).

I.   Implications of a Psychosocial Assessment

Assessments for the elderly, as for all other age groups, touch upon complex psychological and social factors and composites relative to the individual in the context of social environment. For the elderly, there is additionally a precarious and delicate balance of a number of bio-psychosocial components. For instance, particular factors of and responses to time, relationships, losses, and vulnerabilities, as well as entrenched attitudes and a history of experiences, make this balance particularly fragile.

Therefore, a change in any one component is likely to result in a more profound effect upon the others and, in turn, upon the balance than would be expected among the non-elderly. For example, a broken hip that results in temporary hospitalization is more disorienting, alarming, and dependency producing in the elderly than would be the same condition in a non-elderly person and may even lead to symptoms of cognitive impairment and social dysfunction. These consequences, which are most often transient, may lead caregivers to arrange alternative care without including the elderly in the decision process.

Similarly, social changes such as the death of a spouse or changes in a living arrangement may lead to a response (e.g., withdrawal, apprehension, depression, "stubbornness," etc.), which is considered disproportionate and dysfunctional by others. This response may also express itself in physical symptoms (e.g., loss of appetite, sleeplessness, chest pain, fatigue), which may then be interpreted as decrepitude.

Any involvement, therefore, which may imperil the delicate balance is fraught with potential disturbance for the elderly person. Psychosocial assessments are frequently used as a tool. Commonly, an assessment is related to a decision to make a major change in the environment of the elderly person. Rarely does the elderly person seek the assistance of the social worker. More often, family members, health care professionals, facility management, or other service providers instigate the assessment process. Although the assessment is often used by others as an end in itself (i.e., to determine entitlement or access), social workers see assessments as dynamic undertakings, the first part of a process that feeds back on itself as indicated in Figure 3.1.

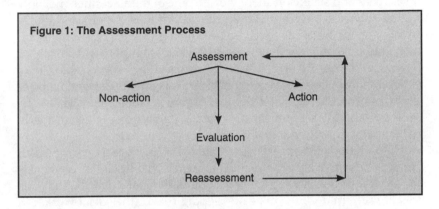

Figure 1: The Assessment Process

II. How to Conduct a Psychosocial Assessment

Social work assessments of the elderly are always guided foremost by the reason for an assessment and the context in which it is being undertaken. Thus, both conducting the assessment and interpreting it requires specialized skills and knowledge on the part of the social worker. Particular attention needs to be paid to the following, which will subsequently be more fully discussed.

A. the purpose of the assessment
B. the circumstances under which the assessment is conducted
C. the capacities and skills of the elderly person and of caregivers
D. cultural factors
E. fears

A. Purpose of the Assessment

The most common reason for the referral of an elderly person to a social worker is to determine "what should be done with her or him"? For instance, there is an external demand to develop, confirm, or negate a plan that has been made for the care of an individual, most often at a time following significant functional or social loss.

Often the assessment is initiated by trusted others, with the purpose being concealed from the elderly person. Although the intent is usually viewed by such concerned persons as necessary and in the "best interest" of the elderly person, the social worker must understand the investment and suspicion about the outcome of the assessment not only for the elderly person but also on the part of these significant others. In this regard, some may wish to be relieved of their responsibilities, while others may view the assessment as an attempt to intrude on, or be critical of, family or institutional caregiving. For example, some children may believe that a psychosocial assessment is an evaluation of their concern for an aging relative, or hospital personnel may believe the same assessment is merely the first step in institutionalizing an elderly patient whose treatment hospital bed they want to free.

In part, both are correct in their perceptions, since one of the major reasons for an elderly person undergoing a psychosocial assessment is to determine his or her capacities to cope and to determine the supports that are required. Thus, the gate-keeping role of the social worker in conducting such assessments is important. It is often on the basis of such assessments that the elderly individual is admitted to institutional care or transferred from one level of care to another.

The purpose of the assessment is frequently missed, identified as "medical" (i.e., part of the prescribed treatment or the consequences of a specific medical condition). Hence, there is often an association of social work assessments of major medical disorders such as strokes, hip fractures, kidney failure, or heart attacks. It is a mistake to link the medical conditions per se with the rationale for assessments. It is rather the impact of the illness on the life situation, on the ability of the individual and his or her environment to cope with the need for new arrangement of interdependencies that inspires such assessments.

B. Circumstances of the Assessment

The circumstances under which the assessments of elderly individuals are conducted are important to understanding the type and meaning of the information that the social worker is able to obtain. Usually the social worker who is attempting to assess the elderly individual will be a stranger to the client, arousing many concerns about talking to strangers, telling family secrets, and revealing the last vestiges of privacy—one's secret thoughts, hopes, and fears—left to the elderly.

Further, it is quite common in institutional settings to disrupt the individual by changing his or her locale for the purpose of the assessment. Well-intentioned relocation to an interviewing room or social work office may result in an individual appearing disoriented. To minimize hurdles in conducting an assessment, the social worker needs to pay particular attention to the problems of personal comfort of the client, including seating comfort (e.g., well-padded chairs that may suit an agile adult will become a trap for the elderly who are unable to get out of the chair), issues of language compatibility (including figurative speech related to era and gender, as well as fluency), and hearing (e.g., although an individual may be able to hear you on a one-to-one basis, the background noises of a hospital, screened out by staff, give garbled auditory input when using a hearing aid) (McInnis-Dittrich, 2002). Also of major importance in conducting such assessments is the significance of the presence, or absence, of caregivers and significant others. Reticence, fear of offending, and allowing others to answer are among the problems inhibiting an honest assessment.

Further, the elderly person may be suspicious about the goals of the assessment, sensing that the results of the assessment may have a profound, yet unspecified, impact on the rest of his or her life. Thus, they may be hesitant to initiate discussion about such issues, retreating instead into passive resistance, which may be missed construed as cognitive and/or personality deficits.

C. Capacities and Skills of the Individual and of the Caregivers

Any psychosocial assessment of the elderly must pay particular attention to the capacities of the individual as well as to any limitations he or she may have. It is tempting to see only the limitations of the elderly and to give these issues inordinate prominence (American Psychological Association Working Group on the Older Adult, 1998). To what degree are the activities of daily living (ADL) managed by the individual and with what type and amount of help? How does this management by this person differ from his or her previous standards and why? These are a few of the more salient questions that could be considered in this regard.

Similarly, it is important to evaluate the skills and capacities of significant others in the life of the client as they relate to possible caring options. For instance, do others provide direct service to the client? What is the nature of the care provided? How able and willing are they to continue to provide these additional services? How does the elderly dependant feel about the care that she or he is receiving and the possibilities for continuing assistance? Has there been, or will there be, a major transfer of assets, and under what conditions? Are there relationship issues being denied or protected by the emotionally, physically, or financially vulnerable elderly person? Is there fear? Is there a realistic plan preferred by the person being assessed?

In many jurisdictions, social workers are among the professionals who conduct capacity assessments. Such assessments are focused on "a person's mental capacity to make decisions about property and personal care" (Ministry of the Attorney General, 2003). Capacity assessment is not limited to older persons but questions of diminished capacity or "incompetence" are raised more frequently in relation among older persons than to other age groups. This type of assessment, while undertaken often by a social worker and formalized to meet legislative requirements, is only one aspect of a total bio-psychosocial assessment.

D. Cultural Factors

The concept of culture of must include socio-economic, geographic, gender, age, racial, religious, minority status, and ethnic components. Such factors are of particular importance to the psychosocial assessment of the elderly and include communication and language, role relationships, and the past and present expectations about aging, including the anticipated behaviour of others.

What needs to be remembered in this context is that both the worker and the elderly person are grounded in his or her own set of age-related cultural values and assumptions. The elderly, often very conscious of these age-generated differences, are often distrustful of the willingness and the ability of the social worker to understand them and, therefore, are frequently not very disclosing. In addition, the current generation of the elderly has a view of social workers and their functions that is quite different (e.g., dispensers of charity, welfare workers, and pryers into privacy) from a professional social worker's in view and practice.

Similar differences may be well disguised within family units, especially between the elderly person and some family caregivers, which may create additional tensions and ambivalence. In addition, there is frequently an overlay of cultural dissonance created by intermarriage and the accrual of extended family members deriving from distinctly different cultures. For instance, in a three-generational situation, these interrelationships are particularly complicated "sandwiched generations" (Imber-Black, 1998).

Finally in this regard, the predominant culture of the agency, in addition to the specific expectations of staff from a variety of cultural backgrounds, further complicates and colours what is expected from the behaviour of the elderly person and from the psychosocial assessment. Such differences may be extreme enough to actually precipitate the request for a psychosocial assessment. Certainly these differences will influence the way in which the assessment is conducted, interpreted, conveyed, and used (Clark, 1997).

E. Fears

Implicit for the elderly person undergoing a psychosocial assessment are a number of fears, often unvoiced, that threaten his or her well-being and may undermine the entire assessment process. Interrelated and interdependent of each other, these fears are truly psychosocial in nature because they represent emotional, practical, relational, and situational changes. They often include the following:

a. displacement (loss of decision making and lifestyle as well as familiar setting);
b. self-doubt (questions raised about memory, cognition, capability, and power);
c. social value conflicts (compromise of social role and image both as perceived by the individual and by others; the sense of being discarded);
d. abandonment (rejection by significant others, not being understood or appreciated, including by the social worker doing the assessment); and,
e. finality (ultimate helplessness and the real beginning to the end of self).

Within the process of the assessment, not only awareness of the worker of these fears is important, but also the opportunity to express and discuss their implications is crucial. Unfortunately, this is an area often shunned by social workers and others. It is difficult for the elderly person to discuss his or her fears, and this is often used as a reason by the social worker for not pursuing them. Excuses such as irrelevance, lack of time, and concern about being hurtful are often used to cover for the potential distress in workers confronting these feelings in others and, significantly, in themselves.

III. Skills

The skills required to evaluate and interpret the information obtained for a psychosocial assessment of an elderly person are in accordance with the best traditions of social work practice and require competent social work practitioners. In short, this is not an area for beginners. In addition to understanding a wide range of theoretical constructs concerning the biological, psychological, and social aspects of adulthood and aging, the social worker must understand the complex cultural and interpersonal structures that transcend several generations.

Although the skills required to undertake the psychosocial assessment of an elderly person are the same skills required in any adult assessment, the vulnerability and fragility of balances for the elderly demand highly competent social workers for obtaining, interpreting, and conveying such information, which reflects an accurate, sensitive, and true picture of the life of these individuals. Particular awareness is required in the obtaining of information and deriving meaning from it, including the need to allocate sufficient time in shorter, more frequent contacts and to grasp the significance of discrepancies and language in communication issues (previously noted).

As well, special sensitivity is needed to explore areas that the elderly often view as sacrosanct (e.g., financial disclosures, family problems, etc.). Elderly persons often believe that problem solving is a matter of honour, something one does on one's own, and the notion of asking strangers for help is viewed as abrogation of responsibility by many [see Chapter 1]. Similarly, the elderly commonly view professionals as possessing authoritative knowledge—"the truth"—and thus may feel obligated to follow the "prescription," even if the options presented are not viewed as necessary or desirable. Self-determination, a cherished social work value, can easily be set aside in such situations.

Many elderly clients assessed by social workers have moved [usually as a result of physical, psychological and social losses] toward increased dependency upon other family members and formal caregivers. Thus, a central theme in any psychosocial assessment becomes at what point in the dependence and independence spectrum the individual finds himself or herself at that particular time and how she or he perceives the exchanges involved in caregiving and getting. For example, the very presence (hovering, answering for, being "betrayed" or offended) or absence of family members (anxiety, lack of confidence) may change the whole tone, course, or even content of an assessment.

The complexity of relationship histories, which are remembered in idiosyncratic ways by the elderly persons and significant others in their lives, produces a potential situation in which the taking of histories is neither straightforward nor subject to objective confirmation. It is how that history is remembered rather than any objective "fact" that is critical to it that becomes the issue. Often, there is mutually agreed to or unilateral "protection" of one or the other of these issues that may distort facts. Thus, the inexperienced social worker is often led by conflicting stories to conclude degrees of memory loss and incompetence on the part of the elderly person when, in fact, it may be evidence of the complexity of perception and the meaning attached for different individuals about the same event. Sorting through these differences in drawing carefully considered professional conclusions is indeed an advanced professional skill.

Conveying the results of psychosocial assessments of the elderly is often more complex than it is for other adults. There is a sometimes an overwhelming temptation to take sides, to advocate for, to wish to protect, and to oversimplify a lengthy history of experiences and relationships. In such situations, there is a need for a skill in succinct reporting of significant conclusions that can and will be read and understood within the framework of the host setting and in the context of the elderly person's actual life situation.

It is important to note that much of the data received by the social worker will not be transmitted to others, but is used to form the basis of the professional assessment. Further, it should be remembered that the transmission of raw, descriptive data, out of context, is potentially more harmful than useful. Sharp, analytic conclusions, briefly documented, are essential in this regard.

In summary, while recognizing the highly refined skills consonant with all social work practice, psychosocial assessments of the elderly demand additional knowledge, sensitivity, and methodology. The fragility of the balance of biological, psychological, and social factors for the elderly is compounded by the fact that such assessments are usually instigated by others and are perceived as leading to major change and loss of self-determination. Differences in the meaning of time, and intergenerational differences in values, expectations, and communications, as well as the lack of understanding or acceptance (by host agencies and involved others) of essential social work values and criteria for making an assessment further complicate the issue. The requirements of a well-trained and highly skilled social worker to conduct such assessments are essential if the profession is to grow and develop in this area.

IV. Role

In a situation where the particular expertise and skills of a social worker are so clearly essential, the actual roles and responsibilities filled by trained social workers vary greatly from setting to setting. The involvement of a social worker in the process of psychosocial assessments of the elderly depends on several factors: (1) whether the past itself, and/or the position of the social worker is community or agency based; (2) whether it is part of an ongoing job description (e.g., intake, discharge planning) or is an occasional part of other expectations; and (3) the status accorded social work in the specific setting, as well as the agenda [official and covert] of those requesting the assessment. Depending on the mandate of the host agency, the assessment process may limit the social worker to:

1. conducting only an assigned part of the assessment, as part of a team, within prescribed criteria, as it delegated assistance to another professional (e.g., psychiatrist, admissions officer, head nurse) or one aspect (e.g., the family, living conditions);
2. a limited time frame for the whole process;
3. reporting within a prescribed format, including a checklist and/or lack of interest in diagnostic or even any written report;
4. *pro forma* performance, with predetermined conclusions, to suit a family or interested agency, with resistance to advocacy or differing recommendations; and,
5. no allowance for follow-up, with the elderly person, family, and/or involved agencies.

Most requests for assessments may come to social workers as a response to a variety of issues.

1. Concern about the functioning of an elderly person, which has been judged to be inadequate or poor, and concern for

the future of the elderly person in his or her present situation based on "observation," complaints, and the value system of the observer who sometimes represents family (or some part of it, not always in agreement with the others), or by a professional, or a "neighbourhood," and a referral is made to a professional or agency with the expectation that a change in situation (e.g., removal to a more protected setting) will be made, preferably quickly.

2. Concern for caregivers based on "observation," complaints, and/or suppositions about "what is best for everybody" or "what is best for the caregivers"; requests made by "other family members" often not the primary caregiver; professional care of a "visitor" (e.g., public health nurse) or social work agency working with all or part of the family; and a referral is made to a professional (e.g., physician) or to an agency expected to admit the elderly person for relief of the family (e.g., a nursing home).

3. As part of a discharge process based on institutional priorities and needs as perceived by identified personnel whose observations and training depend upon disciplines foreign to social work's view of assessment; or by family members who may or may not be aware of relationship, responsibility, and respite issues; and a referral is made to any institution/agency with request for placement/service, preferably quickly (and often directly from hospital).

4. As part of admissions (including transfer) based on decisions usually by family members and/or institution staff often with the approval of a physician and/or other professional care providers; the information on the formal application is often suspect (i.e., "fudged" to insure acceptability of an elderly person); often networking (in all its forms) is used to jump queues or obtain preferred accommodation. Thus, a referral is made directly or by a brokering agency (e.g., placement of coordination service); a reassessment is often made by the accepting agency.

5. To establish competency for legal and financial purposes based on request, usually by family members, or by an interested professional (e.g., physician, lawyer, hospital administrator); often controversial; application often suspect. Then a psychosocial assessment is occasionally made by a lawyer or based on uninvestigated appraisal by

other personnel (e.g., appraisal by a lawyer to determine if someone is competent to sign a power of attorney or to make out a will or appraisal by a nurse of a patient's competency to give medical consent).

6. To remove nuisance and responsibility based on complaints or concerns of neighbours, and a referral is usually to police, church, or visiting professional (e.g., public health nurse) with expectation of quick resolution.

7. Finally, to assess for a course of treatment and/or adjustments in lifestyle based on concern for changing functional ability or life situation by individuals, and a referral is made to a specialized clinic (e.g., gerontological assessment clinic).

V.   Advanced Psychosocial Assessment

Particular assessment difficulties arise in circumstances that may be significantly more fraught with complications for the elderly than for other adult populations. Ironically, many of these involve what appear to be maladaptations to problems or dysfunctions, but are actually ways to maintain an individual's homeostasis, relationships, and/or abilities to function.

Common examples include individuals who live alone in disreputable, unhygienic, and/or dangerous areas, such as abandoned buildings, unserviced apartments, or even outdoors. Elderly persons who talk out loud to themselves or even to unseen others may not be hallucinating but rather merely externalizing the dialogues most people participate in internally or have aloud only in private situations such as driving a car.

Further, in this regard, marriages and companionships that may appear bizarre or even destructive to others may be the product of the well-worn habits and patterns and serve the most important needs of the partners. Often, a sense of propriety or desire to protect the relationship with a spouse, with a child, or other caregivers or with a "buddy" are such that the elderly person denies truths, concocts or colludes in fictions, or purposefully obfuscates. Perceived danger of retribution (even elder abuse), pride, shame, guilt, or desire to deny all may inform what is reported by the elderly person, family members, or other caregivers. Professionals who wish to avoid entanglement or responsibility may participate in hiding or changing such important truths to these elderly clients.

In many cases of persevering and confabulation, the skilled social worker needs to assess the significance of the uses to which these are put and weigh their part of the total biological- and/or psychological-social context. A vital part of every assessment is a consideration of the costs as well as the gains and losses to the elderly of removal or change of those components that comprise their present lifestyle, given their own attachment to them. When such components appear to be linked to the elderly person in a pathological way, it will also require that an experienced clinician make a well-reasoned judgment about the relative costs of intervention. In these situations, the risk of harm is at least as great as the possibility of benefit.

In addition to the acquisition (and practice) of the complex skills required, there are general, realistic, and political issues for the social worker who wishes to engage in legitimate, thorough psychosocial assessments of the elderly. One challenge is to establish the significance of the complexities of psychosocial assessments and move toward changes in understanding and use of the assessment on the part of those with access to them.

Thus, social workers should push for changes in role definitions for social work, including specialized training, authority, status, adequate time, and follow-up allotments. The social worker should always insist that attempts be made for prior involvement of the elderly person, including open discussions of risk, choices, and consequences. Social workers also should be willing to risk the support of social work principles, seeing the elderly person as a client even when this concept is not understood or supported by referring agencies or persons. Finally, social workers should advocate for changes in agencies and community services serving the elderly and their eligibility criteria. They should also participate in creating appropriate policies and innovative community facilities and services as desired and required by the elderly and their caregivers (Fortune et al., 2000).

VI. Case Examples

Case #1

An elderly woman is admitted to hospital following a stroke. She has been left with a functionally useless arm and some difficulty in locating objects in space. At times, she appears to be confused about the time of day and where she is. A social worker is called in to determine where she should go following hospitalization. Prior to her stroke, the lady lived alone in an apartment, which she had shared with her husband of 40 years. He had died suddenly six months before her stroke. Her family had wanted her to leave the apartment at the time of her husband's death, fearing for her safety and her ability to manage on her own. The physician was concerned that the patient's time in acute care was coming to an end since nothing more could be done for her. The nurses, who had become quite fond of the patient, worried about her being alone and about what they viewed as her confusion. The patient wanted to go home to her apartment and appeared not to understand the concerns of the staff or her family: "I've done all right until now and I'll manage just fine."

Case Comments

In this instance, the social worker is required to develop an understanding of this individual in her social context, including the concerns of the significant others in her life. The views of family members, health care professionals, and alternative care providers cannot be ignored. They form part of the environment in which the elderly must function.

Social workers employed in settings providing care for the elderly are engaged in assessing individuals to establish appropriate levels of care and of service provision. For example, social work assessment may play a role in determining intervention programs geared toward improving functioning such as re-establishing ADL skills. Similarly, community-based programs such as Home Care rely on social work assessments in establishing complex in-home care programs. In such cases, the assessment of the environment of the individuals, especially the human environment of the home, will determine not only the suitability of home as the place of care but also the degree to which the home environment can tolerate the intrusive nature of support services that provide direct care.

Generally, social work assessments are called for when the person-in-environment nexus is seen to be either very complex or problematic in the provision of service, which is believed by someone—the client, the family, or any one of a myriad of care providers—as impinging upon, impeding, or preventing the otherwise desired plan of care.

Case #2

Mr. and Mrs. M have lived on the fifth floor of a high-rise, subsidized, senior housing development for 10 years. Mrs. M, a petite woman, speaks no English; although she smiles and nods to neighbours as a greeting, she never invites anyone in nor has she visited anyone in the apartment. Mr. M, a tall, heavy man with a marked limp and awkward gait, speaks a simple, often crude English, and is often loud, argumentative, and, when drunk, belligerent.

Their country of origin is not known, and the Ms have no visitors. Rumour, passed along among neighbours, is that Mr. M use to work at heavy labour, but was badly injured on the job and spent over a year in hospitals and in rehabilitation and has lived for the past 20 years (he is thought to be 70) on disability and old age pension. It is also rumoured that there was a daughter who married, moved away, and died in childbirth.

The superintendent of the building reports that Mr. M has always been angry, bitter, and verbally abusive, but that Mrs. M, when she was with him, could quiet him with a touch or a few soft-spoken words. They always looked immaculately groomed and formally dressed. Lately, however, the neighbours have noted that Mrs. M hardly goes out, and when she does there are spots on her dress, clothing colours do not match, and she seems to stumble. Some neighbours have mentioned to each other that they think she drinks now, too—others wonder whether she's losing vision.

Recently, the neighbours have reported what sounds like loud arguments in a foreign language, occasional weeping, and some loud thuds coming from the Ms' apartment. Unpleasant smells have also been reported on the floor, seeming to emanate from the Ms' apartment. Some neighbours say that Mr. M's drinking has become more frequent than the former regular, monthly binges.

The neighbours held a meeting of tenants without inviting the Ms to discuss them. Some expressed anger and irritation at the Ms. Others expressed concern for Mrs. M's safety and for the possibility of fire threatening them all. Others felt that for the sake of everybody, "the matter" should be looked into. By unanimous vote a call alerting the police was made.

On the basis of the formal complaint of disturbing the peace, two police officers demanded admission to the Ms apartment. They issued a warning and, despite Mr. M's rage, made a referral to Home Care.

Case Comments

The social worker, to make a valid assessment, must acquire basic information about the language, country of origin, and some of the values/customs at the time of Mr. and Mrs. M's youth. Access to the Ms must be made gradually and with their permission if at all possible, especially to counteract the effects of the neighbours' and police intrusions. Help from a compatriot, a public health nurse, or someone who is involved with the disability benefits should be used, if possible, and notice of intended visits (repeated patiently) should always be given.

It is essential, once contact has been permitted, that the assessment includes the nature and nuances of the marital relationship and the investment each has in it. Further, questions about health and safety need to be explored, and the kind of assistance the Ms might be willing to accept (e.g., doctor, nurse, tests, surgery, medication, clinics, pamphlets, etc.) offered, leaving the door open for change.

Assessment should be made with both—and, if possible, separately with each partner—of their perceptions of their present lifestyle and relationships; important changes they see and react to; consideration and preferences for their futures; difficulties they identify for which there may be acceptable solutions, etc., as well as an updated appraisal of their living conditions, interdependencies, attitudes, cognitive function, and emotional liabilities.

References

American Psychological Association Working Group on the Older Adult. (1998). What practitioners should know about working with older adults. *Professional Psychology: Research and Practice, 29*(5), 413–427.

Clark, P. (1997). Values in health care professional socialization: Implications for geriatric education in interdisciplinary teamwork. *The Gerontologist, 37*(4), 441–451.

Fortune, A.E., Keigher, S.M., & Witkin, S.L. (2000). Social work comes of age in the International Year of Older Persons. In *Aging and social work: The changing landscape,* pp. xiii–xix. New York: NASW Press.

Gold, N. (1999). The nature and function of assessment. In Francis J. Turner (ed.), *Social work practice: A Canadian perspective,* pp. 110–131. Scarborough: Prentice-Hall/Allyn & Bacon Canada.

Imber-Black, E. (1998). *The secret life of families.* New York: Bantam Books.

Kazi, M.A.F. & Wilson, J.T. (1996). Applying single-case evaluation methodology in a British social work agency. *Research on Social Work Practice, 6*, 5–26.

McInnis-Dittrich, K. (2002). *Social work with elders: A biopsychosocial approach to assessment and intervention.* New York: Allyn & Bacon.

Ministry of the Attorney General. (2003). *Capacity assessment.* Retrieved from http://www.attorneygeneral.jus.gov.on.ca/english/family/pgt/capacity.asp.

Internet Resources

The American Geriatrics Society
    The premier professional organization of health care providers dedicated to improving the health and well-being of all older adults.
    http://www.americangeriatrics.org
The Merck Manual of Geriatrics
    Merck & Co., Inc. is a leading global research-driven pharmaceutical products and services company.
    http://www.merck.com/mrkshared/mm_geriatrics/home.jsp

Additional Readings

Corcoran, K. & Fisher, J. (2000). *Measure for clinical practice*, volumes 1 & 2, 3rd ed. New York: The Free Press.

First, M.B., Spitzer, R.L., Gibbon, M., et al. (1995). *Structured clinical interview for DSM-IV Axis I disorders, patient education (SCID-P) version 2.* New York: New York State Psychiatric Institute, Biometris Research.

Ramey, D.R., Raynauld, J.P., & Fries, J.F. (1992). The health assessment questionnaire, 1992: Student review. *Arthritis Care and Research, 5*(3), 119–129.

Schneider, L., Tariot, P., & Olin, J. (2000). *Manual of rating scales for the assessment of geriatric mental illness.* Wilmington: Astra Zeneca Pharmaceuticals, LP.

CHAPTER 4

SELECTED PROBLEMS IN COUNSELLING THE ELDERLY

SUSAN BERNIE-MARINO

This chapter outlines five major problems that social workers encounter in counselling the elderly. These are: attitudes and counter-transference in the counselling relationship; the dependence/independence conflict; dealing with issues of loss; intergenerational conflict; and the question of capacity. A discussion of each problem is followed by practice suggestions and a case example. Particular attention is devoted to the multiple nature of problems and high levels of stress in the lives of aging clients. The chapter concludes with a consideration of those counselling interventions that cut across problem areas and practice settings.

I.   Introduction

Counselling the elderly presents social workers with both unique challenges and serendipitous rewards. The rewards come in many ways. There are individual positive experiences in encountering the spirited dispositions of older people who at first glance seem frail and overwhelmed by stress and change. The normal stresses of aging present problems themselves and are always there as undercurrents to the additional crises caused by illness, social circumstances, multiple losses, and relationship conflicts. The challenges too are unique because aging sets up a more complex relationship between life cycle issues, individual psychosocial dynamics, and disease than for younger age groups. The gerontological social worker, therefore, needs to have a way to untangle this web, to assess and respond to what is the most important issue facing clients without denying their other problems.

In this chapter, five major problems experienced by the elderly who are counselled by social workers will be discussed. They were chosen because they are almost always present in some way in all problems brought by the elderly and their families to the counselling process, regardless of the precipitating event. Further, they seem universal in nature and cut across a variety of practice settings. While it is helpful to have an integrated practice model for working with the elderly, there are specific interventions for specific problems. Therefore, the discussion of each problem is followed by some practice suggestions and a case example.

II.   Attitudes, Counter-transference, and the Counselling Relationship

A.   The Problem

As social workers, we are consciously and unconsciously affected by a variety of attitudes toward the aged, which are maintained by our lack of knowledge and life experiences with the elderly. These attitudes often block accurate assessment and diagnosis, the direction of counselling to appropriate goals, and the choice and time frame of interventions. The concept that best explains how one brings these attitudes to the therapeutic relationship is counter-transference.

Counter-transference is the therapist's emotional reactions to a patient, based on the therapist's past relationship history rather than the "real attributes of a patient." These are usually distortions that occur in a worker's perceptions as a result of conflicts within him or herself (Greene, 1986). They are also the result of a set of attitudes workers bring to their roles due to having stereotypic views of a particular client group that causes them to see their clients in biased and incomplete ways.

Aging is associated with decline in all areas of a person's functioning. Social work's belief in the potential for growth and development is challenged and compounded in the struggle to help older clients value themselves in a culture that does not accord them a meaningful place. Often, unconsciously, we agree with this view of aging and react in one of two ways.

We may ascribe helplessness to our clients and rejection by society and thus become inadvertently paternalistic. As well, we may offer solicitous sympathy, believing that they have been abandoned and, therefore, fail to seek out and mobilize the potentially available resources within their families and the larger community. Second, one may deny the impact of older people's functional difficulties and push for a stoic acceptance of their losses, demanding too quickly that they adapt to a compromised existence (at a pace that is sometimes beyond their capacities). These behaviours from social workers can flow from their own anxieties and fears of aging and an unconscious wish to deny its impact. Such attitudes have generally led to unrealistic expectations of rehabilitation of elderly patients, and decisions by professionals to stop treatment when they don't recover quickly enough (Becker & Kaufman, 1988).

Most social workers have not had the benefit of exposure to the special dimensions of life and life review that elders hold by virtue of their position in the life cycle. As well, most workers have probably been trained in professional schools that offer little specific gerontological content in their curricula. Previous social work experience with the elderly is usually insufficient to learn about the unique characteristics and life view of the elderly population. Aging is one life stage social workers have not passed through themselves at the time they practice (Monk, 1986). Younger workers may bring a sense of energy and optimism about life, but it may be difficult to understand those who measure life in terms of "time left" and by past accomplishments (Monk, 1986). Indeed, such notions can feel threatening to a worker's own sense of well-being and feelings of optimism. This altered sense of time is crucial to the elder's preservation of self (Tobin, 1988), for by respecting this life view is in direct contrast to one's tendency to pathologize those who "dwell in the past." It is only in recent years, and by professionals who have learned in clinical relationships with the elderly that the process of life review has been reunderstood as a "legitimate" one. As a consequence, reminiscence has become an essential tool in counselling.

Because aging bears a stigma, so does social work with the elderly. The belief that elders are unable to change usually leads to the assumption that working with elders entails practical resourcing for people, or "supportive" work only, or a "job that no one else wants." Thus, some social workers working with the elderly may unintentionally devalue their work and be reluctant to engage them in psychotherapy directed at change when it is warranted.

Another problem is generated by the medical model inherent in professional social work training, which defines problems as the result of pathology (Miller, 1987). This view is further reinforced by having most services for the elderly as hospital-based ones. Indeed, there are problems caused by disease processes and also problems associated with aging. There are also problems and conflicts that are a reflection of neither—because they are part of a lifelong pattern of coping. Thus, if a worker sees aging as pathological and the problems of aging as being due to disease, his or her ability to separate out the processes of aging from disease and personality and social circumstances is obfuscated.

B. A Practice Framework

Most social workers understand that attitudes and experiences directly affect their work. Social workers with the elderly, however, are more likely not to have had the "corrective experience" related to their own attitudes toward aging prior to entering this field of practice (Greene, 1986). The lack of education/training and lack of personal and professional experience previously noted above are two reasons for this. An additional one is that most attitudes are outside of one's awareness until we experience them within the context of a therapeutic relationship with the elderly themselves, the process in which the concept of counter-transference finds its embodiment.

In this context, social workers need to accept that uncovering such attitudes and feelings is one of the most difficult, and yet most important, aspects of counselling, as it enables them to identify counter-transference issues. As adult children themselves, they also need to be aware of particular opinions they have about dependency and family responsibilities. This will usually protect them from making the error of overidentification with, or judgement of, the adult children of their clients.

Of prime importance in this regard is a social worker's feelings about loss, grief, and dying. "Death anxiety" (Greene, 1986) can affect a worker's assessment and willingness to handle issues such as living wills, pre-arranged funerals, discussions about quality of life, life-threatening illnesses, and spiritual matters, which may be a primary source of support for their clients. The problem presents itself most vividly to the beginning gerontological social worker at a time when she or he is also experiencing the greatest anxiety about bonding with clients and being helpful. Paradoxically, it is such anxiety and discomfort with clients in counselling that are the most useful tools for identifying counter-transference issues.

Supervision is a primary process for identifying counter-transference so that one may see and respond to elderly clients as they really are. More accurate assessments and relevant treatment planning can then occur. Social workers should make this a goal of supervision, if it is available. If not, they should find a colleague in the field whose work, experience, and/or relationships with elderly clients are known to be good and consult them.

As well, social workers can make a special effort to reformulate their understanding of growth and development and client self-determination, and the possibilities for its expression in later years. The recent literature on the psychological tasks of aging can be quite helpful in this regard as it reflects acknowledgement that aging, as different from other stages of the life cycle, includes tasks of integration, finding meaning, and preserving rather than expanding a sense of self (Tobin, 1988).

Further, social workers need to value their work with the elderly and have it valued by their colleagues. They should ask themselves questions such as, "What can I learn from the elderly that no other client group can teach me?" and "What unique role in family and community life do the elderly perform?" They should also spend time with other colleagues in this field who value this practice even if they have to go outside their agencies to do so.

Most importantly, social workers need to consider their clients as their primary teachers. Aging, although it carries some universal themes, has many stages. Subgroups of the young, middle, and frail elderly have decidedly different stresses and adjustment issues (Hartford, 1985), and the experience and reality of aging has particular significance to each individual. Despite our own sensitivity and knowledge, we should not assume that we know what clients have not told us because we failed to ask them.

C. Case Example

Mrs. L, an experienced social worker, began work in a geriatric hospital, a job change of her own choosing. Her first client, Mr. M, a 74-year-old gentleman, had been in long-term care for a year because of an unstable diabetic condition and repeated dizzy spells. His behaviour and self-care in the hospital was erratic and uncooperative. Staff believed he could never be managed outside hospital, although he desperately wanted to live independently. The social worker advocated for an alternative plan to try him living in a nursing home in the community. Finally, the doctor agreed.

Mr. M listened impatiently to the social worker's plan. The social worker cited it as a better alternative to hospitalization and talked of new opportunities available. Suddenly, Mr. M became very angry, accusing her of having no respect for him. Taken aback, the social worker sensed she had missed something. So she apologized, and asked. "You should know better than to tell me what I should like," said Mr. M, "and you should also know that neither I, nor anyone else would want to live in a nursing home."

The social worker wondered how she had missed remembering that no elder ever wants to be institutionalized, and how she had failed to empathize with the loss of self-esteem that accompanies such a move. Later, in discussion with her supervisor, she talked of her eagerness to be helpful and her assumption that her advocacy for discharge would be appreciated by her client. She felt that the "bad" attitudes were held by other team members—not her.

When she examined her own feelings about institutionalization, however, she admitted that they matched Mr. M's. Unable to accept this reality, she was reconstructing an image of new possibilities in nursing home life, so that she would not see herself as an agent in helping the client toward an uninviting future. With this new awareness in her next session with Mr. M, the social worker empathized with his fear of institutionalization and facilitated a discussion of some of the negative aspects of nursing home life. These were compared with Mr. M's experiences of the negative aspects of hospital living. The criteria of continuing care that were crucial to Mr. M's sense of dignity and self-esteem were then identified. Mr. M agreed to visit a number of nursing homes to evaluate them as potential placements on the basis of those criteria. Eventually, he was placed voluntarily in a nursing home that least offended him and his world view.

III. Dependence-Independence Conflicts

A. The Problem

Dependence-independence conflicts are present in some form in almost every counselling situation with an elderly client. This is an issue in the worker-client relationship because many elderly are involuntary clients. Such conflicts can be the primary contributing factor to a client's presenting problem of being faced with growing dependency and the consequent losses of self-esteem and morale needed for recovery. They can also threaten the relationship between the client and his or her caretakers, the family, and the community. They also present ethical dilemmas to the worker who may wish to control and direct treatment plans and, often times, they place a worker in conflict with his or her agency and its mandates.

Western culture values independence, and it is a primary source of self-esteem for persons of all age groups. Productivity and financial self-sufficiency, emancipation from one's parents, and the ability to care for oneself are benchmarks of self-worth. Thus, dependence, vulnerability, and the acknowledgement of such needs are often judged, especially by the elderly themselves, as weaknesses.

Our society has vigorously supported the rights of individuals to maintain autonomy and to retain control of decision-making affecting their own lives. Indeed, the social work ethic of client self-determination is partly founded on this principle. Yet the processes of aging inevitably place elders in a position of growing dependency. For most, beginning with retirement, and/or the death of a spouse, financial resources, especially for women, diminish. Widowhood brings with it the loss of companionship, a caretaker, and the surfacing of "new" emotional needs. Physical and mental illnesses and health decline make it difficult for an elderly person to care for himself or herself independently. In addition, the stresses of loss and changes in the aging process can overwhelm an elder person's capacity to adapt accordingly. They can lower his or her morale and motivation to make use of opportunities to maintain some degree of independence. The lack of fit between an elder person's partial but not totally dependent lifestyle needs (e.g., assisted mobility, "one-stop shopping," simplified bureaucratic procedures for service eligibility, etc.) and his or her environment can cause him or her to withdraw into isolation.

When we are young children, we are expected to be dependent and are supported by institutions of change (e.g., family, friends, church, school system, etc.) to be as such. However, the dependency that accompanies aging is not as facilitative. Faced with the lack of resources to help elders maintain some degree of independent living, the community often feels obligated to turn to institutionalization to solve the problem. Paradoxically, this is the most feared experience for the elderly client, and often the process of institutionalizing a parent causes guilt that tears families apart. What must be understood here is that elders often regress temporarily as the result of the lowering of self-esteem that accompanies loss of, or even partial, dependency.

Helpers, including social workers, may inadvertently reinforce this regression by being overprotective and/or by mobilizing too many services too quickly for their clients. A classic example occurs when families move too soon to institutionalize a parent in difficulty after the death of a spouse as they see their parent's difficulty in coping as a permanent reality rather than a grief or immediate stress reaction. They are frightened by their parent's loss of capacity and feel unable to be their caretakers.

The elderly's resistance to dependency can be functional, as the experience of dependency can be debilitating. Research indicates that institutional living is deleterious and that the less residents have control over their lives the more they tend to lose control of their faculties. Alternatively, the feeling of being in control over what happens in one's life can improve physical and mental functioning (Lowy, 1989). In fact, aggressiveness (seen in younger people as pathological) and unrealistic beliefs in environmental mastery are associated with positive outcomes in the very old in adaptation to stress (Lieberman & Tobin, 1985).

Because of their resistance to dependency, the elderly have become a unique group of involuntary clients. Often they have not initiated contact for help and they do not see a need for services but are pressured to do so by others—usually a family member or health agency (Burstein, 1988). Additional factors are that they have been socialized to see seeking help as a weakness or stigma, and they may have had previous experiences of controlling interventions in their lives. Thus, not used to seeking help, they may be unaware of eligibility for service or become overwhelmed by the maze of bureaucratic tasks involved to gain eligibility (Burstein, 1988). Oftentimes, in this regard, they may truly come to believe that they are without choices.

The social worker then has a dilemma in engaging the elderly at all in the counselling process, not to mention persuading them to utilize services they may need for their own protection and welfare. Additional ethical dilemmas are present for social workers when working with the frail elderly in the community. They are caught between the belief in the client's right to self-determination and the responsibility to protect him or her. Thus, the worker may be ambivalent about his or her own need to be in control of the treatment plan and about being responsible for another person's safety (Burstein, 1988). It may be difficult to decide who the client is in the face of conflicting demands of the elderly client who doesn't want the worker there and the family, who does.

Such problems are made more complex by the fact that there are still no clear guidelines on the issue of rights and freedoms and protective service for the elderly in North America. Traditional medical models of health care delivery emphasize protection and solutions that would be "in the best interests" of patients. Resistance to such orientations is seen as negative. At the same time, the ever-expanding human rights movement in our society emphasizes an adversarial approach, which can pit worker/agency vs. client or the family vs. client, especially in situations of incompetence (Parsons & Cox, 1989). Neither of these approaches offers social workers a viable way to maintain their ethical stance of preserving relationships. In short, the adversarial model does not lessen conflict and can reinforce isolation. The social worker must somehow find a working relationship between the client's right to and need for self-determination, proper social work practice, the mandate of the agency, and the opinions of family members and other professionals working with the client. This is a delicate issue that should not be minimized by practitioners working in this field.

B. A Practice Framework

A worker needs to understand that the elderly must maintain dignity and some control of their lives. Elders must participate, if possible, in all decisions about their present and future circumstances. Even if older people have lost the capacity to do some things for themselves, many still know what they want. Thus, all interventions should include some options.

A social worker's assessment of problems and behaviours should include an attempt to understand what function they play in the maintenance of independence. Even a lack of motivation or interest in coping by a client may be due to his or her belief in a lack of capacity or opportunity for recovery to some level of independence. Behaviours seen as "problematic" among other age groups (e.g., aggression, magical thinking, etc.) must be reassessed in elders as to their functional merit for coping (Tobin, 1988). Thus, an astute assessment of remaining capacities and strengths should be undertaken. As such, initial interventions should be directed toward enlarging a sense of competence and problem-solving abilities (Monk, 1986). Treatment objectives should be simplified and achievable and counselling goals should be aimed at the alleviation of stress rather than personality change.

Engaging elderly clients in counselling requires the use of non-traditional methods and a willingness to be flexible in one's professional role. For instance, home visits rather than office interviews are suggested. The worker must be willing to be patient, to relinquish control, and to begin a therapeutic relationship on the client's "turf" on his or her terms (Burstein, 1988). Helping clients with tasks they choose (e.g., filling out income tax or rent subsidy forms, etc.), even if it does not constitute the worker's purpose in being there, is also recommended. For if the worker succeeds in engaging the client, the worker must be willing to be proactive in a case management as well as psychotherapeutic capacity.

A worker also needs to have thought out the conflict between a client's self-determination and protective service, and be clear about when she or he must intervene despite a client's refusal of service (e.g., extreme self-neglect, malnutrition, suicidal risk, clear danger to others) (Burstein, 1988). The worker should clarify this mandate with the agency for which she or he works and the worker should expect to face many case situations in which the preferred course of action is not clear and be willing to live with such ambivalence. Obtaining support from, and sharing the responsibility with, the agency in this regard is important.

The worker should remember that a client may be incompetent in one area but not in others. Thus, a client may not be competent to care for him or herself, but may be competent to choose who he or she wishes to care for them from among viable alternatives. Assuring integrity in the face of protective service can prevent the spiralling effect of loss of some, but not all, independence.

Paternalistic and adversarial models of conflict resolution about issues in independence should be avoided. Rather, interventions should be directed toward preserving relationships and fostering communication and interaction between elders and others in their lives. Family mediation and helping organizations need to be more flexible to meet elders' needs and wishes is preferable, as it helps elders to maintain rather than be separated from needed ongoing support.

Finally, social workers must be willing to accept elderly clients as permanent clients with fluctuations in service needs. This is the reality of working with the chronically frail elderly in the community—that clients, although stabilized, will return at a later date, when in need, to the agency and worker with whom they are familiar and whom they trust.

C. Case Example

Miss G, 85 years old, was admitted to the hospital due to recurrence of a drinking problem. Medical assessment revealed several physical problems—severe arthritis, malnutrition, and a significant hearing deficit. She had no family and had discontinued attendance at a community day care program three months ago. Doctors, concerned about her frailty, were recommending nursing home placement. Miss G adamantly refused. She was referred to the hospital social worker for discharge planning. The social worker was advised that doctors were considering a declaration of incompetency in order to place her.

After initial assessment, the social worker concurred that Miss G was becoming too frail to live on her own much longer. In the absence of family, no one was available to help on a regular basis and Miss G did not have the financial means to hire a part-time caretaker. The social worker, lacking time and a mandate to provide ongoing support, could not be involved beyond Miss G's hospital stay.

Miss G refused to sign the applications for nursing home placement, which she said would also deny her financial independence because of the high cost of care. The social worker decided to "buy time" and deferred placement planning. Further discussion with Miss G revealed that the pain of her arthritis had demoralized her and she had started drinking again to cope with the pain. She had stopped going to day care because of social problems arising from her hearing deficit. The social worker persuaded the doctor to refer Miss G to a pain clinic. Medications were prescribed that relieved the pain and improved her mobility. A hearing aid was obtained with the help of a government subsidy.

Subsequently, Miss G's morale improved and she was more than ever determined to return home. The grounds for incompetency decreased with her improved functioning and her doctor had no choice but to discharge her home. Before she left hospital, the social worker proposed that Miss G visit several nursing homes in her area as a preparation for the future possibility of being unable to live independently. Surprisingly, Miss G agreed to this plan and also to return to the day care program she had previously attended.

In this case, the social worker's initial assessment indicated a need for institutional placement. The client's strong resistance moved the worker to alternative interventions, which improved the patient's competence and the chances of a better quality of life wherever she would ultimately reside. The social worker's efforts to delay adversarial action (declaration of incompetency) were productive. Creative solutions not present in the initial assessment arose and the need for placement against the client's wishes was lessened.

IV. Dealing with Issues of Loss

A. The Problem

As indicated in Chapter 1 loss is a central theme of aging. It is intrinsic to other stages of life, but is experienced differently when successful grieving can more easily lead to new roles, relationships, and opportunities. Loss for the elderly is much more difficult. Aging is characterized by a multitude of changes, matched in number and intensity probably only to those experienced in childhood. Changes are stressful at any age, and in later years many changes are experienced as loss. These losses often follow each other in rapid succession, such that the elderly have little time to adapt to one before they face another, creating a "domino effect" with one impacting the next. While many elderly have learned to adapt to change throughout their lives, they are often without the resources, vigour, and supports that were available to them in earlier years.

Some losses lead to other losses. For example, the death of a spouse (loss of companionship, intimacy) can lead to a reduction in income and a change in residence (loss of familiar surroundings, lifestyle), especially for women. If the spouse was also a caregiver, his or her death may lead to the institutionalization of the widow(er) (loss of home, financial flexibility, privacy, independence). For young elderly, the experience of initial losses, especially in physical functioning, may precipitate an awareness of aging, expectations of impending frailty, and fears of future losses. Some of these fears are realistic; others are not. In any event, these fears can be immobilizing.

Grief reactions are different for the elderly. Grieving for prior losses may not be complete before additional loss is experienced. Further, loss provokes memories of earlier losses and additional grieving tasks. Grief and loss reactions in the elderly can be so pervasive that they precipitate other problems—depression, excessive preoccupation with self, ill health, self-imposed isolation, and, in some cases, even death by suicide or "failure to thrive" (Garrett, 1987). This is sometimes referred to as "bereavement overload"—overwhelming grief reactions related to multiple successive losses with little or no separate grieving time (Garrett, 1987). Losses experienced by the elderly may be categorized according to five main areas outlined as follows (Freeman, 1984).

Loss of some physical and mental functioning is experienced by most elders at some time. Physical losses can be life-threatening (e.g., cancer, heart conditions, etc.), or those whose chronic nature necessitate living with ongoing pain, diminished energy, and mobility and the curtailment of some social activities (e.g., arthritis, sight and hearing loss, etc.). These losses may represent the onset of old age, the end of usefulness, depletion of strength and vigour, and result in a lowering of self-esteem.

Mental losses include loss of cognitive abilities (memory, concentration, ability to integrate new learning) and are most often due to stroke or senility. In this regard, the diagnosis of organic brain syndrome (e.g., Alzheimer's disease) is the one most feared by the elderly. Its significance is indeed profound, for this disease inevitably leads to a loss of memory, orientation, perception, communication, and ultimately a loss of identity and all forms of independence. The reality of this diagnosis is different from the fear of it. A primary defence for the maintenance of hope and self-esteem for cognitively impaired individuals facing further deterioration is denial. Paradoxically, this attitude is functional through the phase of the illness when the patient is aware of his or her impaired capacities and is a defence against depression. The fear of senility is another matter. It is not uncommon for depressed elderly to suffer memory problems and to resist treatment because of the fear of the diagnosis of senility. Residing in treatment facilities and institutions with cognitively impaired individuals generally compounds this fear.

Losses in status and role in aging occur with retirement and changing marital and family role, e.g., when the last child leaves home or with the chronic illness of a spouse. These have significance for many elderly persons.

Losses of relationship are profoundly felt because relationships are the primary source of connectedness, for the expression of caring and fulfilment of needs for companionship and intimacy (Powell, 1988). Opportunities for close relationships are lost through death, separation, divorce, the relocation of friends, colleagues, neighbours, and adult children. One of the most painful losses is the death of one's child, as it is experienced as a "death out of time" (Conway, 1988).

Loss of lifestyle and familiar surroundings occur when one is no longer able to participate in activities formerly enjoyed due to physical decline, or reduction in income or relocation occur. Such losses are compounded if the elderly person has no choice in these changes and is unable to maintain a sense of continuity during a move.

Loss of hope and self-esteem are usually the consequence of multiple losses and the meaning attributed to these losses. They can occur if one's identity is primarily tied up in a lost relationship or role, or if the loss seems to signal decline and further losses.

The intensity of these loss experiences varies with the individual and his or her place in the late life cycle—whether one is in the early, middle, or later stages of aging (Hartford, 1985). For instance, the younger elder responds by adapting quite well. Of those who experience difficulties some become depressed but respond quite well to treatment. It is the frail elderly and, for the most part, those in institutional care who have experienced the most losses, are isolated, and present more serious emotional and behavioural problems. The most common fears of loss held by the elderly are the fear of losing independence, the fear of loss of one's mind through senility (mentioned earlier), the fear of abandonment and isolation, and the fear of dying, particularly of dying alone.

Normal grief reactions of elders may seem quite pervasive. Grieving may initially be overwhelming for many and they may find even the most basic activities difficult to do. This is not a permanent incapacity as much as it is the initial response of anxiety. In turn, they may withdraw temporarily, experience somatic complaints, or express anger toward family members or friends. Further, they may seem unduly resistant to problem-solving and to making even the smallest, practical change or to accept new opportunities. These grief reactions are normal and stem from the need to minimize change and maintain continuity in their lives in the aftermath of loss. Generally, grieving for elders takes longer than for younger people, often for a period of up to two years.

Some grief reactions are more serious and require radical and prompt intervention. These include rapidly deteriorating physical health, alcohol and substance abuse, excessive feelings of unworthiness and guilt, refusal to eat, a pervasive and prolonged sense of hopelessness, and/or anxiety that prevents the person from functioning at all. These are also symptoms of clinical depression, which if left untreated can be life-threatening.

Finally, some of the influences affecting an elder person's ability to cope with grief are his or her age, the number of losses within a short period of time, past experiences coping with loss, the existence of other relationships and a support system, the ability to maintain control over related factors, one's state of health, and belief in a power greater then oneself (Garrett, 1987).

B. A Practice Framework

Helping the elderly deal with loss involves four main practice principles: (1) a comprehensive assessment; (2) mobilization of resources to reduce stress, minimize change, and maintain continuity during the grieving process; (3) assisting in grief resolution; and (4) instillation of hope.

The assessment of loss includes its perceived and real consequences to the griever. A history of previous losses should be obtained with information about how such losses were dealt with in the past. As well, fears of future losses should be uncovered. The extent of a person's support system should be explored — including the state of health, financial and social resources, and the attitudes and availability of family, friends, and other caregivers. Attempts should be made to understand the person's belief system about loss, what causes it, how one is "expected" to cope and express grief, and what is necessary for resolution, e.g., religious beliefs and/or ritual, etc. A "before loss" picture of the person's personality and lifestyle should be obtained in this regard.

An evaluation of the person's grief reactions should be undertaken, and assessment as to whether they seriously impede the person's capacity to function or not should occur. Even some bizarre behaviours (e.g., acting as if a dead person is there, repeated and numerous gravesite visits, etc.) should be tolerated. Particular attention should be given to the potential presence of clinical or acute depression.

As indicated previously, social workers need to explore their own feelings and reactions to loss and be aware of attitudes and feelings they bring with them to the counselling relationship. This will allow them to identify issues of counter-transference and to more sensitively and accurately respond to the client's reality rather than their own.

Initial interventions should be aimed at reducing stresses and minimizing change. Most behaviours of the elderly associated with coping with loss are directed toward preserving self-esteem and continuity of lifestyle. What is most needed is to maintain connectedness with others. All interventions, especially initial ones, should be in concert with these goals. This means that interventions should be scaled down to the minimum to solve immediate problems caused by the loss (Monk, 1986). Because self-esteem is so closely tied to the issue of independence, those interventions that will allow an elder as much choice and autonomy as possible are recommended. There are exceptions, of course, but very few. Even faced with the necessity of institutionalization, an elder can be offered some options and some involvement in decision-making, which are crucial to successful adjustment. If possible, no major life changes should be contemplated at the initial stage of grieving, especially against a person's will.

Efforts should also be made to communicate with family members and to encourage them to refrain from moving too quickly to assume control of an older person's affairs. In this context, the family needs to understand that an elder's incapacities provoked by loss are often normal grief reactions and temporary. The social worker should understand that the family's own stress load may make it difficult for them to become primary caregivers. Social workers can mediate between the conflicting sides of adult children and their aging parents or relatives and point out alternative sources of support for both the grieving elder and his or her caretakers.

Models of grief resolution have been presented by experts in death and dying. Most more or less follow the stages outlined by Kübler-Ross (denial, anger, bargaining, depression, acceptance). These models are helpful in assisting elders with grief resolution. However, the grieving process does not always occur the same way for elders. In some cases, only partial grief resolution is possible if losses occur in rapid succession. Sometimes, final resolution is delayed, for example, in the case of the institutionalized widow(er) whose spouse is institutionalized or of a marital partner who becomes the caretaker of a chronically ill spouse over a period of several years.

Special counselling interventions may include:

a) *Normalizing grief:* Helping the elderly understand that their grief, associated anxiety, fears, and impulses are normal and are not pathological and, that they are not "crazy." Helping them express feelings of anger and guilt are important, especially for a spouse caretaker who may have felt exhausted and resentful during the long illness of his or her partner.

b) *Separating present losses from the fear of further ones:* This process sometimes reduces the overwhelming nature of current adjustment tasks. Discussions of fears can identify realistic from unrealistic worries and pave the way for later counselling aimed at preparation for future losses. Interventions for cognitively impaired individuals differ in this regard. It is not always advisable to directly challenge their impaired perceptions because of their inability to integrate reality and recover accurate memories. Empathizing with feelings and responding to the purpose behind their behaviours is preferable.

c) *Reviewing present and past losses:* Discussing the significance of these attachments is a useful way to identify their meaning and value in the life of an elderly person. This process affirms their past and contributes to a sense of worth. Such review should include a gentle uncovering and validation of both positive and negative aspects of those relationships. Loosening bonds with the past only occurs when it can be accepted in its true perspective (Schwartz-Borden, 1986).

Social workers should learn about the transformational possibilities of loss experiences in order to communicate hope to their clients. This includes exploring existential dimensions of loss and grieving. Petersen (1985) has identified spiritual counselling as a crucial component to grief resolution. Grieving involves spiritual dimensions as well, and such faith can provide a solution to the dilemma of guilt, a means to maintain a sense of worth beyond what one can do, and provide a sense of love and relatedness beyond loss. Older people often refer to their faith as a source of hope for grief recovery.

Social workers without the appropriate training should not act as experts in pastoral matters. However, they need to respond with some understanding and compassion to reflections about faith as a support in the face of loss. Information and workshops for professionals working in death and dying are prolific and are good sources of counselling support.

C. Case Example

Mr. P's 45-year-old son called a family counselling agency for help with his 73-year-old father. Mr. P had relocated a year ago to be closer to this son. However, he had been miserable since the move and was becoming excessively demanding of his son's time. Ever since a heated argument between them a week ago, Mr. P had been hallucinating but refused to see a doctor.

A social worker visited Mr. P in his apartment. During their first interview, she discovered he had suffered a series of major losses over the past ten years, beginning with the death of his wife and followed by the death of two siblings and the deaths of two other adult children. Consequently, he had moved to town to be closer to his only remaining son. The relocation had involved the sale of his home of 40 years and leaving his church congregation, which constituted his main social network.

The move had not gone as positively as he had hoped. His adolescent grandchildren in the new setting were uninterested in him. Unsure of his way around, he was dependent on his son for transportation everywhere. After their argument the previous week, he had been seeing his dead wife in his apartment at night. Believing his father was psychotic, his son had suggested he be admitted for psychiatric treatment.

Mr. P refused the social worker's suggestion of a joint interview with his son to discuss his feelings and the issue of dependency. The social worker, therefore, met alone with Mr. P's son, identifying the issues of loss and grief. She agreed to remain involved and Mr. P's son agreed to delay a referral for psychiatric treatment if his father would attend a day care program. Mr. P reluctantly agreed to a referral for day care for three months and began attending.

During the next eight weeks, the social worker undertook individual counselling sessions with Mr. P. An extensive review of his losses was carried out. Mr. P had a very close relationship with his deceased wife. He acknowledged that probably he had "imagined her presence" in the nights that followed the argument with his son, as she had always been a support to him. The social worker explained this as a grief reaction and affirmed that he was not crazy. Mr. P also talked of the years following his first son's death, during which he helped to raise his grandson, and felt proud of his contribution as a grandparent. The social worker affirmed Mr. P's close bond with his grandson and encouraged him to correspond with him.

Mr. P's hallucinations disappeared. He began to take an interest in day care activities. Alternative ways of solving his transportation and shopping difficulties were organized through community agencies so that Mr. P would not be so dependent on his son for daily outings. Mr. P transferred to a church-based activity group from the day care program. His son reported that their visits were more amicable.

However, Mr. P continued to resist discussing any conflict issues with his son for fear of alienating him and losing the relationship with his only remaining child. The social worker did not push him to do so, but reminded him of her availability to mediate should conflict arise in the future. After two months, visits were decreased to monthly contact and Mr. P continued to function well.

V. Intergenerational Conflicts

A. The Problem

Every family has within an issue of aging. This statement has emerged in recent years as a reminder to social workers, and especially family therapists, of the impact of aging on family life. The social work literature generated from practice experience is emphasizing the changing nature of intergenerational relationships occurring in families as a result of people living longer and pointing to new problems experienced between these generations.

Because of technological advances that have increased life expectancy and population behaviour patterns begun earlier in the century, the nature of the extended family has changed. The lower average age of marriage, earlier parenthood, and the decrease in the number of large families in that mothers are younger when they have their last child have contributed to the advent of the four- and sometimes five-generation extended family (Miller, 1981). There are often generations in childhood, early adulthood, middle age, those in their early to middle elder years, and elders at an advanced stage of frailty.

These generations, for the most part, live separately and studies of the very old indicate that they prefer it this way (Berman, 1987). However, numerous studies are validating the existence of, the importance of, and the frequency of contact between these generations. It is well known that family members turn to each other first for economic and financial help, emotional and social support, and assistance in crisis situations (Miller, 1981).

The myth that families abandon the elderly, or are alienated from them, has been put to rest. It is known that family members are the primary caretakers for the elderly, and particularly significant are findings that emotional involvement with others may increase in relative importance after the middle years, probably because losses in aging remove other sources of gratification (Brody, 1974). As well, the mental health of older people is linked with family relations (Kirschner, 1985). While generational ties are strong, there are new stresses and strains between the generations, which underlie family problems presented to the gerontological social worker.

In life cycle terms, one of the primary reasons for conflict is that the developmental tasks and needs of each generation are no longer complementary. In the aging family, the most prevalent tensions occur between the elderly and their adult children. The middle aged, or young elderly, are facing major changes in their own lives—including preparation for, or adjustment to, retirement. Their adolescent or young adult children may not quite be independent. If they have successfully launched their children from home, they face adjustment to the "empty nest" and attendant changes to their marital relationships. The young elderly are faced with the task of placing some boundaries between themselves and their adult children, which is difficult for parents whose primary source of identity and satisfaction was found in raising their children. Problems at this stage are mediated by the energy and wellness of most young elders who have opportunities for new freedom and the pursuit of new interests. They also gain new roles as grandparents. In this regard, conflict occurs if children have difficulty leaving the parental home or if their parents cannot let them go. In recent years, a new problem has been presented to the young elderly by the returning home of their adult child, often with their own young children, after separation or divorce.

Early widowhood of a parent often presents adult children with first concerns about the potential dependency of their parents. A common reaction is for these children to mobilize prematurely to take control of their parent's lives, unaware that their own fears and grief are affecting their judgement about the ability of their remaining parent to adjust successfully to living alone.

The most prevalent conflicts, however, occur because of the real and increasing dependency needs of frail elderly parents and the high stress load already being carried by their middle-aged adult children. Terms such as "the sandwich generation" (Miller, 1981) and "women in the middle" (Brody, 1981) explain the particular dilemmas of this middle-aged generation who become caretakers of their parents. Most studies have revealed that the bulk of caring is by women—adult daughters, daughters-in-law, a female spouse—often a single woman, unmarried or divorced and, therefore, is seen as the one most able to provide support. The sons and daughters of these elderly are in the middle, squeezed by the competing demands for their resources and caregiving to generations above and below them, to their spouses, and by their responsibilities to work outside the home. This problem is particularly felt by women, many of whom have returned to the workforce. They highly value the care of the elderly as a family responsibility, and also their financial contribution to the marriage and the new opportunities for personal development and freedoms their own children's departure from home has brought them. The culture in which they were raised assigned to the daughters the principal caregiving role, yet their ability to carry this out is profoundly affected by lifestyle changes. The strain is usually felt in terms of competing roles, financial resources, fatigue, and personal relationships (Brody, 1981).

The particular position of adult children becoming caregivers to their frail elderly parents is not helped by the fact that there are no models for behaviour for the aging multigenerational family because it is a relatively new phenomenon. In addition to problems created by competing interests for time and resources, there are individual emotional issues experienced by each generation—both the givers and receivers of help.

As well, there is a culturally supported notion that "one has a duty to one's parents." Indeed, one of the prevalent dilemmas facing adult children is their belief that they "can never do enough" for their parents, indebted as they are for the gift of life and the care they received as children (Berman, 1987). Most adult children do what they can do willingly and out of love for their parents, but the issue of "what is enough" usually causes them significant anguish as they make decisions about how to, and how much to, care for their frail parents. Certainly, it is a guilt-inducing dilemma, and because adult children have difficulty negotiating this conflict, they are often unable to place limits on their caretaking and present to social workers as suffering from extreme exhaustion and stress.

Their elderly parents, on the other hand, are suffering themselves. They have probably experienced a series of irreplaceable losses (e.g., health, spouse, work, home) and come to their children with additional losses in hope and self-esteem (Berman, 1987). In turn, they feel guilty at not being able to maintain themselves independently and may be afraid of losing the support of their children because of their immediate needs. Some authors are predicting trends whereby it will not be unusual for adult children to share their home with a frail parent despite their desire to live independently (Berman, 1987; Parsons et al., 1989). In one study, frail elderly women living with their adult children reported most frequently their wish not to be a burden (Parsons et al., 1989). Elders may, therefore, be afraid of openly discussing their problems with adult children for fear of alienating them, and as a result may become more isolated. In addition, the frail elderly have fewer opportunities to reciprocate the care given by adult children, and thus their sense of usefulness diminishes.

Some mention must be made of the vulnerability of this particularly stressful relationship to elder abuse. The problem of elder abuse is now recognized as a family issue whose victims are both the elderly and their exhausted caretakers. In this context, some elderly feel the only thing they have left to give is money, and the risk of adult children in financial need taking financial advantage of their parents, or being perceived as doing so, is well known.

How can adult children and their parents resolve their own personal emotional conflicts in the shifting balance of dependency as their parents grow old? A new relationship is needed, and it is inadequate to explain the change in terms of role reversal that children need to become parents to their parents, or parents need to become children to their children (Brody, 1974). The concept of filial maturity attempts to explain this relationship shift, suggesting that it is a maturational task of the adult child to be depended upon, to relinquish childhood roles, and to decide, without extreme guilt, how much they can do, and that it is enough. Their ability to do so generally depends upon many factors—facing their own fears of aging, accepting separation from and the future death of their parents, and resolving or putting aside previous conflicts with their siblings and parents. The onset of the dependency of aging parents is certain to reactivate old wounds among all family members. Frail parents need to be willing to depend upon their children and to accept that there are limitations to their children's resources.

Conflicts are most dramatically evident in families facing the crisis of institutionalizing a parent. Paradoxically, at this time, it is the giving up of the caregiving role, rather than maintaining it, which can be the problem. Also, at this time, the parents' fears of abandonment and the children's sense of guilt are exacerbated because of the attendant losses in relationships that are anticipated. Unfortunately, institutionalization is often considered an urgent matter by families, hospitals, and placement agencies by whom social workers are employed, affording little time to carry out the interventions that result in a successful adjustment process.

B.   A Practice Framework

Most families who seek help from gerontological social workers are coping with the issue of intergenerational conflict arising out of the perceived or real increasing dependency needs of an older, sometimes frail, member. More often, it is the adult children who initiate the referral rather than the elderly person themselves. Sometimes, the problem is not initially presented as a family issue but as an individual referral by a hospital or health agency concerned about the ability of an elderly person to care for himself or herself.

Some professionals suggest the utilization of a family systems approach to all issues facing the elderly because of the belief that problems in one generation inevitably affect other generations. In my experience, there are problems facing elderly individuals and couples that should be treated individually, and the boundaries between the generations should be honoured. However, as standard practice, all assessments of elderly problems should include an inquiry about the nature of the extended family network, their availability for support, the relationships among the generations, and whether changes in the life of one generation have had an impact on the problem presented for help (e.g., divorce, death, financial setbacks, or illness of adult children). As well, the importance of relationships with grandchildren should not be ignored.

It is particularly important in cases of elderly spouses where one is a caretaker to inquire about the emotional and other support they receive or do not receive from other friends, relatives, and adult children. In addition, in all cases where problems of an elderly person involve increased caretaking or alternative placement needs, a strong effort should be made to contact and involve other family members. Other relatives may already be providing support and need to have their effort confirmed. It is important to remember that caretakers, especially siblings, may have differing perceptions about the problem and personality of their parent, and this difference is a reflection of their own relationship history and the stresses and strains of caretaking they may be experiencing. For example, reports of an elder's uncooperativeness may be exaggerated because of current relationship stress.

Adult children, faced with making decisions about care for their parents who don't want to, often need help to understand the dependence/independence conflict and loss and grief issues from the elder's point of view. Further, they should be helped to refrain from assuming control over their parents' lives unless they really need it, and encouraged to become willing to assume a nurturing role. Helping adult children to know about community support services for themselves and their parents, and how to access them, is useful counsel.

As a matter of course, major decisions involving competence and institutionalization should involve meetings with all the adult children, even if it entails them coming from considerable distances. Adult children need to feel consulted and invited to contribute to such major changes in their parents' lives. Further, a family gathering gives the social worker the opportunity to assess family dynamics. Family meetings reveal the existence of conflicts and supportive networks and the family's style of problem-solving. Children should be invited to share their fears about their parent's frailty and the stresses they are experiencing in their own lives related to their capacities and motivation to assume responsibilities.

At such family meetings, it is the social worker's responsibility to have assessed the functioning of the parent and to have some opinion regarding his or her capacities and needs, especially related to placement in an institutional setting or the potential for continued independent living. These issues should be realistically interpreted to the family. Social workers should be aware of the tendency of families to assign the caretaking role to a particular member—often a daughter or the sibling living closest—and for that person to assume it. It is here that work can be done to prevent the future problems of resentment, exhaustion, and caretaker breakdown that occur when one family member carries the total responsibility. All siblings should be encouraged to offer help, even if they live at a distance.

Problem-solving and family cooperation is the primary goal of family meetings, not the resolution of previous long-standing relationship issues (Parsons & Cox, 1989). The presence of conflict should be identified and recognized as legitimate suffering, but family members should be encouraged to put this aside for the time being. The elderly parents should be present if possible. They should *always* be asked to contribute their opinions and be involved in decision-making if they are competent. If the social worker has time, subsequent counselling can be offered to individual family members to help them understand and resolve rivalry and conflicts arising from their earlier history.

Special problems arise around decisions of competence and managing finances. Adult children are very sensitive to the issues of disenfranchisement and inheritance, and if a parent's finances are to be managed by one or more of their adult children, they must have a relationship of trust and cooperation and the blessing of the rest. Otherwise, a third party trustee is advisable.

Social workers also need to help adult children identify how much care is enough and empathize with the guilt and sense of loss that is felt by them, especially if the need is for institutionalization. Helping elders and their children find a suitable placement acceptable to both, interpreting institutional care issues, and mediating between families and staff during the initial phase of placement when adjustment problems are most prevalent are important counselling tasks. Social workers can be of great assistance in helping institutions understand that families' initial complaints about care are often a reflection of their grief reactions and in finding ways for families to continue in a supportive role in caretaking after placement.

The elderly, especially the frail elderly, may have a more difficult time resolving conflict with their adult children if they perceive them as abandoning them or not doing enough. Thus, they must be encouraged to refrain from making them feel guilty. Individual counselling; utilizing life review aimed at recovering one's history as parent and grandparent; validating and finding meaning in these roles, past and present; and identifying feelings of failure and needs for forgiveness is very helpful in this regard. It is also important to remember that the elderly and their adult children yearn for reconciliation, and sometimes joint sessions can be arranged to provide both the opportunity to ask for and offer forgiveness. Finally, parents provide counsel and emotional support to their children at all stages of the life cycle. Social workers can be creative in helping both generations identify ways the elderly can continue to be parents, even in the last stages of life.

Case Example

Mrs. G, a 79-year-old widowed woman, lived alone and seldom went out. She was visited regularly by her 50-year-old daughter, B, and a public health nurse who was concerned about her failing memory. During one of her visits, the public health nurse found Mrs. G in bed crying. After much effort, she was finally able to determine that Mrs. G had had an argument with her daughter, whom she said had shouted and pushed her. The public health nurse contacted a social worker at a psychogeriatric outpatient clinic, which had a mandate to investigate concerns of elder abuse. The social worker and nurse visited Mrs. G together. After a prolonged interview, the social worker determined that Mrs. G had extensive cognitive problems. She then contacted B, her daughter.

Over the phone, B burst into tears. She told of how she had been visiting her mother three times a week for two years, looking after her banking, meals, laundry, and housekeeping. She wanted her mother to see a doctor because of her memory problems, but Mrs. G refused. On the night of the quarrel, Mrs. G accused B of stealing her money and was refusing to pay her rent. B admitted to exhaustion, frustration, and fear of losing control again with her mother's lack of cooperation. An office interview with B allowed the social worker to determine in more detail Mrs. G's history of progressive mental deterioration, the probability that she was not competent, and that it was unsafe for her to continue living alone. A family meeting including B and two siblings, a brother and sister living in towns nearby, was subsequently arranged. At the meeting, B's brother accused B of wanting to institutionalize their mother and of being an unwilling caretaker. The younger sister expressed guilt at her unavailability to help out because of job and family responsibilities.

The social worker explained Mrs. G's problem as one of possible senility and not neglect. She outlined B's great caretaking efforts and explained the phenomenon of caretaker stress. She suggested that placement in a nursing home was probably required, pointing out how difficult this process is for adult children and their parents. A plan was suggested whereby Mrs. G would be referred immediately for respite care and a psychiatric assessment undertaken to clarify questions of diagnosis, competency, and further ability to live independently. Mrs. G was unable to participate in the family meeting because of her confusion. The family agreed to this plan. Respite care was organized. A psychiatric assessment revealed the probability that Mrs. G was suffering Alzheimer's disease and required nursing home placement.

Three weeks later, a second family meeting was held. The social worker discussed the diagnosis of Alzheimer's disease and its implications for further mental deterioration, providing the family with written educational information about the disease. All three siblings outlined their inability to take their mother into their own homes. The social worker advised placement and offered to assist. The siblings agreed to visit several nursing homes and to return to the social worker with their selections and for assistance with the application process.

At this meeting, the question of Mrs. G's money management was also raised as the psychiatric assessment indicated financial incompetence. The siblings decided to apply for committeeship together and to delegate B to make day-to-day decisions regarding spending to which B agreed. Unfortunately, Mrs. G was not well enough to participate in the planning. She was advised of the plan and given an opportunity to share her wishes, which she was unable to do. During her weeks in respite care, she remained very confused but seemed more secure. She could not understand why she was unable to return home and was unable to participate in the placement process.

After Mrs. G was admitted to a nursing home, the social worker met with the family again to talk about institutional care, to encourage all to visit regularly, and to offer suggestions about communication strategies with nursing home staff. She also provided information about Alzheimer support groups. During the next year, B remained the primary adult child involved in her mother's life. She called the social worker from time to time for advice and to gain support for her feelings of loss as her mother gradually became unable to recognize her. A year later, all three adult children were able to decide together on issues of heroic measures after their mother was admitted to general hospital.

V. The Question of Capacity

A. The Problem

Specific issues about capacity and risk assessment of the elderly thread their way throughout this chapter. This topic deserves its own discussion for many reasons. Social workers are increasingly involved in legal assessment roles, are consulted for opinions about capacity and risk, and provide leadership in mediating opinions and finding solutions while participating in multiple counselling tasks and maintaining therapeutic relationship with their clients.

The problem is indeed complex, posing questions that when first experienced seem impossible to answer. For instance, how do we maintain therapeutic alliance with elderly clients who cannot manage independently but are determined to do so when we may be a direct agent in depriving them of their right to continue to make their own choices? Where do we stand on borderline situations of risk, in the ethical dilemma between autonomy and protection from harm? What guides us to make decisions and develop skill?

A social worker's dilemma is increased if job roles conflict with either our professional or personal values. We most often experience this in the context of working in jobs where scarcity of resources and time make it very difficult to provide supports to enable elderly to maintain independence longer, or in others' attitudes that define being elderly as a condition of infirmity. Bissell (1996) suggested that social workers must avoid colluding with role prescriptions that promote the gap between how others see an older person and his/her true worth. He argued that when in role, we cannot keep our personal morality for private life. The literature on ethics and health care has shown that one consequence of experiencing this dichotomy is "moral residue," which significantly promotes stress and affects work performance if we witness or act in ways that compromise our integrity. "The experience of compromised integrity that involves the setting aside or violation of deeply held (and publicly professed) beliefs, values, and principles can sear the heart" (Webster & Baylis, 2000, p. 221).

Furthermore, earlier this chapter identified that social workers too are influenced by their subjective opinions of who and what is "old" and "frail." We may inadvertently practice ageism in well-intended but unconscious ways. Recent research suggests that our subjective assessment of the elderly's mental and physical functioning influence our assessment of risk and, in turn, recommendations for care. Clemens and Hayes (1997) found that health care professionals vary significantly in their threshold for risk tolerance of elderly clients. These authors named one group "snap decision makers" who judge risk, make decisions, and recommend action quickly. Another group, "the agonizers," withdraw from crises to assess client wishes and resources more carefully, but "agonize" over decisions about risk and practice recommendations. The "agonizers" are more likely to be social workers who adopt a process-oriented approach. But both groups are likely to use positive or negative character labelling strategies to legitimate their plans of care, and thus mediate their ethical dilemmas. The result may be risk assessment that is highly subjective and reflective of a practitioner's professional and work culture (Clemens & Hayes, 1997).

Social Work's Codes of Ethics directs us to act first and foremost in the interests of our clients. This is always the first principle from which all others flow. These ethical principles are further embedded in the practice guidelines of our professional colleges and licensing bodies and remind us to be aware of the potential for liability. The standards are explicit about the privacy of client interests, but they still do not tell us how we determine those interests (Clemens & Hayes, 1997). Social workers, then, do experience significant ethical conflicts in jobs that involve deliberating about issues of capacity and risk with the elderly.

B.   A Practice Framework

Good counselling skills are informed by knowledge and enhanced by professional experience. They are also developed by the practice of *discernment*—the specific skill of integrating what we know with what we value and learning how to make choices.

When we work with elderly clients at risk, we are informed by law, our professional ethics and guidelines, our process-oriented approach to assessment, therapeutic relationship building, and problem-solving. These are valuable tools and guide us more than we may realize.

We should know the laws that define capacity and substitute decision-making and how they are determined in our respective provinces or states. It is true that such laws do not always offer unanimity or definitions or precision re-operational tests (Kapp, 1988). However, some venues are becoming clearer in law. For example, the test for capacity under three laws in Ontario, Canada, *The Substitute Decisions Act, 1992, The Health Care Consent Act*, and *The Mental Health Act*, is a cognitive one. Capacity is specifically defined as the ability to *understand* information required to make decisions, and *to appreciate* the consequences of a decision or lack of a decision. Capacity is mental capacity, not a clinical condition or diagnosis. Furthermore, it is task-specific. A person can be incapable in one area and capable in others. Who is designated as legal assessors (social workers are included in SDA, 1992), who has the right to be substitute decision-makers, and how they are to act is further defined by law (Wahl, 2003).

In addition, the principles that inform legal definitions and tests of capacity, and guide appeals are often articulated and available to us. Among the most predominant are: (1) persons can make risky decisions if they know what they are doing; (2) substitute decision-making should be a last resort; (3) a person's values, goals, and preferences are respected in laws that define how capacity is determined and how substitute decision-makers should carry out their responsibilities.

There are arguments that our codes of ethics and practice guidelines should be more explicit to help us make decisions in ambiguous situations of risk. However, even if they were, they could not resolve the inevitable gap between our ethics and the complexities of practice. "The occupational rules which cover every possible situation have yet to be written" (Bissell, 1996, p 3).

Perhaps it is to our advantage that these guidelines are not so prescriptive. We are thus forced to think more deeply to discern what is really in the interests of our clients. In the process we become creative, finding solutions that hitherto we did not perceive. Facing uncomfortable decisions often takes us to our learning edge. We can do this when we accept the reality of ambiguity—there is a cost to autonomy and a price for paternalism (Moody, 1998).

Nevertheless, there are some helpful guidelines available. Professional practice with the elderly has generated a number of agreed-upon principles in working with the elderly at risk:

1) Competency should be set at a decent level of functioning rather than the optimum level, one that can provide a safety net below which persons are not permitted to fall. This supports the principle of least intrusion (Kapp, 1988).

2) Social workers should manipulate environmental barriers to maximize elders' decision-making capacity and remember that the elderly are capable of *assisted* decision-making (Kapp, 1988).

3) Social work interventions should focus on motivating capacity for decision-making, on prevention, and rehabilitation efforts that delay the onset of frailty (Lewis, 1984).

4) Promoting elderly clients' perceptions and experiences of empowerment, i.e., having some control over their lives and environment, will enhance competency and self-esteem (Neeman, 1995).

5) Social workers can employ the ethics of dignity and respect in therapeutic relationships; how we carry out our work is as important as the decisions we make (Moody, 1998).

6) Elderly clients particularly benefit from social work's process-oriented approach to assessment, treatment planning, and intervention. This process asks us to stand back, to take time to see the whole, to understand future consequences of our decisions for many players including family members. This allows us to mediate and reconcile relationship conflicts that prevent further loss and social isolation of elderly clients.

7) Finally, social workers need to develop a tolerance for some risk for our elderly clients. This threshold is supported and enhanced when we share the responsibility for decision-

making with others—our clients, families, and other professionals who know them.

Case Example

Bradley is the social worker on an outreach geriatric mental health team providing services to Mrs. W, 72 years old, who lives independently in a senior's apartment. She has no family. Although well physically, Mrs. W has a history of alcoholism and bi-polar illness. Over several years, the team has established a good but fragile therapeutic link with her and Mrs. W no longer drinks, and now co-operates with visits to review her medication regime and general wellness. However, residual brain damage from her alcoholism and ongoing mood fluctuations continue to cause her erratic functioning. She is fiercely independent.

Over the past year, the social worker has become more concerned about Mrs. W's financial capacity. Rent cheques have bounced, Mrs. W spends most of her income at the beginning of each month, and now gives all her financial correspondence and income tax forms to Bradley to "help" her complete. The mental health team is worried that Mrs. W now may have an early dementia, but she refuses to participate in a dementia assessment. The social worker believes that according to strict legal criteria, Mrs. W would probably fail a legal financial capacity test.

A crisis arises when Mrs. W signs a contract to buy a computer that she cannot use and obligates her to a substantial monthly payment that she cannot afford. The social worker's assessment reveals Mrs. W misunderstood the terms of the contract and the cost.

He is very concerned and experiences emotional turmoil. Mrs. W's vulnerability to exploitation is now an issue. What are his professional obligations? He believes that the fragile therapeutic relationship with Mrs. W will be lost if he recommends assessment for financial legal guardianship, yet her needs for support and the protracted negotiations required to maintain her co-operation are taxing his time and resources.

The social worker brings the problem to the care team. As he leads them through a discussion of relevant facts, he realizes that there is additional information available to help them decide on a course of action. He finds himself articulating legal and practice principles, which help guide their deliberations. They realize that Mrs. W's actions have not yet significantly compromised her personal safety. Her clear wish is for autonomy rather than protection from possible future risk. Her basic security needs are still met. Allying on behalf of her insistence for financial autonomy will enable them to maintain the therapeutic relationship with Mrs. W, which has taken years to develop. Consequently, the team may be able to continue to provide other supports that will significantly help Mrs. W maintain capacity in the immediate, if not distant, future. They conclude that these latter interventions are "the least intrusive measure."

The team decides not to recommend assessment for legal guardianship of Mrs. W's financial affairs at this time. They assure the social worker that they share with him responsibility for this decision and its consequences. Together, the team realizes that they will likely revisit their decision in the future, at which time other factors such as a relapse of Mrs. W's psychiatric illness or deterioration in her physical health may necessitate a different course of action.

The social worker experiences satisfaction with the team's deliberation. He is aware that sharing both his risk assessment and decision for action with the team has significantly diminished his anxiety. In his next visit with Mrs. W, after obtaining her permission, he contacts the computer company and persuades them to rescind the sale. He suggests to Mrs. W that she might wish to consult him before signing financial contracts in the future. He also finds renewed energy and enthusiasm for working with this client.

Among other things, this case illustrates the ambiguity and anxiety social workers often experience when working with the elderly at risk. Knowing when to consult with others, and remembering to reflect on what we may already know are two very important skills to bring to this counselling problem.

VI. Concluding Remarks

It is evident from the preceding that, while specific problems require a special focus, many counselling interventions with the elderly transcend the boundaries of practice settings and problem areas. This is because all elders are coping with the experiences of aging, which challenge their capabilities to adapt to multiple changes and diminished opportunities, especially in the later years. As such, all problems of the elderly are experienced within this context. Regardless of the specific manifestations of difficulty, their paramount motivation is to maintain continuity, identity, and self-esteem as they reluctantly move in the direction of dependency.

Because of the complex nature of these problems, initial counselling interventions with an elderly person should be aimed at the assessment and reduction of stress in his or her life. This process often calls on the gerontological social worker to have and assume a variety of case management functions in addition to counselling. The complex interplay of difficulties of an aging person also affects the timing of social work interventions and expectations for recovery. Treatment goals should be realistic and achievable and, where dependency is an issue, oriented to the minimum amount of change needed to solve the problems at hand. At the same time, social workers should persist with assistance and rehabilitation efforts beyond the time required for younger populations to recover.

Aging is a family affair, and families are primary caretakers of the elderly. They suffer in a complementary fashion and need to be consulted, involved, and supported. The processes of life-review and reminiscence are gaining widespread acceptance in individual, marital, and group work with the elderly. These counselling tools offer special therapeutic qualities of bringing one's history to the present and affirming continuity, meaning, and identity in one's life. While the methods of life review have developed with special reference to the elderly, they may prove to be a gift to the work with other client populations as well.

Social workers, especially at the beginning stages of their gerontological practice, should become consciously aware of their own attitudes and feelings about aging, loss, dependency, and family responsibility. Doing so will ensure that they respond more accurately and sensitively in therapeutic relationship with the elderly and their families. Finally, when confronting the dilemma of capacity and risk, they need to accept the reality of living with some anxiety, seek consolation, and practice discernment.

References

Becker S. & Kaufman, S. (1988). Old age, rehabilitation and research: A review of the issues. *The Gerontologist*, 28(4), 459–468.

Berman, H.H. (1987). Adult children and their parents: Irredeemable obligation and irreplaceable loss. *Journal of Gerontological Social Work*, 10(1/2), 21–33.

Bissell, G. (1996). Personal ethics in social work with older people. *International Social Work*, 39, 257–263.

Brody, E.M. (1974). Aging and family personality: A developmental view. *Family Process*, 13(1), 23–37.

Brody, E.M. (1981). Women in the middle and family help to older people. *The Gerontologist*, 21(5), 471–480.

Burstein, B. (1988). Involuntary aged clients: Ethical and treatment issues. *Social Casework*, 69(10), 518–524.

Clemens, E.L. & Hayes, H.E. (1997). Assessing and balancing elder risk, safety and autonomy: Decision-making practices of health care professionals. *Home Health Care Services Quarterly*, 16(3) 3–20.

Conway, P. (1988). Losses and grief in old age. *Social Casework*, 69(11), 541–549.

Freeman, E. (1984). Multiple losses in the elderly: An ecological approach. *Social Casework*, 65(5), 287–296.

Garrett, J.E. (1987). Multiple losses in older adults. *Journal of Gerontological Nursing*, 13(8), 8–12.

Greene, R.R. (1986). Counter-transference issues in social work with the aged. *Journal of Gerontological Social Work*, 9(3), 79–88.

Hartford, M. (1985). Understanding normative growth and development in aging: Working with strengths. In G. Getzel & J. Mellor (eds.), *Gerontological social work practice in the community*. New York: Haworth.

Kapp, M.B. (1988). Forcing services on at-risk older adults: When doing good is not so good. *Social Work in Health Care*, 13(4), 1–13.

Kirschner, C. (1985). Social work practice with the aged and their families: A systems approach. In G. Getzel & M. Mellor (eds.), *Gerontological social work practice in the community*. New York: Haworth.

Lewis, H. (1984). The aged client's autonomy in service encounters. *Journal of Gerontological Social Work*, 7(3), 51–63.

Lewis, H. (1984). Self-determination: The aged client's autonomy in service encounters. *Journal of Gerontological Social Work*, 29(2/3), 111–127.

Lieberman, M.A. & Tobin, S.S. (1985). *The experience of old age*. New York: Basic Book.

Lowy, L. (1989). Independence and dependence in aging: A new balance. *Journal of Gerontological Social Work*, 13(3/4), 133–145.

Miller, D. (1981). The sandwich generation: Adult children of the aging. *Social Work*, 26, 419–423.

Miller, L. (1987). The professional construction of aging. *Journal of Gerontological Social Work*, 10(3/4), 141–153.

Monk, A. (1986). Social work with the aged: Principles of practice. In C. Meyer (ed.), *Social work with the aging*, 2nd ed., pp. 9–16. Silver Spring: National Association of Social Workers.

Moody, H.R. (1998). The cost of autonomy, the price of paternalism. *Journal of Gerontological Social Work*, 29(2/3), 111–127.

Neeman, L. (1995). Using the therapeutic relationship to promote an internal locus of control in elderly mental health clients. *Journal of Gerontological Social Work*, 23 (3/4), 161–176.

Parsons, R.J. & Cox, E.O. (1989). Family mediation in elder caregiving decision: An empowerment intervention. *Social Work*, 34(2), 122–126.

Parsons, R.J., Cox, E.O., & Kimboko, P.J. (1989). Satisfaction, communication and affection in caregiving: A view from the elder's perspective. *Journal of Gerontological Social Work*, 13(3/4), 9–19.

Petersen, E. (1985). The physical, the spiritual: Can you meet all of your patients' needs? *Journal of Gerontological Nursing*, 11(10), 23–27.

Powell, W. (1988). The ties that bind: Relationships in life transitions. *Social Casework*, 69(11), 556–562.

Schwartz-Borden, G. (1986). Grief work: Prevention and intervention. *Social Casework*, 69(8), 499–505.

Tobin, S.S. (1988). Preservation of self in old age. *Social Casework*, 69(11).

Tobin, S. & Gustafson, J. (1987). What do we do differently with elderly clients? *Journal of Gerontological Social Work*, 10(3/4), 109–121.

Wahl, J. (2003). Consent and capacity/substitute decision-making: The basics. www.advocacycentreelderly.org/pubs/poa/Consent-and-Capacity-basics.pdf. Last updated 06/06/03.

Webster, G.C. & Baylis, F.E. (2000), Moral residue. In S.B. Rubin & L. Zoloth (eds.), *Margin of error: The ethics of mistakes in the practice of medicine*, pp. 217–231. Hagerstown: University Publishing Group.

Internet Resources

Advocacy Centre for the Elderly (Canada)
    A community-based legal clinic for low-income senior citizens.
    http://www.advocacycentreelderly.org/
CASW National Scope of Practice Statement
    http://www.casw-acts.ca/Practice/RecPubsArt1.htm
NASW Code of Ethics, 1998
    http://www.socialworkers.org/pubs/code/code.asp
Ontario Ministry of the Attorney General
    The Capacity Assessment Office: Questions and Answers
    http://www.attorneygeneral.jus.gov.on.ca/english/family/pgt/
    capacityoffice.asp

Additional Readings

Disch, R.B., Dobrof, R., & Moody, H.R. *Dignity and old age.* (1998). Binghamton: Haworth Press.

Hunink, M. & Glasziou, P. (2001). *Decision making in health and medicine.* Cambridge: Cambridge University Press.

Reamer, F.G. (1990). *Ethical dilemmas in social service,* 2nd ed. New York: Columbia University Press

Rubin, S.B. & Zoloth, L. (eds.). (2000). *Margin of error: The ethics of mistakes in the practice of medicine.* Hagerstown: University Publishing Group.

Schmidt, W., Jr. (ed.). (1995). *Guardianship: Court of last resort for the elderly and disabled.* Durham: Carolina Academic Press.

CHAPTER 5

MEDICATION UTILIZATION PROBLEMS AMONG THE ELDERLY: IMPLICATIONS FOR SOCIAL WORK PRACTICE

VINCENT J. GIANNETTI

The improper use of medication can frequently threaten the health and well-being of elderly persons. This chapter alerts social work practitioners to the possible dangers of drug utilization among the elderly and explains the factors commonly associated with the inappropriate use of drugs.

I.   Introduction

Demographic trends in the United States over the past century have necessitated shifts in the emphasis of the health care system to accommodate the special needs of increasing numbers of people surviving beyond age 65. One area of health care delivery to the elderly that has received increased attention is the use of medication. Older people frequently suffer from multiple chronic diseases and they are often prescribed several medications. Elderly patients account for 30 percent of all medication consumption and consume significant amounts of over-the-counter medications while only accounting for 12.6 percent of the population (Koch & Knapp, 1985). Medication usage increases substantially with age (Miller, 1973; Stewart et al., 1991) resulting in medication-related problems responsible for 25 percent of nursing home admissions and 17 percent of hospitalizations.

The social work practitioner working with elderly clients may be confronted with a variety of medication-related problems. These problems may manifest themselves as exaggerated or less-than-optimal responses to medication, symptoms of drug-induced illness, and a lack of therapeutic response to medication. The increased risk for drug-related problems in the elderly can be summarized in Table 5.1.

In general, medication utilization problems common among the elderly may be divided into four basic categories: (1) problems related to over-prescribing; (2) dose-related complications caused by the unique manner in which drugs are metabolized by and distributed in the body of the elderly patient; (3) adverse drug interactions related to a lack of coordination among the prescribing practices of the medical professionals treating the elderly; and (4) self-medication regimens, which may result in the exacerbation of illness.

II.   Over-prescribing

The elderly are at increased risk for drug related problems due to the greater number of medications consumed and tend to have atypical presentation of drug-related symptoms that often are attributed to the aging process itself (Golden et al., 1999). For example, there is an extensive list of medications that can cause cognitive and behavioural changes that can be mistaken for "senility" (Medical Letter of Drug Therapy, 1998). Thus, complete review of medication history should be completed before making any assumptions about cognitive and behavioural changes in the elderly. The extent to which medication is over-prescribed for the elderly is difficult to precisely analyze because the appropriateness of a particular drug regimen is related to individual factors and dependent on the individual physician's clinical expertise. However, U.S. federal Medicare regulations require a review of drug regimens in extended-care facilities, and the results of drug utilization reviews by clinical pharmacists offer some evidence that a tendency toward over-prescribing exists in regard to the institutionalized elderly.

Estimates of the use of medication among elderly people in institutions have revealed that an average of seven to eight drugs are taken per patient and that 33 percent of this population receive eight drugs daily (U.S. Dept. of Health, Education and Welfare, 1976b; U.S. Senate, 1975). In a study reported by Cheung and Kayne (1975), 122 potential adverse reactions to drugs were identified and corrected as a result of a drug utilization review conducted by clinical pharmacists and this prevented the development of more serious illness among nursing home residents. In another study, a decrease from 6.8 to 5.6 prescriptions per month was realized per patient after a drug regimen review (Hood et al., 1975). Other evidence of over-prescribing has been offered. During a review of 13,081 medical charts at ten skilled nursing facilities, clinical pharmacists identified 928 potential or actual medication problems, which represented 7.1 percent of all the prescriptions reviewed (Witte et al., 1980). Approximately 60 percent of these problems stemmed from the prescription of medication without reference to a patient's laboratory test results or other documented indications for the drug or a lack of data concerning a medication's effectiveness.

In a study conducted over an eight-year period in three long-term care facilities, Strandberg and his associates have also described some indications of over-prescribing (Strandberg et al., 1980). As a result of consultation in the facilities by clinical pharmacists who reviewed 4,004 medical records, a significant decrease took place in the number of prescription drugs taken, accompanied by a reduction in dosage for selected drugs. An interesting by-product of the pharmacists' review was a reduction of 28.9 percent in medication costs per patient after adjustments had been made for inflation over the eight years. In addition, the findings of an epidemiological study suggested the overuse of psychotropic medication in nursing homes (Ray et al., 1980). Finally, limited evidence for excessive dosing of elderly patients in office-based medical practice has been suggested (Manning et al., 1980).

III. Dose-Related Complications

The second category of medication utilization problems among the elderly relates to improper dosage. The absorption and distribution of drugs in elderly people and their elimination or clearance from the body are altered as a result of specific physiological changes that take place during aging. These changes place the elderly at higher risk than younger people of developing various adverse reactions to drugs. One such change is a modification in the ratio of fat to lean tissues, which is altered significantly in aging. The fat content of tissues doubles in elderly men and increases by 1.5 percent in elderly women. This significant change in fat composition affects the concentration of fat-soluble drugs in the elderly because it increases the storage of such drugs in fat tissues, thereby making them less immediately available in the blood. Because the elderly also lose approximately 10 to 15 percent of the water in their bodies as a result of aging, the distribution of water-soluble drugs is also affected. Specifically, the reduction of water in the body increases the concentration of such drugs in the blood.

The clearance of drugs in the elderly is also changed as a result of aging. The kidney and liver basically accomplish the clearance of drugs in the body. Because of changes in the liver's ability to modify drugs, total drug clearance may be affected in elderly people. Furthermore, the glomerular filtration rate, the rate at which the kidney filtrates and secretes substances, tends to decrease with aging, thus slowing down the rate at which drugs are excreted by the kidney. This can also result in higher levels of drugs in the bloodstream.

Finally, when in the body, some drugs tend to bind to proteins. Because of the decline in plasma albumin in elderly people, it is hypothesized that when such a drug is taken by an older person, there may be an increased amount of unbound, protein-binding medication in his or her bloodstream. This may increase the likelihood that the individual will develop adverse reactions and that drug interactions will take place (Schmucker, 1979; Vestal, 1982).

Other changes in the physiological status of older people have also been suggested as possible factors affecting drug distribution in the body. Because cerebrovascular disease results in reduced blood flow to the brain, anti-hypertensive agents that cause hypotension (or reduced blood pressure and blood flow) may also cause cerebral hypoxia (a lack of oxygen to the brain) in elderly persons with cerebrovascular disease. Both coronary artery disease and decreased cardiac output in the elderly may reduce blood flow to organ systems and thus affect the distribution of drugs to target areas. Elderly people who have chronic respiratory disease may also be especially vulnerable to medications that depress the respiratory rate. Finally, changes in intestinal function and motility in the elderly may result in changes in the rate at which drugs are absorbed if their primary site of absorption is the intestines (Wallace & Watanabe, 1977).

Although all these changes in drug distribution in the elderly may be caused by aging or by chronic illnesses common in aging, the disposition of any particular drug in the body is dependent on many complex factors. Some of these pertain to the specific physiochemical properties of the drug; others pertain to patient-related variable such as the individual's body composition and weight, the presence of disease, altered physiological functions, and other drugs present in the body. The field of clinical pharmacokinetics is specifically concerned with the distribution and disposition of drugs in the body and is a subspecialty within the pharmaceutical and medical sciences. Many hospitals are now developing clinical pharmacokinetic services to assist physicians in prescribing medication for special populations, such as children and the elderly, and certain drugs whose range between therapeutic and toxic levels is extremely narrow, such as digitalis and theophylline. It has been suggested that physicians in general do not receive adequate training in the special pharmacokinetic considerations important in prescribing medication for elderly patients and tend to prescribe for the elderly as they would for younger patients, thus increasing the possibility that medication-related problems may develop (National Academy of Sciences, 1978).

One example of drug-related problems affecting the elderly is the use of benzodiazepines, or tranquillizers, including Valium and Librium. The use of these drugs is not without difficulties for older people. Certain types of benzodiazepines have been associated with an increase in the frequency of drowsiness (specifically, diazepam and chlorodiazepoxide) and with impaired psychomotor performance (specifically, nitrozepam) in the elderly. These reactions are apparently caused by heightened central nervous system depression, which occurs among elderly as compared to non-elderly subjects who are administered these drugs at equal doses, and which leads researchers to caution against the drugs' use with the elderly (Bender, 1979; Wilkinson, 1979). Mental confusion and falling may already be problems for some elderly people, and the use of certain benzodiazepines may exacerbate these problems and create a potentially dangerous situation.

However, in a survey in Great Britain of drug-prescribing patterns for the elderly, 50 percent of the psychotropic medications prescribed were found to be one of the benzodiazepines (Freeman, 1979). In 40.5 percent of the cases, psychological conditions such as anxiety, insomnia, depression, and drug habituation were cited as the primary reason for prescribing the medication. Interruptions in social functioning caused by such factors as bereavement, marital problems, and a seriously ill spouse and nonspecific ailments such as headache, dizziness, and general malaise were given as the reason for the prescription in 20 percent of the cases. Organically related problems such as cardiovascular disease and musculoskeletal ailments were the primary factor in 39.5 percent of the cases. In addition, in a study of the use of tranquillizers by elderly people in Texas, an increased use of both tranquillizers and sleeping pills was influenced by social stress caused by such factors as unemployment, divorce, widowhood, inadequate income, and loneliness as well as by a lack of social supports (Eve & Friedsam, 1981). Although this study used secondary data and was based on a non-random sample, which limits the extent to which its findings can be generalized, it did suggest that the use of psychotropic drugs varied directly with the number of stresses related to health, social, and emotional problems in the elderly person's life. In light of findings indicating that the use of benzodiazepines and other tranquillizers is not uncommon among the elderly, it should be repeated that the efficacy and wisdom of the pharmacological management of complex psycho-social problems with tranquillizing drugs have been frequently and widely criticized (Illich, 1975; Koumsian, 1981).

IV.   Drug Interactions

In addition to drug-related problems having to do with the physiological processes of aging, drug interactions can be a major problem for the elderly. Older people living in the community may be taking many different medications while under the care of various physicians who may not coordinate their prescribing practices for chronic diseases, and the risk of adverse drug interactions is increased under such circumstances (Lamy, 1980). Also, because many elderly people medicate themselves with over-the-counter (OTC) drugs, there is an increased risk of interactions taking place between these drugs and prescribed medications (Lamy, 1980).

Both the extent and the pharmacological complexities of drug interactions in the elderly are well beyond the scope of this chapter. However, two specific problems may be discussed here: drug-related hypothermia and self-medication among the elderly.

Each year, many thousands of elderly people die from accidental hypothermia, the loss of body heat leading to illness or death. The elderly are especially vulnerable to hypothermia because they have decreased physiological capabilities that result in reduced blood circulation and because they are often subject to financial constraints that cause an inability or reluctance to use enough heat to keep warm in severe weather. Certain psychotropic medications that are commonly used by the elderly can increase the risk of hypothermia. The phenothiazines, minor tranquillizers, and tricyclic anti-depressants affect the central nervous system in such a way as to decrease the perception of cold. Moreover, alcoholic beverages will potentiate the effects of these drugs in addition to increasing heat loss by the body. The use of alcohol in combination with any of the drugs described can therefore significantly increase the risk of hypothermia for elderly individuals. In addition, vasodilating agents used in the treatment of cardiovascular disease will inhibit vasoconstriction, which is the body's normal response to cold and which is intended to decrease peripheral radiant heat loss and increase internal temperature. The elderly who live alone, who are having financial difficulties, and who may be using any combination of the drugs mentioned should be considered at risk for accidental hypothermia (Avery, 1982).

Self-medication is fairly common among the elderly, and a variety of problems involving over-the-counter drugs may result from this practice. For example, aspirin in high dosages is often used by elderly people who have rheumatoid arthritis. If taken in large enough doses, aspirin may cause toxicity that is manifested as confusion, irritability, tinnitus or ringing in the ear, blurred vision, vomiting, and diarrhoea. Moreover, aspirin taken in combination with alcohol can result in gastrointestinal bleeding. Because the long-term use of aspirin may result in bleeding of this kind, elderly patients with a history of anemia may exacerbate their problem if they medicate themselves with large doses of aspirin.

Antacids are another kind of OTC preparation whose use by the elderly can lead to unforeseen difficulties. Antacids may cause constipation and may interfere with the absorption of certain drugs by causing acid-base imbalances in the intestines. Also, because many antacids have a high sodium content, they may cause problems for elderly patients who must restrict their intake of salt. Cough and cold preparations contain alcohol (the content of some is 40 percent) and may expose the elderly who use them to drug-alcohol interactions, such as those in which the effects of sedatives, barbiturates, and tranquillizers are heightened. Many products also have high sugar content, and this can be a problem for elderly diabetics or other elderly persons who should restrict their intake of sugar. The use of laxatives can result in harm as well. Reliance on laxatives may be frequent among the elderly because of common misconceptions concerning irregularity and the necessity of a daily bowel movement. Overuse and dependence on laxatives can cause constipation by reducing muscle tone and reflexes in the large bowel, whereas many non-pharmacological approaches to the treatment of constipation can be effective. Increased dietary fiber in the form of such foods as bran, whole grains, fresh vegetables and fruits, an increased intake of water, and increased activity and exercise have all been suggested as methods for overcoming constipation. Vitamins are another substance whose use by the elderly may entail complications. Self-medication with high doses of vitamins, especially fat-soluble vitamins, can lead to adverse reactions such as vitamin toxicity and organ damage (Lamy, 1980).

V.   Non-compliance

Non-compliance represents a final category of medication utilization problems among the elderly. Both the sophistication of pharmaceutical technology and the individual physician's expertise are of little value if the patient does not take medication that is prescribed or fails to take it correctly. Non-compliance may lead to the exacerbation of illness as the patient consumes dosages insufficient to prompt a therapeutic response or suffers toxic reactions from taking unprescribed drugs in dosages that are too high.

Estimates indicate that non-compliance in the ambulatory population may vary from as much as 25 to 50 percent (Blackwell, 1973). Because of various physiological, social, and psychological processes common in aging, many elderly people may tend not to comply with medication regimens and may consequently be subject to negative effects on their health. In addition, financial constraints may lead a number of older people to delay seeking treatment while medicating themselves, to share medication with other elderly friends, or to save leftover medication for another episode of illness when taking the full prescription of the drug is indicated. Overall, five primary factors are associated with non-compliance among the elderly:

1.   *Polymedicine:* As the older person is prescribed an increasing number of drugs with different purposes and dosing schedules, the probability increases that he or she will fail to take medication or will confuse instructions (Fletcher et al., 1979; Haynes et al., 1980; Hulka et al., 1976; Wandless & Davis, 1977).
2.   *Inadequate knowledge:* Communication among physicians, pharmacists, and elderly patients regarding the purpose and proper use of drugs tends to be incomplete. Furthermore, many elderly people do not ask questions of health care

provers concerning the use, purpose, and side effects of medication (Lunden, 1980; Lunden et al., 1980; Schwartz et al., 1962).

3. *Financial constraints:* Delays in filling and refilling prescriptions, premature discontinuance of drug therapy, and the saving of medication for subsequent self-medication may result from the inability of many elderly people to afford drugs (Brand et al., 1977; Smith, 1976).

4. *Poor memory:* Because of the effects of aging, a number of older people may have difficulty remembering instructions regarding medication (Waugh et al., 1978).

5. *Social isolation:* Many of the elderly lack a significant other who expresses concern about their medications or monitors whether they are following regimens.

VI.   Social Work Implications

As indicated in the preceding, problems involving the usage of medication can significantly affect the health and well-being of many of the elderly. Because social work practitioners work with elderly clients in both institutions and the community, they should have a basic knowledge of both medication-related problems that are common among older people and the ability to refer clients for medical intervention. This ability is especially critical for the social worker in the community, for in many cases the worker comes into contact more often than any other health care professional with the older person who is living in the community. This places the social worker in a unique position for monitoring drug-taking behaviour and adverse effects among elderly clients, and it may be helpful for workers to familiarize themselves with the variety of sources of information available on drug utilization problems.

Although physicians are generally accustomed to consulting with pharmacists and nurses about the medication problems of patients, they are not accustomed to doing so with social workers. Traditionally, the social worker has not been trained to act as a source of information on drugs. However, it would be within the worker's recognized province to play the role of advocate for the elderly by recognizing medication-related problems and helping to resolve them and by encouraging health practices that could reduce medication utilization problems. For the past decade, publications in the social work literature have begun to emphasize basic knowledge regarding medications for the social work practitioner (Bentley & Walsh, 1997). Knowing the right questions to ask with a basic understanding of adverse drug reactions can often cue medical practitioner to explore further the nature of medication problems.

The Medication Appropriateness Index (MAI) is a standardized rating scale that allows practitioners to evaluate the appropriateness of medication therapy and ask critical questions. While the scale is designed for calculating a score using assigned weights and operational definitions, the ten questions comprising the scale can be used as a guide for the elderly in utilizing medication, and social work practitioners asking questions regarding drug therapy. The contents of the scale are summarized in Table 5.2 (Hanlon et al., 1992).

Because periodic reviews of drug regimens are essential for coordinating the prescribing of drugs for elderly patients, it may be beneficial for social workers to encourage the elderly to patronize pharmacies that keep medication profiles of their clients and that screen these profiles for drug interactions and other medication-related problems. A medication profile is a list of medications that an individual is taking, and many pharmacies compile such lists, often computerizing them. Elderly people may tend to patronize pharmacists on the basis of the prices they charge for drugs and may therefore not consistently use one pharmacy that offers medication profile reviews as a service to clients. If at all possible, the elderly should be helped to choose a pharmacist with whom they can communicate and who offers consultation and medication reviews, even if they must pay slightly higher prices for their medication. If maintaining a medication profile in a pharmacy is not possible for an individual, s/he should be encouraged to keep a record of all prescription and non-prescription medications taken on a regular basis. Ideally, physicians should take a drug history before prescribing new medications for a patient, and when the elderly person visits a physician who changes a prescription or initiates new medication, s/he should inform the physician of any medications being taken and the medical conditions for which they are being prescribed.

Elderly people who live alone should be closely monitored for medication utilization problems and for compliance with drug regimens (Sloane et al., 2002). Social workers can take an active role in this important area. It would not be inappropriate for workers to speak with physicians and pharmacists about the medications their clients are taking. In this way, they can become familiar with standard dosages, major side effects, and adverse reactions, which in turn would help them monitor drug regimens more effectively. For instance, if non-compliance or medication-related complications are suspected, most physicians would appreciate being informed of this by the social worker. In such cases the worker can simply state the problem and ask for intervention by the physician. Examples of such problems would include: a client's complaints of tiredness and lethargy after the initiating of diuretic therapy, symptoms of depression after the initiation of steroid therapy, or increased episodes of falling and dizziness after psychotropic medication has been prescribed. Observing and interviewing elderly clients about the medication they take and applying basic knowledge on drugs or consulting with a pharmacist should enable workers to detect medication-related problems.

In addition, social workers can adopt a number of specific strategies for reducing non-compliance with medication regimens among the elderly. For example, in many cases in which financial considerations may be contributing to non-compliance, generic drugs can be substituted for more expensive brand-name drugs. Although there is considerable controversy concerning bioequivalency and bioavailability of generic drugs, pharmacists and physicians who are knowledgeable about them and whether they are as effective as their brand-name counterparts can evaluate their appropriateness for the individual and recommend quality products that can reduce costs for the elderly patient. This debate is currently typical in North America as we are witnessing politicians, drug companies, physicians, and the elderly trying to reconcile this double-edged cost vs. quality sword (Bates et al., 1997).

A variety of procedures can also help reduce confusion for the older person taking more than one medication. Typewritten instructions in large type can be developed, and colour-coded charts matching the pills taken and showing the amount prescribed and time of day of consumption can be particularly helpful when multiple medications are involved. Ideally, the elderly patient should understand the disease being treated, how the prescribed medication alleviates or controls the disease, what the major side effects of the medication are, the proper manner of taking the medication, any special instructions for the storage of the medication, and what adverse effects should be reported to the physician. The social worker can help elderly clients become well-informed consumers by encouraging them to ask questions of physicians and pharmacists and by telling them where they can obtain further information about drugs. In some instances, if properly trained, social workers can undertake educational efforts with elderly clients regarding certain diseases and the proper use of medication.

Finally, older people should be encouraged to take a written list of their current medications with them when they are purchasing OTC drugs. Buying OTC preparations should be done in consultation with a pharmacist who knows about the medications an elderly person is taking. Pharmacists are trained to assist their clients with the selection of non-prescription medication and with the identification of the symptoms of serious disease and this may be particularly important for an older person who is experiencing distressing symptoms. Non-prescription medication is frequently not indicated for the serious symptoms of disease, and self-medication may actually mask these symptoms or cause a delay in the seeking of treatment. For example, it is not uncommon to interpret the chest pain of angina as an upset stomach and through self-medication with antacids to delay the diagnosis and treatment of potential heart disease.

By acting as an advocate for the coordination of prescribing practices for the elderly in the community, as a resource for monitoring medication utilization problems, and as an educator of patients, the social worker can greatly increase his or her effectiveness in the delivery of health and social services to the elderly. The advocacy role is especially critical in work with elderly people living alone, who may not see a physician or pharmacist regularly and whose contact with helping professionals other than the social worker may be limited. In filling this gap in service delivery, social workers can become an important resource for the elderly in need.

Table 5.1: Factors Associated with Adverse Drug Reactions in the Elderly

- Increased incidence of chronic disease
- Lack of coordination and case management among prescribing physicians
- Tendency to self-medicate and share medications
- Non-adherence due to economic and psychosocial and physical limitations
- Inadequate or lack of effective patient education for both prescription and over-the-counter medications
- Age-related physical changes that alter drug metabolism

Table 5.2: Medication Appropriateness Index

1. Does the drug have a specific indication for use?
2. Is the medication effective for the specific condition?
3. Is the dosage correct?
4. Are the directions correct?
5. Are the directions understandable and practical?
6. Are there significant drug interactions?
7. Are there significant drug-disease interactions
8. Is there unnecessary duplication with other drugs?
9. Is the duration of therapy acceptable?
10. Is the drug the least expensive alternative compared to others of equal utility?

References

Avery, W.M. (1982). Accidental hypothermia, drugs and the elderly. *American Pharmacy*, 2, 14–16.

Bates, W., Spell, N., Cullend, D.J., et al. (1997). The costs of adverse drug events in hospitalized patients. *Journal of the American Medical Association*, 277, 307–11.

Bender, A.C. (1979). Drug sensitivity in the elderly. In J. Crooks & I.H. Stevens (eds.), *Drugs in the elderly: Perspectives in geriatric clinical pharmacology*, pp. 147–153. Baltimore: University Park Press.

Bentley, K.J. & Walsh, J. (1997). *The social worker & psychotropic medication: Toward effective collaboration with mental health clients, families, and providers.* Belmont: Brooks/Cole Publishing Company.

Blackwell, B. (1973). Patient compliance. *New England Journal of Medicine*, 237, 49–63.

Brand, F., Smith, R.T., & Brand, P.A. (1977, January–February). Effect of economic barriers to medical care on patient compliance. *Public Health Reports*, 92, 72–78.

Cheung, A. & Kayne, R. (1975). An application of clinical pharmacy services for extended care facilities. *California Pharmacist*, 22–26.

Eve, S.B. & Friedsam, H.J. (1981, April–June). Use of tranquilizers and sleeping pills among older Texans. *Journal of Psychoactive Drugs*, 13, 165–173.

Fletcher, S. et al. (1979). Patient understanding of prescribed drugs. *Journal of Community Health*, 4, 183–189.

Freeman, G.K. (1979). Drug prescribing patterns in the elderly: A general practice study. In J. Crooks & I.H. Stevens (eds.), *Drugs in the elderly:*

Perspectives in geriatric clinical pharmacology. Baltimore: University Park Press.

Golden, A.G., Preston, R.A., Barnett, S.D., et al. (1999). Inappropriate medication prescribing in homebound older adults. *Journal of the American Geriatrics Society,* 47, 948–953.

Hanlon, J.T., Schmader, K.E, Samsa, G.P., et al. (1992). A method for assessing drug therapy appropriateness. *Journal of Clinical Epidemiology,* 45, 1045–1051.

Haynes, R.B., Sackett, D.L., & Taylor, D.W. (1980). How to detect and manage low compliance in chronic illness. *Geriatrics,* 35, 91–97.

Hood, J.C., Lemberger, M., & Stewart, R.B. (1975). Promoting appropriate drug therapy in a long-term care facility. *Journal of the American Pharmaceutical Association,* 15, 32–34.

Hulka, B. et al. (1976). Communication, compliance, and concordance between physician and patients. *American Journal of Public Health,* 66, 847–853.

Illich, I. (1975). *Medical Nemesis.* London: Clader and Bayers Ltd.

Koch K. & Knapp D.A. (1985). *Highlights of drug utilization in office practice. National ambulatory medical care survey.* Vital and health statistics, no. 143. DHHS Publication No. (PHS) 87-1250. Hyattsville: National Center for Health Statistics.

Koumsian, K. (1981). The use of valium as a form of social control. *Social Science and Medicine,* 15E, 245–250.

Lamy, P.P. (1980). *Prescribing for the elderly.* Littleton: PSG Publishing Co.

Lunden, D.V. (1980). Must medication be a dilemma for the independent elderly? *Journal of Gerontological Nursing,* 4, 25–27.

Lunden, D.V. et al. (1980) Education of the independent elderly in the responsible use of prescription medications. *Drug Intelligence and Clinical Pharmacy,* 14, 46–71.

Manning, P.R. et al. (1980). Determining educational needs in the physician's office. *Journal of the American Medical Association,* 244, 1112–1115.

Medical Letter of Drug Therapy. (1998). Drugs that cause psychiatric symptoms. *Medical Letter of Drug Therapy,* 40(1020), 21–24.

Miller, D.R. (1973). Drug surveillance utilizing epidemiologic methods. *American Journal of Hospital Pharmacy,* 30, 584–592.

National Academy of Sciences. (1978). *Aging and medical education.* Washington: National Academy of Sciences.

Ray, W.A., Federspiel, C.F., & Schaffner, W. (1980). A study of antipsychotic drug use in nursing homes: Epidemiologic evidence suggesting misuse. *American Journal of Public Health,* 70, 489–491.

Schmucker, D.L. (1979). Age-related charges in drug disposition. *Pharmacological Reviews,* 30, 445–456.

Schwartz, D. et al. (1962). Medication errors made by elderly, chronically ill patients. *American Journal of Public Health,* 52, 3018–3029.

Sloane, P., Zimmerman, S., Brown, L., Ives, T., & Walsh, J. (2002). Inappropriate medication prescribing in residential care/assisted living facilities. *Journal of the American Geriatrics Society,* 50(6), 1001–1011.

Smith, M.C. (1976). How drug costs affect compliance. *Drug Therapeutics,* 6, 12–15.

Strandberg, L.R. et al. (1980). The effects of comprehensive pharmaceutical devices on drug use in long-term care facilities. *American Journal of Hospital Pharmacy,* 37, 92–94.

Stewart, R.B., Moore, M.T, May, F.E., et al. (1991). *Age Aging,* 20, 182–188.

U.S. Department of Health, Education and Welfare. (1976a). *Drugs and the elderly* (Publication No. (NIH) 78-1449). Washington: National Institute on Aging.

U.S. Department of Health, Education and Welfare. (1976b). Physicians' drug prescribing patterns in skilled nursing facilities (Publication No. 76-50050, p. 27). Rockville: Office of Long-Term Care.

U.S. Senate, Subcommittee on Long-Term Care of the Special Committee on Aging. (1975). Drugs in nursing homes: Misuse, high costs and kickbacks (mimeographed).

Vestal, R.F. (1982). Pharmacology and aging. *Journal of the American Geriatrics Society,* 30(3), 191–202.

Wallace & Watanabe. (1977). Drug effects in geriatric patients. *Drug Intelligence and Clinical Pharmacy,* 11, 597–603.

Wandless, I. & Davis, J.W. (1977). Can drug compliance in the elderly be improved? *British Medical Journal,* 359–363.

Waugh, N.C. et al. (1978). Retrieval time from different memory stores. *Journal of Gerontology,* 33, 718–724.

Wilkinson, G.R. (1979). The effects of aging on the disposition of benzodiazepines in man. In J. Crooks & I.H. Stevens (eds.), *Drugs in the elderly: Perspectives in geriatric clinical pharmacology,* pp. 103–116. Baltimore: University Park Press.

Witte, K.W. et al. (1980). Drug regimen review in skilled nursing facilities by consulting pharmacists. *American Journal of Hospital Pharmacy,* 37, 820–824.

Internet Resources

Canadian Society of Hospital Pharmacists
    Position Statement on Monitoring Drug Therapy in the Elderly.
    http://www.cshp.ca/advocacy/elderly.html

Drug Information by RxList
　　Drugs and Medications Fuzzy Search Brand Generic Cross Index.
　　http://www.rxlist.com/
MEDLINEplus: Drug Information
　　Information on thousands of prescription and over-the-counter
　　medications.
　　http://www.nlm.nih.gov/medlineplus/druginformation.html

Additional Readings

Alliance for Aging Research. (1996). Will you still treat me when I'm 65? *The national Shortage of geriatricians*. Washington: Government Printing Office.

Beers, M. & Berkow, R. (eds.). (2000). *The Merck manual of geriatrics*, 3rd ed. White House Station: Merck Research Laboratories.

Delofuente, J.C. & Stewart, R.B. (2001). *Therapeutics in the elderly*, 3rd ed. Cincinnati: Harvey Whitney Books Company.

Duthrie, E.H., Jr. & Katz, P. (eds.). (1998). *The practice of geriatrics*, 3rd ed. Philadelphia: W.B. Saunders Corp.

General Accounting Office. (1996). *Prescription drugs and the elderly: Many still receive potentially harmful drugs despite recent improvements*. Washington: Government Printing Office.

McLeod, P., Huang, A., Tomblyn, R., & Gayton, D. (1997, February). Defining inappropriate practices in prescribing for elderly people: A national consensus panel. *Canadian Medical Association Journal*, 156(3), 385–391.

CHAPTER 6

SOCIAL POLICIES THAT INFLUENCE PRACTICE WITH THE ELDERLY[1,2]

DONALD R. LESLIE AND

MICHAEL J. HOLOSKO

This chapter's purpose is to identify social policies in North America related to the elderly and suggest ways that social workers can be more directly and actively involved in policy formulation and implementation. It discusses the complexities involved in understanding the relationship between macro policy and front-line practice; a comparison of social welfare policies for the elderly in Canada and the United States; and practice and policy development issues in terms of an advocacy-in-action model. The profession's Code of Ethics and practice values espouse the importance of social policy development, and the authors contend that social workers have a responsibility to do something more than simply being aware of policies related to the client groups they serve.

I.   Introduction

Our intention in this chapter is to unravel some of the complexities inherent in a consideration of social policy so that practitioners may be better informed about what policy has to do with practice as it relates to the elderly. Thus, some generalizeable issues about the nature of social policy need to be addressed so that the more substantial practice issues can be understood. These general issues relate to: (1) its definition; (2) its rationale; and (3) its evolution in the field of social work practice.

Every text or literature source that attempts to convey information about social policy defines it differently [while reviewing literature for this chapter, we found some 64 different definitions of social policy]. The reasons for this are less important than the resultant question, which is, what definition should practitioners use? A fairly simple consensus definition is: social policies are directives (which are usually written) that are the basis to provide services for people's needs. As such, social policies are intended to reflect social welfare programs or services within a framework of humanistic values (Barnes, 1983).

Social policy in this perspective may be considered on a continuum from macro to mezzo to micro. For instance, at the macro level, some authors explicitly maintain that social policies require formal authority or legitimating and are solely social legislative acts or regulations. At the mezzo level, social policies are guidelines, procedures, or mandates that human service organizations use to operationalize their missions. At a micro level, policies may be formal or informal ways of doing things on the front line by direct service practitioners. In this regard, all social policies eventually start at an external source, e.g., either through laws, acts, mandates, operational procedures, policy manuals, and trickle down to front-line practitioners and eventually to the clients they serve. Thus, as one might assume, most policy changes are effected at administrative levels beyond the day-to-day concerns of direct service practitioners (Titmuss, 1974).

While tabling some of these definitional issues, it is important to note that social policies are distinct from, yet interrelated to, economic and political policies. Further, all social policies are derived from or are the result of broader and more prioritized economic or political agendas. This usually renders such policies and their related social welfare concerns to a vulnerable power-dependency relationship in most Western world countries. For instance, it is well known by students of policy science in many fields (e.g., economics, public policy, political science, law, etc.) that social policy initiatives are usually based on the residuals left over after taking care of economic and/or political concerns. Some Western countries, most notably Sweden, Norway, Canada, and West Germany, have attempted to push social concerns to the forefront of their national priorities, but the reality is that economic and political imperatives, their infrastructures and power positions in society, supersede and generally inhibit the potential for social policies and programs to become prioritized as such.

There are basically four rationales (some more altruistic than others) for the formulation of social policies in North American society. The first is that policies are developed in order to respond to needs (e.g., child abuse, domestic violence, income maintenance, etc.). As we well know, however, there are more social needs than policies, needs often change, and common sense tells us that one would be naive to assume that all social needs are being met by social policies [just look around you].

The second rationale for social policy formulation relates to the humanitarian and universal notion that social policies are developed in order to close the gap in society between the "haves" and "have nots," that is, reduce social inequalities. This redistribution notion, couched in a social responsibility imperative, has been questioned by numerous authors and theorists in the fields of economics, political science, business, and social welfare. Their consensus conclusion is that social policies do indeed help some groups of "have nots," e.g., through income supplementation, in-kind services, or programs, but they *do not* reduce the social inequalities existing in our society, they perpetuate them! (Mullaly, 2002; Schiller, 1989). [See Cloward and Piven, 1971, for a good example of how public welfare serves as a social control mechanism to regulate the poor, and Leslie (1997), for a comparison of outcomes between American and Canadian health care systems.]

The third rationale for the development of social policies has to do with the fact they attempt to provide guidelines, regulatory mechanisms, plans of action, and/or criteria for social welfare concerns. Social policy analysts stress that the content of these policies should be examined in terms of: the rationale for the policy; how it was formulated; what it says; how it will be interpreted and implemented; and who will be affected by it. Such questions are not trite and oftentimes serve as the impetus for policy change, modifications, revisions, amendments, and clarifications. Clearly, this rationale reminds one both about: (1) the importance of understanding the policy-making process and whether those who formulate policy understand the needs of those who implement it (Majchrzak, 1984); and (2) the content of the actual policies themselves, e.g., intents, acts, legislated policies, regulations, service documents, implicit vs. explicit policies, etc. (Delaney et al., 2003).

The finale rationale for how social policies emerge in our society is that they are the direct result of appeasing a political agenda. A study of some of the more profound social policies in North America that have emerged in the past 100 years would suggest that many of these have been largely politically motivated. That is, individual politicians or political parties have been the driving force behind their formulation. The consideration of social policy in a political context as such certainly causes one to be mindful about the larger sociopolitical context of policy formulation. For instance, at a very simple level, front-line practitioners may ask, "How can the needs of my clients get to the agenda of policy-makers?" At another level, one may certainly wonder about whether political agendas mesh with the social welfare concerns of citizens. In any event, to try and understand social policy without a consideration of the political context is erroneous.

The history of the social work profession has been intertwined with social policy throughout its evolution (Lubove, 1973). Essentially, both the practitioners and educators of social work consider social policy as the cornerstone impetus for the development of the profession. Indeed, the profession's inception was deemed to have occurred when the Elizabethan Poor Laws (in Britain) in the 16th century set down a series of legislative acts to help the poor, sick, and indigent. With these laws, the church, state, and charitable organizations became recognized as the main institutions of social welfare. Thus, social policy determined the character of social welfare practice as much then as it does today. However, as history reminds us, the profession was (and is) more concerned and better able to implement policies than it is to influence, develop, or analyze them (Lubove, 1973).

Schools of social work in North America virtually gave lip service to the study of social policy science until about 1960, at which time there was both a proliferation in social policy development (in society at large), as well as a shift in social welfare service delivery (from the voluntary to the public sector). The working definition of practice, espoused by the National Association of Social Workers (NASW) in 1958, implicitly acknowledged the importance of policy in the configuration of social work practice (Bartlett, 1958). In addition, the profession's subsequently revised Code of Ethics had three sections (IV, V, and VI) explicitly operationalizing policy concerns affecting all practising social workers (National Assocation of Social Workers, 1980). A recent re-examination of the working definition of social work saw attention focused upon social policy issues as part of the process of determining "whether or not the working definition of social work really works" (Cassano & Leslie, 2003). As well, both North American accrediting bodies for social work education, the Council on Social Work Education (U.S.A.), and the Canadian Association of Schools of Social Work (Canada) presently require that policy courses be taught in all BSW programs of study. In this regard, social work educators have finally "claimed" social welfare policy science as their domain and have moved beyond the previous awareness and policy consciousness stages into more proactive, educational concerns such as ways to influence policy formulation, implementation, and analyses.

We [the authors] are particularly optimistic and encouraged by the profession's (both practitioners and educators) investment in social policy issues and concerns to date. Indeed, the primary assumption put forward in this chapter is that social work practitioners have a responsibility to ensure that they are not only aware of social policies directly related to the elderly, but also have a role to play in developing and implementing such policies.

The purpose of this chapter is to provide a framework for understanding social welfare policies in Canada and the United States that guide the provision of income security, medical care, and social services to the elderly. The content of these policies in terms of how benefits are allocated, what benefits are provided, how services are delivered, and how benefits are finances are discussed. The value assumptions underlying the development of social welfare policies are also presented and the policies in both countries are compared. In the final section, the relationship between social work practice and policy development is explored.

We as social workers need to first understand the "process" of becoming a client in social welfare organizations. For instance, the elderly may be made to feel confused or humiliated by bureaucratic red tape and procedures established by the government agencies that implement social welfare policies. Although worthy of assistance by virtue of their past contributions to society, some elderly may not be treated with the respect they deserve when they attempt to obtain income or medical assistance.

We also need to realize that there is a wide difference between policy and practice in government programs (Armitage, 1988). For example, social welfare legislation often reflects the conflicting goals and values of a number of interest groups in society. The resulting policies are not always beneficial to the elderly, but may prove to reflect the policy preferences and values of other interest groups as well (such as the medical profession or corporations). In addition, biases or difficulties can arise since policies may be implemented by government bureaucrats in a discretionary manner (Delaney et al., 2003; Lipsky, 1980). Many services are designed to be standardized by legislative mandate, and this can result in elderly persons having difficulty obtaining services to meet their needs. By understanding the content of these policies and the value assumptions that contribute to the design of social welfare programs for the elderly, we as social workers can develop the capacity to help elderly consumers gain access to the benefits to which they are entitled. Our knowledge, as to the impact of various policies on the elderly people we serve, can also be utilized to successfully intervene in the policy development process in order that programs are effective, equitable, preserve self-determination, and enhance the quality of life for senior citizens.

II. Comparing Social Welfare Policies in Canada and the United States

Social workers often use policy models to examine the content of social welfare policies and the effect of these policies on the consumers of service. Such models offer specific frameworks for analyzing policies (Delaney et al., 2003). For example, Gilbert and Specht (1986) identified several characteristics common in all social welfare policies. These are: (1) allocation (Who receives the service?); (2) provision (What benefits are offered?); (3) service delivery (How are the services delivered to clients?); and (4) financing (Who pays for the service?) (p. 37).

In examining social welfare policies related to the elderly, each of these characteristics is important in understanding the manner in which these policies interact with the needs of elderly consumers. More specifically, allocation of resources can be made either on a universal basis (almost every citizen has access to the benefit) or a selective basis (specific groups of citizens having special needs). As a consequence of resource allocation decisions, social welfare organizations may establish eligibility criteria that exclude clients without specific needs or income above a specified level from the service delivery process. Government programs in North America have historically selected beneficiaries based on their "moral worth," and people needing assistance have been categorized as: (1) the worthy poor (children, the disabled, and others who cannot be expected to work for benefits); and (2) the able-bodied or undeserving poor (people who could work if jobs were available and are regarded as choosing not to work).

As well, benefit provision may involve compensation for past contributions to the workforce (social insurance) or income assistance (welfare) for the very poor. However, welfare participation often carries a stigma, in that recipients may be viewed by other members of society as incapable of helping themselves. Generally, people will be more likely to apply for a benefit regarded as a universal "right" based on past contributions in the workforce than a benefit associated with socially stigmatized groups of people (the unemployed, low-wage earners) who have been "selected" as requiring a special service (Hasenfeld, 1985; Rein, 1983). Postmodern theories and approaches go well beyond identifying these difficulties as resulting in stigma. At the least, many social policies are seen as disempowering the elderly (Cox, 1999), or as resulting in outright oppression (Mullaly, 2002).

Although the elderly have primarily been perceived as "worthy" to receive social welfare benefits, income security programs seldom provide equal benefits to all elderly citizens. Programs for the elderly almost always differentiate between those eligible for adequate levels of social insurance benefits based on past work contributions and others who need additional assistance to meet their needs. The Old Age Security (OAS) program is the only program for the elderly in North America that provides an equal monthly cash benefit for all Canadian residents age 65 or over. However, this is somewhat misleading since from the early 1990s (as shown in Table 6.1). Old Age Security payments have been clawed back through income tax provisions for high-income earners. Service delivery also reflects assumptions about worthy vs. unworthy beneficiaries. Benefits can be provided in ways that enhance the dignity of recipients (direct bank deposit of social insurance cheques) or in a manner that reinforces the social stigma associated with assistance—a cumbersome application process and a long wait for service (Chambers, 1993; Dolgoff et al., 1997). Further, the use of a "means-test" to determine who will receive the service often requires that applicants submit proof of income, living expenses, and savings. Such procedures often discourage applications and are associated with income assistance rather than social insurance programs.

The financing of the program also determines how the benefit will be allocated, provided, and delivered. For example, a benefit system funded through past contributions of recipients will be more generous than one funded through general tax revenues and is less vulnerable to government cutbacks (Chambers, 1993; Starr, 1988). Although government expenditures for both income security and medical care rose rapidly during the 1970s and 1980s in both Canada and the U.S., government policy-makers have been relatively unsuccessful in limiting the growth of social insurance programs. These programs provide benefits to almost all adults over 65 years of age and have a much larger political constituency than programs targeted specifically to the poor. Income-assistance programs, on the other hand, are more likely to be subject to reductions in government funding and consequently attempts have been made to contain costs by decreasing access to services for all but the most needy.

In addition to the examination of policy content, policy analysis also requires that policies be evaluated in terms of specific social values. Social workers may ask whether policies as implemented promote such key social work values as confidentiality, client self-determination, and equality (Chambers, 1993; Flynn, 1987). Government's purpose in establishing new programs or restructuring current programs may be to reflect changing societal attitudes about program operation and beneficiaries. For example, the U.S. Medicare program, first implemented in 1965, was designed to provide equal access to hospital and medical services. However, after the election of conservative president Ronald Reagan and a tremendous growth in program costs, the government began to emphasize medical cost containment (Starr, 1986). Thus, "efficiency" in service delivery became a primary policy value.

Rein and Van Gunsteren (1985) have identified two value criteria primarily associated with social welfare policies for the elderly: equity and adequacy. Equity is associated with social insurance programs in which benefit levels are proportional to the past work-related contributions of beneficiaries. Adequacy refers to whether the benefit is sufficient to meet the needs of recipients. In both Canada and the U.S., adequacy is assessed in terms of the "poverty line," or the amount of income considered sufficient for individuals, couples, or families to meet minimum basic needs. Income assistance programs are primarily designed to help low-income people increase their total income to an amount equivalent to the poverty line.

Income assistance programs for the elderly were developed in both Canada and the U.S. as a consequence of the design of social insurance programs. Social insurance programs were never intended to "lift" retired wage earners out of poverty, but to provide income to supplement retirement savings and private pensions (Burtless, 1986). Consequently, both the U.S. and Canada developed three-tiered income security policies that emphasized self-reliance on income from wages, insurance to supplement lost income during retirement, and income-assistance programs to help the elderly poor obtain an adequate income. [Canada also has a fourth tier, the Old Age Security program providing universal and equal benefits to all residents over the age of 65 (Health and Welfare Canada, 1988; Social Security Administration, 1990)].

Although most elderly social welfare beneficiaries have made a contribution to social insurance programs, benefits are not always sufficient to provide adequate support. In Canada, benefits provided through the Canadian Pension Plan are equivalent to only 25 percent of the individual's pre-retirement earnings (Human Resources Development Canada, 1998). Length of work history and employment determine work-related contributions and future benefit levels. Thus, minimum-wage workers will not receive the Canadian Pension Plan or U.S. Social Security benefits equivalent to individuals with a greater amount of income from work. Further, women who have remained out of the workforce while raising a family will also receive lower benefits based on their own work history or will receive benefits by virtue of their marital status that may not be equivalent to that of the male wage earner (Eichler, 1987).

Programs such as Supplement Security Income and Food Stamps in the U.S. and Guaranteed Income Supplement and Spouse's Allowances in Canada are designed to help people obtain an adequate level of benefits. Because these programs are means-tested and selective, access to benefits often proves difficult for some elderly consumers.

Social welfare policies for the elderly in the U.S. and Canada deal primarily with two types of benefits: income security and medical care. The content of income security policies (allocation, provision, access and service delivery, and financing) and the values underlying these policies are illustrated in Table 6.1 (Social Insurance) and Table 6.2 (Income Assistance). Social insurance programs are not only clearly differentiated from income-assistance programs in terms of basic value assumptions and the universal/selective dichotomy, but also vary significantly in terms of access. Verification of past work contributions and age are the only requirements for participation in social insurance programs. That is, assistance program applicants must often supply proof of income, marital status, assets (home, savings account, investments), and living expenses. Access to services also varies greatly by country. U.S. residents are subject to more stringent income and asset tests than Canadians, suggesting that income security is much more likely to be regarded as a "universal entitlement" in Canada than a selective program provided only for the neediest (or least worthy) citizens.

Medical programs in the U.S. and Canada are described in Table 6.3. Again these programs are dichotomized as social insurance and medical assistance for the poor or "medically needy." Canada's health program

Table 6.1: Social Insurance, United States and Canada

Policy	Date	Allocation	Provision	Service Delivery and Access	Financing	Basic Assumptions	Values
Social Security (OADSI) (U.S.A.) See (a) below	1935	Individuals 65 or over. Previous work-related contributions, surviving or divorce spouses at age 62, or disabled surviving spouses between ages 50–60. Retirees between ages 62 and 65 can receive 80% of their monthly benefit. Late retirees can receive increased benefits. Ten-year minimum contribution required for participation.	Monthly cash benefit. Amount determined by past contributions, age, and quarters of coverage. Adjustment annually for cost of living.	Application at age 65 or upon disability, death of spouse, or early retirement. Verification required: birth certificate, proof of recent earnings, and surviving spouse's proof of the worker's death. Medical verification of disability for surviving spouses, ages 50–64.	Worker and employer contributions from payroll taxes. Income tax on 50% of Social Security benefits for beneficiaries receiving income from other sources over $25,000 per year.	Supplements retirement income for contributors; income protection for low-income wage earners.	Equity; universal coverage.

Table 6.1 (continued)

Policy	Date	Allocation	Provision	Service Delivery and Access	Financing	Basic Assumptions	Values
Old Age Security Program (Can.)	1952	Age 65 or over and Canadian citizen or landed immigrant who has lived in Canada for 10 years past the age of 18. Employment history is not a factor in eligibility. Retirement is not a requirement.	Monthly cash benefits for cost of living quarterly. Maximum: $343/mo (1990). Partial benefits for those who have lived in Canada less than 40 years after the age of 18. (1/40 of full pension for each year of residence.)	Application at age 65. Proof of age and Canadian residency. Portion of benefits to be taxed or clawed back for persons with income over $50,000/year. No income or asset test.	Consolidated revenue fund. Federal government.	All seniors should have a minimum level of income to meet their needs. Compensation for past social and economic contributions.	Adequacy equality; universal coverage. Full implementation of the clawback change will make the program selective in intent, means tested.

Table 6.1 (continued)

Policy	Date	Allocation	Provision	Service Delivery and Access	Financing	Basic Assumptions	Values
Canada Pension Plan and Quebec Pension Plan See (b) below.	1965	Age 65 or anyone over 60 who has ceased pensionable employment and who has made at least one valid contribution above minimum. Surviving spouses, divorced spouses split credits earned by both spouses.	Monthly cash benefit equal to 25% of contributor's average monthly pensionable earnings. Maximum $543 (1988). Benefit decreases if taken before age 65 and increases if taken after age 65. Surviving spouses over 65 receive 60% of the worker's pension. Benefits adjusted annually for inflation.	Application at age 65, disability, death of spouse. Proof of age (birth certificate or baptismal record).	Worker, employer, and self-employed make contributions.	Protection against loss of income due to retirement, disability, and death. Supplements private pensions and savings.	Equity; universal coverage.

(a) The U.S. maintains separate pension systems for federal government employees and railroad workers.
(b) Both Canada and the U.S. provide pension benefits and medical services for veterans.

Table 6.2: Income Assistance, United States and Canada

Policy	Date	Allocation	Provision	Service Delivery and Access	Financing	Basic Assumptions	Values
Supplemental Security Income (SSI) (U.S.A.)	1972	Individuals or couples, 65 and older. Any adult who is blind or disabled. Individual assets many not exceed $2,000. A couple's assets may not exceed $3,000 (2002). Assets do not include home, a car, burial plots, or funds.	Monthly cash benefits. Maximum: $386/mo. for individuals and $579/mo for couples. Reduced if beneficiaries have other income or are living in institutions. Additional benefits are provided in 26 states.	Application through Social Security office. Verification: birth certificate, income assets, living expenses (mortgage, rent, food, utilities). Changes in income must be reported annually.	General revenues, federal government.	Minimum monthly benefit to needy aged, blind, and disabled people. Uniform benefit standard in all 50 states.	Adequacy; Selective assistance program, means testing.

Table 6.2 (continued)

Policy	Date	Allocation	Provision	Service Delivery and Access	Financing	Basic Assumptions	Values
Food Stamp Program (U.S.A)	1964	Households with less than $3,000 in disposable assets if one member is age 60 or over (in two-person households). Net household income cannot exceed 100% of the poverty line after deducting mortgage, rent and utility costs.	Coupons that are to be used to purchase food. Benefit level is determined by household size, income, and expenses. Average monthly benefits: $50.04/person.	Households in which all members receive SSI or Social Security may file Food Stamp application at their local SS Office. All other households must apply through state public assistance offices. Households with elderly or disabled members may be certified for Food Stamps over the phone or through office visits once the application h as been received. Verification: income, assets, medical expenses, proof of mortgage or rent, and utility payments. A new application is required each year.	General revenues, federal government.	Diet supplements for low-income households. Recipients are expected to use one-third of their income exclusive of Food Stamps to purchase food.	Adequacy; selective assistance program, means testing.

Table 6.2 (continued)

Policy	Date	Allocation	Provision	Service Delivery and Access	Financing	Basic Assumptions	Values
Guaranteed Income Supplement (Can.)	1966	Persons who receive Old Age Security Pension and little or no other income.	Monthly cash benefit. Amount determined by marital status and combined net income for couples. Maximum benefit is $407/mo. for a single person or a married person whose spouse does not receive OAS payments or spouse's allowance and $263/mo. for each married person whose spouse receives OAS payments or spouse's allowance. Benefits indexed quarterly at full rate of inflation. Benefit may be increased for people receiving partial OAS benefits.	Beneficiary must reapply each year. Proof of marital status. Applications are mailed to all OAS beneficiaries by Health and Welfare Canada each January. Eligibility based on previous year's income. No asset test. Benefits are not taxable.	General revenues, federal government.	To compensate those whose only source of income is OAS.	Adequacy; selective program, means testing.

Table 6.2 (continued)

Policy	Date	Allocation	Provision	Service Delivery and Access	Financing	Basic Assumptions	Values
Spouse's Allowance (Can.)	1975	All low-income widows and widowers or spouses of pensioners age 60 to 64. Must be a Canadian resident for at least 10 years after age 18.	Monthly cash benefit. Amount based on combined yearly income of both spouses exclusive of OAS and GIS benefits. Maximum: combination of full OAS and GIS at the married rate. Indexed to inflation quarterly. Benefit cases when spouse reaches 65, leaves the country for more than six months, or is separated or divorced.	Beneficiary must reapply each year. Proof of marital status.	General revenues, federal government.	Designed to recognize difficulties of couples living on the pension of one spouse and widowed persons.	Adequacy, selective program, means testing.

Table 6.2 (continued)

Policy	Date	Allocation	Provision	Service Delivery and Access	Financing	Basic Assumptions	Values
Provincial supplements to GIS (Can.)	Varies by province.	Top up benefits to OAS/GIS/SPA beneficiaries. Available in Alberta, British Columbia, Manitoba, Nova Scotia, Saskatchewan, Yukon, and Northwest Territories. Alberta also provides assistance to widows and widowers age 55–64. Manitoba provides supplemental benefits to low-income individuals age 55 and over. Pensions aged 65 and over who are ineligible for OAS/GIS because of residency requirements can receive enhanced income assistance under regular social assistance legislation in all provinces.	Monthly cash benefits. Amount varies by province but is less than $100/mo. Nova Scotia provides one lump sum payment each May. Maximum: $219. Cost of living adjustments are made on ad hoc basis.	Automatic eligibility for OAS/GIS/SPA beneficiaries. Annual application for federal programs are necessary. Application must be made in Alberta and Manitoba by persons not categorically eligible. Nova Scotia also requires a separate application for lump sum payments. All provincial supplement are nontaxable. Income reduction rates are similar to GIS rates.	Provincial general revenue funds.	Ensures that income of the elderly does not fall below minimum levels.	Adequacy.

Table 6.3: Medical Care, United States and Canada

Policy	Date	Allocation	Provision	Service Delivery and Access	Financing	Basic Assumptions	Values
Medicare, Part A (U.S.A.)	1965	Age 65 and older who have made payroll contributions. Spouse, divorced.	Hospital insurance. Reimbursement for in-patient care after beneficiary pays an annual deductible ($592 for first 60 days, 1990). Skilled nursing facility for up to 100 days. Beneficiary pays co-insurance of $74/day for 21–100 days of skilled care. Unlimited approved home, health, and hospice care.	Benefits automatic at age 65 for Social Security beneficiaries. Individuals who continue to work after age 65 or government employees must apply for benefits. Prospective payment system limits the length of hospital stay.	Worker and employer contributions through payroll taxes. Non-contributors may buy into the system ($175/mo. in 1990).	Partial payment of hospital expenditures for the aged. Increased access to health care. Cost containment.	Equity efficiency.

Table 6.3 (continued)

Policy	Date	Allocation	Provision	Service Delivery and Access	Financing	Basic Assumptions	Values
Medicare, Part B (U.S.A.)	1965	Age 65 and older. Anyone is eligible for hospital insurance. (Part A) Previous Social Security credits not necessary for enrolment.	Medical insurance. Reimbursement for 80% of doctor's services, out-patient hospital services, home health visits, and other medical services and supplies after $75 deductible (1989).	Beneficiaries pay a monthly premium of $28.60. Must also be enrolled in Part A. States must pay premiums and deductibles for people with incomes at/ below 100% of the poverty line by 1993.	Partial payment of medical expenses for the aged. Increased access to health care. Cost containment.	Equity efficiency.	

Table 6.3 (continued)

Policy	Date	Allocation	Provision	Service Delivery and Access	Financing	Basic Assumptions	Values
Medicaid (U.S.A.)	1965	Based on state discretion. Elderly persons assessed by the state to be SSI eligible. At state option, persons needing long-term care and medically needy individuals and households who spend down to Medicaid eligibility through accumulation of medical expenses that reduce income below income guidelines. 1990 Medicare provisions permit elderly couples to retain up to 50% of income and their homes while qualifying for Medicaid coverage for nursing home care for one spouse.	Basic, medical, doctor, and hospital services. Many services such as intermediate care services for the aged are state optional.	Reimbursement for services is made to providers. States may limit hospital stays or number of doctor visits per year. States may also cap provider reimbursement levels. This can result in Medicaid patients being transferred to low-cost hospitals. Inner city and rural hospitals have also been forced to shut down due to high number of Medicaid patients and unrealistic reimbursement levels.	General revenues, federal and state government. Federal government paid between 50–78.5% of state medical costs and 50% of administrative costs. Wealthier states are reimbursed at lower levels. States required to pay for Medicap coverage, i.e., Medicare premiums and deductibles for individuals and couples with incomes at or below 90% of the poverty line.	Federal/state partnership to provide medical services to the needy. Cost control.	Adequacy, selective program, means testing.

Table 6.3 (continued)

Policy	Date	Allocation	Provision	Service Delivery and Access	Financing	Basic Assumptions	Values
Canada Health Act 1) Hospital Insurance and Diagnostic Service Act 2) Medical Care Act (Can.)	1957 1966	Federal mandate to provide comprehensive hospital and medical insurance to 90–95% of the population in each province and territory at little or no cost to the consumer.	Hospital and medical services, including: medically necessary services in nursing homes, homes for the aged and hospitals, portion of ward costs in nursing homes, physician services, rehabilitative services, home care, ambulance services, prescription drugs, and medical devices. Some services are provided at provincial discretion. For example, Ontario's insurance program (OHIP) covers only prescription drugs for the elderly.	Provinces pay insurance premiums for the elderly, social assistance recipients and other low-income individuals. Some individuals pay own premium if not covered through employer plans. Specialized services such as coronary care may not be available in some localities. There may also be a waiting period for some services. Available services are often supplemented by the purchase of private health plans by individuals and employers.	Employers pay insurance premiums for most employees. Provinces pay premiums for low income or elderly. Some individuals buy into the system. Under the Established Program Financing Act, provinces receive federal block funding for health care. Canada Health Act (1984) prohibits extra billing by physicians for services rendered. Co-payments are required for some services such as nursing home care.	Health services should be universal and accessible to all.	Equality of access.

provides universal access to medical and hospital insurance for nearly all Canadian residents regardless of income. Although premium payments are required from members of the workforce, all Canadians age 65 and older receive free medical services (some co-payments are required for nursing home care). The U.S. insurance program provides medical care only for those elderly who make premium payments both prior to and after retirement. Co-payments and deductibles are required for most services, and nursing home care is not covered under this program. Many of the elderly must apply for medical assistance from state Medicaid programs to cover the costs of nursing home care. Applicants are subject to a means test, and eligibility is determined by the proportion of an individual's or couple's income spent on medical care. A focus on cost-containment in both Medicare and Medicaid programs has reduced the accessibility of medical services for many beneficiaries regardless of income (Marmour, 1988). U.S. federal and state governments now ration services with the use of prospective payment systems that limit the amount of money paid to hospital and physicians for services to individual clients. Similarly, Canada has also initiated cost containment measures resulting in the rationing of some specialized medical services.

A final category of social policies for the elderly involves the actual provision of social services. Social services, designed to help seniors remain independent, are funded by federal governments in both Canada and the U.S. The Canadian Assistance Plan (1966) provided 50 percent of the funding for counselling, homemaker, food, and other social services for every individual over 65 in each of the provinces and territories. These services are now provided directly by the provinces and territories with some funding subsidy through the Canada Health and Social Transfer Program. The funding level has been reduced significantly from the original 50 percent subsidy.

The Older Americans Act (1965) provides federal funding to state governments for community programs like: Meals-on-Wheels, ombudsman, legal assistance, employment training, congregate dining, transportation, recreation, and other social services to income-eligible people over 65 or others receiving benefits through the Supplemental Security Program (SSI). These services are oriented toward promoting the betterment of health, social networks at the community level, and increasing access to information on health and healthy lifestyles (Torres-Gil & Villa, 2000).

III. Social Welfare Practice and Policy Development: "Advocacy in Action"

For many social work practitioners, the connection between policy and practice is unclear. Policies seem to be made by government officials with little input from social workers' advocacy groups or the people they serve. Social workers are the essential linkages between policy-makers and the people served by government programs, however. Not only do social workers have direct knowledge of how policies impact on their clientele, they are also responsible for the implementation of many government policies in both public and voluntary social welfare organizations. Further, social workers often develop policy in the course of everyday practice. Dolgoff (1981) defined one of the primary social policy roles of social workers as the: "individual discrete decisions by workers [that] are policy choices that affect, for the time being, only the immediate situation and are ideological choices determining sources or plans of action." Individual decision-making by front-line workers also contributes to the formulation of agency policies. Social workers help to influence community policies and practices through networking with other social workers, helping professionals, consumer groups, and government officials. Social workers also engage in social action in order to change macro level policies (pp. 288–289).

Pierce (1984) identified a number of policy roles for social workers. For instance, outreach workers, advocates, and brokers help link clients with needed resources. Social workers can also be catalysts, organizers, or activists working with community groups to effect change. Social workers may undertake research to document existing problems, engage in community planning and networking to develop programs, and work as administrators and evaluators of programs. In addition, social workers may provide testimony at public hearings, analyzing the effects of legislation on client groups (p. 178).

Many of the social work roles defined by Pierce are familiar to social workers as part of the profession's commitment to advocacy. Thus, policy practice can be thought of as advocacy on behalf of individual clients or client groups. According to Sauber (1983) there are two basic types of advocacy: (1) general case advocacy and follow-up services by staff; and (2) consumer advocacy education and investigation of complaints (p. 386). *Case advocacy* involves increasing client access and utilization of social welfare services. Consumer advocacy, on the other hand, involves the use of influence or the mobilization of pressure to achieve changes in service quality. Case advocacy is provided by professional social workers who have obtained information about social welfare policies and benefits. Thus, the social worker acts as a broker, linking people with available resources. However, advocacy in social welfare organizations is often confined to action on individual cases rather than addressing the root causes of the problem (such as government policies or organization practices). Organizations (and individual workers) may also choose not to practice advocacy due to the commitments of time and resources required to sustain such activities (Lipsky, 1980).

In consumer or *self-help advocacy*, the involvement of service consumers and the dissemination of information about services are essential to the advocacy process. Self-help advocacy has been associated with efforts to increase access to services for the mentally or physically disabled (Ardinger & Gould, 1988; Rose & Black, 1985). Self-help advocacy can also be used as a strategy to help powerless groups obtain other assistance such as emergency food, shelter, welfare benefits, or social insurance payments. This type of intervention requires not only that the social worker provides information to client groups about service availability and social welfare policies, but also assists them in learning the skills necessary to obtain benefits from public organizations (Cassano et al., 2001). The purpose of self-help advocacy is to empower clients by developing their capacity to advocate for themselves. Solomon (1976) argued that empowerment should be the goal of any social work intervention because "power and control are energizing magnets, drawing the client into the redefinition of his own self-worth, competence, and ability to affect his social and physical worlds" (pp. 342–343).

A third type of advocacy commonly practiced by social workers is *legislative advocacy* or lobbying for laws or regulations that will benefit either the profession or service consumers. Legislative advocacy is conducted not on behalf of individuals, but involves issues affecting a group or class of individuals having similar needs (Paul, 1977). For instance, a caseworker may find it necessary to help several people receiving income assistance who have problems meeting their basic needs by organizing a legislative campaign to increase income assistance grant level.

Dear and Patti (1975) defined legislative advocacy as an attempt "to influence the course of a bill or legislative measure" (p. 108). Kramer (1981) identifies four such advocacy activities: securing tax exemptions or benefits for clientele; obtaining voluntary agency funding; improving governmental service programs; and, influencing legislation or regulations (p. 214). Legislative advocacy requires the utilization of a number of social work skills: defining problems and needs, research to document needs, community organization to build public support, development of recommendations for changes in service delivery or policy, testimony at public hearings, and lobbying public officials.

Mayer (1982) stated that advocacy practice on the part of social workers is insufficient to shape the development of social welfare policies:

> The mission of the profession and the methods in which its recruits have been trained tend to focus on changing the public agenda or the ends to which public programs are directed. This mission is consistent with the profession's involvement in social reform.... From such a perspective, the concern for how one achieves those reform goals, or for assessing the availability of resources for their attainment is defined as the responsibility of other professions. (p. 58)

Mayer believed that social workers should be involved in the development of social welfare policy. Thus, not only do social workers have access to information about the impact of policies on clients, but they also have the power to implement policy at the agency level. The value base of social work (our emphasis on equality, self-determination, and confidentiality) makes it preferable that social workers formulate policy rather than economists, public administrators, or government officials (Au & Holosko, 1996).

In this regard, Specht (1968) identified eight policy formulation tasks that correspond to social work roles. These have transcended some 35 years of practice and still hold true today.

Social workers as *practitioners, researchers, community organizers, planners, legislative analysts, advocates, educators, and administrators* can influence the development of social welfare policies at the case, agency, or governmental level. Policy development requires the identification and analysis of problems, providing information to the public and building support, the development of policy goals, the approval of legislation, program implementation and evaluation of the program (achievement of policy goals). The role of the direct service practitioner is crucial in the policy development process. Practitioners help define the needs of the people they serve and can communicate these needs to policy-makers in agencies and government bureaucracies. For instance, our involvement in the policy development process is essential if programs for the elderly are to promote the dignity and independence of all senior citizens. Current efforts by the federal governments in both Canada and the United States threaten to dismantle current programs and limit access to both income security and medical services for many elderly.

These social and political pressures, along with new methodologies in social work practice, identify an emerging trend and need for social workers to contribute to the process of policy analysis in a new way from a different perspective. As social work practitioners have developed and honed their skills in the areas of empowerment practice, structural social work, and anti-oppressive practice, a shift from attention on individual problem focus to the impact of social domination has occurred (Breton, 1999; Gingrich, 2003; Mullaly, 1997). It is now clear that both social institutions and related social policies can have the impact of creating and sustaining barriers that restrict the ability of vulnerable populations, including the elderly, from experiencing and realizing their maximum potential. It is still necessary to analyze and contribute to the development of social policies through the various methods and levels listed above. However, it is also necessary to adopt a point of perspective that allows social work practitioners to exercise due diligence in understanding the impact of the policies upon the very populations they are intended to serve.

Social work practitioners have long been aware of the need to ameliorate the effects of ageism in the forms of discrimination against and undervaluing of the older person [see Chapter 2]. These issues have also become central to the social policy arena as we see the elderly being depicted as an unworthy or at best an unproductive and therefore undeserving group (Cox, 1999). This negative view and its consequent impact are being exacerbated further by the changing socio, economic, and political ideologies, which are placing more emphasis upon cost efficiency and reduced services (Breton, 1999). The negative attention being focused upon the elderly can be explained only in part by a shift to a neo-conservative ideology. In addition, there is an apparent backlash to the success experienced by various vulnerable populations, including the elderly, in establishing a voice in the process of meeting their needs. Breton (1999) stated "one of the main characteristics of change in the political context is the brutal negative reaction to the empowerment of previously disempowered people and the consequent and often successful attempts to dismantle the policies, programs and services which empowerment had helped to bring about" (p. 222).

Postmodern approaches are proving to be useful in assisting social work practitioners in their efforts to help the elderly establish a new and more positive sense of meaning for themselves and their lives in later years. These same techniques of deconstructing, positioning, realizing client expertise, constructing a different story, and broadening the vision can be important tools for social workers in their efforts to identify oppressive features and systemic barriers embedded in social policies (O'Connor, 2003). However, rather than using only the understandings gained through the policy analysis process to influence the development and implementation of such policies, social work practitioners must accept the responsibility to inform and educate the vulnerable population itself. The dominant bio-medical narrative, traditionally used to understand the elderly, unduly emphasizes their limitations while ignoring their strengths. A well-informed cohort of elders can and will be a strong social and political source quite capable of speaking for itself. Policy analysts must redefine their target populations to include this significant and powerful group who have formally been viewed only as clients in need.

IV. Concluding Remarks

Social workers have to become more concerned with understanding the relationship between policy formulation, implementation, and practice and how this affects the clients they serve. This chapter does not attempt to minimize the complexities involved in this issue, but discusses how workers can better serve their elderly clients if they move beyond an awareness level of policy consciousness to a more proactive "advocacy-in-action" orientation. After a comparison of policies that influence practice with the elderly in Canada and the United States, we presented a three-tiered advocacy model for practice, which involves case advocacy, self-help advocacy, and legislative advocacy. Each type of advocacy is not beyond the roles and responsibilities of front-line practitioners—indeed, we contend they should be part of their practice. Our ability to empower our clients rests clearly with our ability to empower ourselves in the policy process. The sooner we understand how to assist elderly clients in this regard, the better we will be able to serve them.

Notes

1.   We would like to acknowledge the assistance of Donna Hardina, PhD, and Robin Perry, MSW, in the preparation of this chapter.

2. Social insurance programs in both Canada and the U.S. provide low-income wage earners with benefits that are proportionately larger than their past contributions. High-wage earners receive slightly less in benefits proportionate to past contributions. Hence the programs somewhat adjust for disparities in past income.

References

Ardinger, R. & Gould, M. (1988). Self-advocacy. *Journal of Voluntary Action Research,* 17, 46–53.

Armitage, A. (ed.). (1988). *Social welfare in Canada: Ideals, realities, and future paths,* 2nd ed. Toronto: McClelland & Stewart.

Au, E. & Holosko, M.J. (1996). Social and public policy analysis: A niche for social work practice. *Journal of Health and Social Policy* 7(3), 65–73.

Barnes, J. (1983). *Welfare: An overview.* Windsor: University of Windsor Press, The Research and Development Unit.

Bartlett, H. (1958, April). Toward clarification and improvement of social work practice. *Social Work,* 3(2), 3–9.

Breton, M. (1999). Empowerment practice in a post-empowerment era. In W. Shera & L.M. Wells (eds.), *Empowerment practice in social work: Developing richer conceptual foundations,* pp. 222–233. Toronto: Canadian Scholars' Press.

Burtless, G. (1986). The policies of elderly Americans. In S.H. Danzinger & D.H. Weinberg (eds.), *Fighting poverty: What works and what doesn't.* Cambridge: Harvard University Press.

Canada Information Office. (2000). *Government of Canada services for you,* Cat. No.PF4-2/2000. Ottawa: Public Works and Government Services Canada.

Cassano, R., Holosko, M., & Leslie, D.R. (2001). How service users become empowered in human service organizations: The empowerment model. *International Journal of Health Care Quality Assurance* 14(3), 26–132.

Cassano, R. & Leslie, D.R. (2003). The working definition of social work practice: Does it work? *Research in Social Work Practice,* 13(3), 366–375.

Chambers, D.E. (1993). *Social policy and social programs,* 2nd ed. Boston: Allyn & Bacon.

Cloward, R.A. & Piven, F.F. (1971). *Regulating the poor: The functions of public welfare.* New York: Vantage Books Inc.

Cox, E.O. (1999). Never too old: Empowerment—the concept and practice in work with frail elderly. In W. Shera & L.M. Wells (eds.), *Empowerment practice in social work: Developing richer conceptual foundations,* pp. 178–195. Toronto: Canadian Scholars' Press.

Dear, R. & Patti, R. (1975). Legislative advocacy: One path to social change. *Social Work, 20,* 108–114.

Delaney, R., Graham, J.R., & Swift, K.J. (2003). *Canadian social policy: An introduction,* 2nd ed. Scarborough: Prentice-Hall/Allyn & Bacon Canada.

Dolgoff, R. (1981, May). Clinicians as social policymakers. *Social Casework, 62,* 284–292.

Dolgoff, R., Feldstein, D., & Skolnik, L. (1997). *Understanding social welfare,* 4th ed. New York: Longman.

Eichler, M. (1987). *Families in Canada today.* Toronto: Gage Education Publishing Company.

Flynn, J. (1987). *Social agency policy.* Chicago: Nelson Hall Publishers.

Gilbert, N. & Specht, H. (1986). *Dimensions of social welfare policy.* Englewood Cliffs: Prentice-Hall.

Gingrich L.G. (2003). Theorizing social exclusion: Determinants, mechanisms, dimensions, forms, and acts of resistance. In W. Shera (ed.), *Emerging perspectives on anti-oppressive practice,* pp. 3–24. Toronto: Canadian Scholars' Press.

Hasenfeld, Y. (1985). Citizens' encounters with welfare state bureaucracies. *Social Service Review, 59,* 623–635.

Health and Welfare Canada. (1988). *Senior citizen's financial benefit programs in inventory of security programs in Canada,* Cat. No. H75-161 1988E ISBN 0-662-17178-9. Ottawa: Minister of Supply and Services, Canada.

Human Resources Development Canada. (1998). *Old age security Canada pension plan,* Cat. No. MP90-3/1-5-1997E. Hull: Income Security Programs.

Human Resources Development Canada. (1998). *Retirement pension,* Cat. No. MP90-3/1-1-1997E. Hull: Income Security Programs.

Human Resources Development Canada. (1998). *Survivor benefits,* Cat. No. MP90-3/1-2-1997E. Hull: Income Security Programs.

Human Resources Development Canada. (1999). *Old age security pension,* Cat. No. H76-58 /1999E. Hull: Income Security Programs.

Human Resources Development Canada. (1999). *Spouse's allowance and widowed spouse's allowance,* Cat. No. H76-55 /1999E. Hull: Income Security Programs.

Human Resources Development Canada. (2001). *Disability benefits,* Cat. No. MP90-3/1-4-1997E. Hull: Income Security Programs.

Human Resources Development Canada. (2002). *The allowance and the allowance for the survivor,* Cat. No. H76-55/1999E. Hull: Income Security Programs.

Human Resources Development Canada. (2002). *Guaranteed income supplement,* Cat. No. H76-56/2001E. Hull: Income Security Programs.

Kramer, R. (1981). *Voluntary agencies in the welfare state*. Berkeley: University of California Press.

Leslie, D.R. (1997). Health and poverty in Canada. In M. Holosko & M.D. Feit (eds.), *Health and Poverty*, pp. 65–88. New York: Haworth.

Lipsky, M. (1980). *Street-level bureaucracy: Dilemmas of the individual in public service*. New York: Russell Sage Foundation.

Lubove, R. (1973). *The professional altruist*. New York: Harvard University Press.

Majchrzak, A. (1984). *Methods for policy research*. Beverly Hills: Sage Publications Inc.

Marmour, T. (1988). Coping with a creeping crisis: Medicaid at twenty. In T.R. Marmour & J.L. Mashaw (eds.), *Social security: Beyond the rhetoric of crisis*, pp. 119–148. Princeton: Princeton University Press.

Mayer, R. (1982). Social planning as social work practice. *Administration in Social Work, 9*, 49–60.

Mullaly, R.P. (1997). *Structural social work: Ideology, theory, and practice*, 2nd ed. Toronto: Oxford University Press.

Mullaly, R.P. (2002). *Challenging oppression: A critical social work approach*. Toronto: Oxford University Press.

National Association of Social Workers. (1980). *Code of ethics*. Washington: National Association of Social Workers.

O'Connor, D. (2003). Anti-oppressive practice with older adults: A feminist post-structural perspective. In W. Shera (ed.), *Emerging perspectives on anti-oppressive practice*, pp.183–202. Toronto: Canadian Scholars' Press.

Paul, J. (1977). A framework for understanding advocacy. In J.L. Paul, G.R. Neufeld, & J.W. Pelosi (eds.), *Child advocacy within the system*, pp. 11–31. Syracuse: Syracuse University Press.

Pierce, D. (1984). *Policy for the social work practitioner*. New York: Longman.

Rein, M. (1983). *From policy to practice*. New York: Armonk.

Rein, M. & Van Gunsteren, H. (1985). The dialectic of public and private pensions. *Journal of Social Policy, 14*, 129–149.

Rose, S. & Black, B. (1985). *Advocacy and empowerment: Mental health care in the community*. Boston: Routledge & Kegan Paul.

Sauber, R. (1983). *The human service delivery system*. New York: Columbia University Press.

Schiller, B.R. (1989). *The economics of poverty & discrimination*, 5th ed. Englewood Cliffs: Prentice-Hall.

Social Security Administration. (1989). Social security programs in the United States. *Social Security Bulletin, 52*. Washington: Department of Health and Human Services.

Social Security Administration. (1990). *Social security facts and figures.* Washington: Department of Health and Human Services.

Social Security Administration. (2002). Food stamp facts. Available from http://www.ssa.gov/pubs/10101.html.

Social Security Administration. (2003). Fact sheet: Social security. Available from http://www.ssa.gov.

Solomon, B. (1976). *Black empowerment.* New York: Columbia University Press.

Spears, G. (1990, March 21). Benefit gains offer hope to the elderly. *Detroit Free Press.*

Specht, H. (1968). Casework practice and social policy formulation. *Social Work,* 12, 42–51.

Starr, P. (1986). Health care for the poor. In S. Danzinger & D. Weinberg (eds.), *Fighting poverty: What works and what doesn't,* pp. 119–148. Cambridge: Harvard University Press.

Starr, P. (1988). Social security and the American public household. In T. Marmour & L. Mashaw (eds.), *Social security,* 177–199. Princeton: Princeton University Press.

Titmuss, R. (1974). In B. Abel-Smith & K. Titmuss (eds.), *Social policy: An introduction.* New York: Pantheon Books.

Torres-Gil, F.M. & Villa, V. (2000). Social policy and the elderly. In J. Midgely, M.B. Tracy, & M. Livermore (eds.), *The handbook of social policy,* pp. 209–220. Thousand Oaks: Sage.

Internet Resources

Canadian Association for Retired Persons (CARP)
  An organization providing information to those over 50 years.
  http://www.50plus.com/carp/about/main.cfm
Human Resources Development Canada
  http://www.hrdc_drhc.gc.ca
Law Commission of Canada
  Studies and reviews the law of Canada and its effects on society.
  http://www.lcc.gc.ca
Ministry of Health and Long-Term Care
  http://www.health.gov.on.ca
National Center for Policy Analyses
  Aims to develop and promote private alternatives to government regulation and control, solving problems by relying on the strength of the competitive, entrepreneurial private sector.
  http://www.ncpa.org

Population Council: Population and Social Policy
    Seeks to marshal social science expertise toward the better
    understanding of population problems.
    http://www.popcouncil.org/ppdb/ppo.html
United States—Social Services Site
    http://www.ssa.gov

Additional Readings

Abelson, D.E. (2002). *Do think tanks matter? Assessing the impact of public institutes.* Kingston: McGill Queen's University Press.

Carmiol, B. (1995). *Case Critical*, 4th ed. Toronto: Between the Lines.

Jansson, B. (2003). *Becoming an effective policy advocate: From policy practice to social justice*, 4th ed. Pacific Grove: Brooks/Cole/Thompson Learning.

Jurkowski, E. & Tracy, M. (2000). Social policy and the aged: Implications for health planning, health education, and health promotion. *The Health Education Monograph Series 2000*, 18(2) 20–26.

Lightman, E. (2003). *Social policy in Canada.* Toronto: Oxford University Press.

Sidell, N. (1998). The politics of Alzheimer's special care units: Lessons to be learned from the demented? *Journal of Health and Social Policy*, 9(3), 29–43.

Wharf, B. & Mackenzie, B. (2004). *Connecting policy to practice*, 2nd ed. Toronto: Oxford University Press.

CHAPTER 7

IDENTIFYING THE ELDERLY ALCOHOLIC: A NICHE FOR GERONTOLOGICAL SOCIAL WORK PRACTICE[1]

MICHAEL J. HOLOSKO AND

MELANIE GALLANT

This chapter presents a case for social workers practising in this field to become more actively involved in the assessment and detection of alcoholism among the elderly. The chapter rests on the assumption that early detection and assessment serves as a perfect niche for gerontological practice. This issue is discussed from the standpoint of: (1) the profile of the elderly alcoholic; (2) prevalence rates; (3) methodological issues; (4) early identification issues; and (5) direct practice suggestions.

I.   Introduction

Alcoholism is a multi-faceted problem, both for the addicted individual and society at large. Many elderly citizens who could be potentially enjoying their "golden years" are caught in the web of alcohol addiction, and instead lead lives of misery and unhappiness (Aims Media Source, 1990). Social workers are in an ideal position to help identify elderly alcoholics as the nature of social work is helping persons to cope and adjust to their life situations in timely and effective ways.

This chapter begins by providing a profile of the types of elderly alcoholics identified in the literature and some examples of prevalence data. Identification of elderly alcoholics remains somewhat of a professional enigma as the gerontological social worker must have specific assessment knowledge and skills in order to ask the right questions. She or he also needs to identify the various aspects associated with treating addicted clients in this age group. Our experience has shown that there is an opportunity for both direct and indirect social work practitioners to be effective in this field; however, this ability rests foremost on developing a specialized approach to performing assessments that are reliable and valid. This chapter builds upon Chapter 3 (by Watt and Soifer) and makes a case for showing how the assessment and detection of problems of the elderly are inextricably linked to treatment. In short, good assessment makes for the likelihood of good treatment.

II.   Profile of the Elderly Alcoholic

In the early 1970s researchers in this field differentiated older problem drinkers into early-onset and late-onset/reactive categories (Schonfeld & Dupree, 1991). While these two typologies remain widely accepted today, other researchers and clinicians maintain that not all elderly persons with problematic drinking patterns fit one of these categories. For instance, an early- or late-onset diagnosis is based solely on age of onset, whereas those proposing additional typologies also take other factors into account.

A.   Early Onset

The early-onset elderly alcohol abuser typically begins an excessive drinking pattern in mid-life and has managed to survive to old age. Usually concerns about drinking are not new to them, as they have had significant alcohol-related problems for many years (Schonfeld & Dupree, 1991). Further, earlier onset has been related to a family history of alcoholism and more severe alcohol problems (Graham, 1993). When compared to late-onset drinkers, they generally have more psychological problems: higher levels of depression, greater trait anxiety, and lower levels of life satisfaction (Graham, 1993; Schonfeld & Dupree, 1990). As well, Zimberg (1984) has suggested that early-onset drinkers have personality characteristics that are similar to younger alcoholics.

Other variations found between the early- and late-onset groups are the quantity and frequency of drinking as well as their receptiveness to treatment. Generally, the early-onset group also consumes more liquor on a typical day of drinking and has twice as many drinking days as late-onset drinkers (Wetterling et al., 2002). They are also more resistant to treatment with a 56 percent dropout rate, compared to 26 percent for late-onset individuals (Schonfeld & Dupree, 1990).

B. Late Onset or Reactive

In contrast to the early-onset alcoholic, the late-onset drinker usually reacts to the stresses of aging with a pattern of heavy drinking (Rigler, 2000). Typical age-related stressors include depression, bereavement, retirement, loneliness, marital stress, and physical illness (Zimberg, 1984). In general, one-third of elderly alcoholics are reactive drinkers, but the distribution varies across study or region. For example, in Toronto, the Community Older Persons Alcohol Program reported a prevalence rate of 29 percent to 68 percent in programs for older people (Graham, 1993). Ironically, no empirical evidence of late-onset alcoholism was reported in elderly skid row communities, as a study of alcoholic patients in private hospital found 88 percent had begun excessive drinking later in life (Atkinson, 1984). There is also some evidence to suggest that late-onset alcoholism is more common among women and persons of higher educational attainment and socioeconomic status (Council on Scientific Affairs, 1996; Graham, 1993). Apparently, although late-onset alcoholics have less emotional and social problems than early-onset drinkers, they also tend to have more physical problems (Gulino & Kadin, 1986).

Recent research focusing on the similarities between the two groups warrants some acknowledgement at this point. Although age of onset has been used as a distinguishing factor separating types of drinkers, antecedents for current drinking behaviour have been found to be similar for both groups. Specifically, "most were steady drinkers, who drank at home and alone, and in response to such negative emotional states as sadness, loneliness, depression, and boredom" (Schonfeld & Dupree, 1990, p. 7). Further, many of them were widowed, divorced, retired, and had a limited social support network. These authors, among others, have suggested that the early-onset drinkers may have caused some of their losses by drinking, whereas the late-onset alcoholics drank in response to such losses.

C. Additional Typologies

Age for late-onset alcoholism is not clearly defined or agreed upon. Age and history of drinking behaviour and/or dependence have both been used to define the so-called "late drinker" (Johnson, 2000; Liberto et al., 1992). The U.S. Department of Health and Human Services however, classifies "late drinkers" as those 60 years of age or older (U.S. Department of Health and Human Services, 1995). As gerontological practitioners acknowledge, there is a generation of difference between mid-life and old age. For instance, at a national conference in Toronto, Graham (1993) presented data that differentiated drinkers into three "age-of-onset" categories. In this typology, early-onset drinkers, those who began before age 40, represented 38 percent of the elderly alcoholics who showed up in treatment. Mid-life onset drinkers were those who began drinking between ages 41 and 59, and made up 47 percent, while the remaining 15 percent were in the late-onset group, or those who began drinking after age 60 (Graham, 1993). These figures may lead to a much clearer picture of cohort differences, lifestyles, and reasons for drinking than the previous two-age differentiation dichotomy.

Others have proposed alternate typologies to differentiate elderly alcoholics. A study in Ontario used the early- and late-onset model, as well as a category for persons with inter-related alcohol abuse and cognitive/psychiatric problems (Graham et al., 1990). Persons in this category were mainly young-old women who displayed irrational thinking patterns, denied excessive drinking, and could not comprehend that drinking might be related to their physical, psychological, and/or social problems. Further, some had long histories of drinking and others had begun as a reaction to grief (Graham et al., 1990). Finally, in this regard, Sumberg (1985) proposed a third type of alcoholic, the binge drinker, as one who abstains between periods when drinking gets out of control. His evidence suggests the notion that assessment may be more complex than slotting all "other alcoholics" into either one of two traditional groups. More recently, a fourth type has been added that includes individuals with a history of heavy drinking who became problem drinkers in response to retirement stress and age-related loss and grief (Mellor et al., 1996). Despite all of these typologies, the clinical diagnosis of alcohol dependency in elder people still remains problematic (Johnson, 2000).

D. Prevalence Rates

While it is commonly accepted that rates of drinking among elderly cohorts are lower than those of younger populations studied (Graham, 1986), it is difficult to determine the scope and nature of the problem of alcoholism among the elderly population. Some reports suggest there is little cause for concern, while others contend that alcohol abuse affects a high proportion of elderly persons. (The reasons for variation in these statistics will be examined in a subsequent subsection of this chapter that addresses the applicability of current screening instruments when applied to this population.)

The Addiction Research Foundation's (ARF) (1991) statistics for the province of Ontario indicated that 27.5 percent of people age 65 and over reported consuming five or more drinks at a single sitting and 3.6 percent had two or more alcohol-related problems. In a comprehensive review of cross-sectional population studies of drinking patterns of people over age 60 living in the community, significant variance in prevalence of problem drinkers was found by ARF. When the threshold criteria of "heavy" drinking was consumption of 12 to 21 drinks per week, 3 percent of these older persons were considered to have "problematic" drinking behaviour. Dropping the classification criteria down to five to seven drinks per week resulted in identifying 11 percent to 25 percent of the older population as so-called "heavy" drinkers. Similarly, in a study of one-month prevalence rates that used the *Diagnostic and Statistical Manual of Mental Disorders, Third Edition Revised (DSM III-R)* criteria, 3.1 percent of men and 0.4 percent of women were considered to be "problem" drinkers (Liberto, Oslin, & Ruskin, 1992). More recently, Canadian statistics suggest that 6 percent of men and 3 percent of women surveyed were excessive drinkers. Excessive drinking is this case was defined for men as consuming 14 or more drinks per week and for women as consuming 9 or more drinks per week (Statistics Canada, 1996–1997).

In an earlier study that reported the overall prevalence of alcoholism in the population over age 21 to be 19 per 1,000, elderly widowers' rates were the highest of all groups at 105 per 1,000 (Zimberg, 1984). Although these data are limited, it appears that elderly hospital and nursing home residents have increasingly high rates of alcohol-related problems. For instance, prevalence of alcoholism was reportedly as high as 40 to 60 percent for nursing home residents in a study by Gulino and Kadin (1986). Among older hospital patients, some research reported rates of 17 percent, while others ranged up to 63 percent (Blazer &

Pennybacker, 1984). The variation in these rates was explained as the result of different clinical samples (i.e., medical wards, mentally ill patients and veterans' hospitals) used as a basis for such research.

Canada's shifting demographic profile of elderly persons, if nothing else, will result in increased rates of alcoholism among elderly persons. From all accounts it appears that the problem may become even more predominant in future years. Alcohol consumption patterns vary within cohorts, and today's elderly tend to view drinking with more restrictive pre-Prohibition mores (Graham, 1986). For instance, those elderly who recently became late-onset alcoholics were found to already have moderate habitual drinking patterns prior to later life, and since those cohorts who approach old age usually have a higher incidence of moderate drinking patterns (Holzer et al., 1986), we anticipate seeing problematic drinking, particularly the late-onset type, become an increasing concern in the future.

III.   Methodological Issues

The variation in prevalence rates indicates that there are factors, other than actual drinking patterns of elderly people, that distort the picture of what is really happening in the lives of many of these older men and women. Although these are research-oriented concerns, they are intertwined with practice realities and interventions. A critique of methodological issues related to assessment makes it obvious that social workers need to learn to ask the right questions when conducting psychogeriatric assessments, and that they should not necessarily take statistical data at face value when planning interventions or services for such clients.

A.   Operational Definitions

There is no apparent consensus on operational definitions for "elderly" or the older "alcoholic," hence how each researcher individually defines these terms in the literature is different. As a result, such data are not readily comparable. The prevalence rates cited in this chapter are extrapolated from studies that used either age 60 or 65 to define elderly. As gerontological social workers are aware [see Chapter 1 of this text], the within group variability of elderly cohorts presents its own particular practice dilemmas. Coupled with this, the lack of a singular operational definition for "alcoholism" [a long-standing and perennial problem in the addictions field] results in the use of differential identification criteria, which compounds data interpretation of incidence, occurrence, or prevalence. Traditional criteria frequently used to define alcoholism among the elderly are: quantity, frequency and volume of drinking, social and behavioural problems, tolerance and withdrawal symptoms, and physical health problems (Blazer & Pennybacker, 1984). Addictions workers are mindful that these criteria in and of themselves present an incomplete operational definition.

B. Variations in Measurement Instruments

Closely related to the definitional dilemma is the lack of a consistent measurement instrument used to identify alcohol abuse among the elderly. Rigler (2000) noted that the DSM uses fairly stringent criteria to diagnose alcoholism per se but that such criteria may be difficult to apply to older adults (e.g., tolerance levels, repeated absences, or poor work performance and neglect of children). Other common instruments used are *The CAGE Assessment* (Saunders & Conigrave, 1990), *The Michigan Alcoholism Screening Test (MAST)*, and its shorter version (Gulino & Kadin, 1986). Unfortunately, all of these rely on younger males as a normative reference group to determine alcohol abuse. However, the effects of alcoholism on social, behavioural, or psychological functioning (Liberto et al., 1992), factors that are usually relevant to elderly persons, are not normally considered in such assessments.

Measures more sensitive to the contextual lives of older adults have been designed. The Short Michigan Screening Test-Geriatric Version (SMAST-G) (Blow et al., 1992) is an adapted form of the MAST, which contains questions specific to the experiences of older people (i.e., Have you increased your drinking as a result of experiencing a loss in your life? and Does alcohol make you feel sleepy so that you often fall asleep in your chair?). The Alcohol-Related Problems Survey (Fink et al., 2002). It classifies elderly drinking as either harmful, hazardous, or non-hazardous based on alcohol intake, physical and mental health status, and medication use. Both of these measures have been described as adequate short screening measures for use with older adults (Fink et al., 2002).

C. Quantity and Consumption Measures

Although overall rates of "heavy" drinking are lower (than the general population) for elderly persons, it does not mean that drinking among the elderly is any less of a problem. Indeed, physiologically, alcohol consumption may decrease because of disabilities related to aging or due to increased effects of alcohol related to a poorer ability to metabolize alcohol (Graham, 1986). Further, many medications are seriously contraindicated when alcohol is consumed concurrently, and the effect of alcohol is amplified (Willenbring & Spring, 1990). Thus, alcoholism detection can be obscured by using gross quantitative measures of drinking. In this regard, Sumberg (1985) offered an example where an elderly client repeatedly insisted she had only two drinks of vodka a day. It was only when she was asked what size the glass was, and she produced her eight-ounce tumbler, that her alcohol problem was uncovered.

D. Self-Report Data

Similarly, Graham (1986) pointed out the unreliability and invalidity of standardized questionnaires when indiscriminately applied to elderly persons. For instance, most valid instruments require a degree of self-report, and such data rely on an accurate memory and a willingness to provide truthful information. For many elderly, without jobs to structure their days or concurrent drug use that may impair their mental ability, our experience has shown that they may be confused about reporting drinking behaviours. Additionally, given that denial is part of the pathology of alcoholism, many elderly often do not respond accurately on self-report or inventories. Atkinson and Ganzini (1994) suggested that denial may be more prevalent among elderly people due to cognitive deficits in memory, shame over alcohol dependence and/or abuse, reluctance to change drinking behaviour, and scepticism about treatment effectiveness

E. Health Criterion

Alcohol-related health problems are easily confounded with those that are a natural consequence of aging (Deblinger, 2000; Graham, 1986). While alcoholism normally intensifies physiological changes of the aging process, signs of alcoholism, such as slurred speech, poor coordination, and visual disturbances, are different from specific age-related changes (Gulino & Kadin, 1986). Even when elderly alcohol abusers formally enter the health care system, their addiction is frequently undiagnosed because it is not the presenting problem. According to Menninger (2002), elderly patients presenting to health care facilities with symptoms of alcohol abuse (e.g., insomnia, anxiety, memory loss) are more likely to be diagnosed with disorders commonly associated with geriatric disorders. In general, diagnoses using health indicators do not focus on those health problems that are exclusively alcohol related in elderly patients (Blazer & Pennybacker, 1984).

F. Lifestyle Data

Indicators of alcohol abuse on standardized questionnaires (e.g., employment difficulties, spouse abuse, drinking and driving, etc.) often do not realistically reflect the lifestyle issues of elderly persons. For instance, these questionnaires are not only biased toward younger, active, employed persons, but they also tend to characterize a male gender bias (Graham, 1986). Further, the elderly are less likely to enter the legal system because of public disturbances, arrests, drunk driving, or the social/behavioural consequences of drinking, which are ways many alcoholics become detected (Blazer & Pennybacker, 1984). In short, often times due to their lifestyles (i.e., not working; isolated from family, friends, or neighbours; not driving, etc.) the elderly are less likely to exhibit problems with alcohol that could be readily detected.

IV. Early Identification Issues

The point of departure for this chapter rests on the commonsense and well-known social work assumption that early identification and assessment leads to more effective treatment. Therefore, social workers have a vital role to play in that they often serve as the gatekeepers to the variety of institutional and community-based settings (see Section II of this text) in which the elderly are treated. It is necessary for the profession to realize its potential and act more proactively in providing prudent early identification of this problem. The role of the social worker in this early identification process will be discussed with respect to: (1) assessment, (2) dispelling myths, (3) transference and counter-transference, and (4) using support systems.

A. Assessment

Weinberg (1983) clearly stated the importance of assessment to uncover alcohol problems among adult clients, and his warnings should be heeded by the social workers practising in this field:

> The most important potential contribution that social workers might make in the treatment of alcoholism would be to move from intellectual recognition that alcoholism is a prevalent problem to direct application of appropriate helping strategies in clinical practice. First and foremost, social workers should systematically screen all adult clients, prior to launching into treatment of the presenting problem, to see whether they can rule out a diagnosis of alcoholism. The alcoholic will derive little or no benefit, and much time will be wasted if his treatment focuses on secondary or interdependent individual, family, or marital problems. (pp. 209–210)

If accurate diagnosis is not made, there is little, if any, chance that either the problem drinker or the members of the family will be helped by any subsequent interventions (Ehline & Tighe, 1977). Indeed, it has been well acknowledged that "assessment is the cornerstone of good psychogeriatric care. Careful, systematic examination is essential for accurate diagnosis and appropriate treatment decisions" (Health and Welfare Canada, 1988, p. 8). Acknowledging that alcoholism is a problem facing many elderly and that often it is the social worker who is responsible to uncover its presence leads to the issue of scrutinizing the assessment process as a whole.

Social workers may facilitate such awareness by routinely conducting comprehensive bio-psycho-social intakes and assessments where they become acutely aware of the many physical symptoms, which may appear to be age-related but are associated with drinking, and by asking direct and detailed questions about drinking-related behaviours (Sumberg, 1985). When a problem is suspected at intake, one of the simplest and most frequently used instruments is *The CAGE Assessment*. This acronym is derived from four questions: "Have you felt you should Cut down on your drinking?" "Have people Annoyed you by criticizing your drinking?" "Have you felt Guilty about your drinking?" "Have you ever had a drink first thing in the morning (an Eye-opener) to steady your nerves or get rid of a hangover?" (Jacobson, 1989, p. 22). *The CAGE Assessment* has high face validity and sensitivity in that it purportedly identifies 76 percent of positive cases and has a specificity rate of 94 percent among general populations of various adult age groups (Health and Welfare Canada, 1988). Among elderly populations it has proved effective in identifying 70 percent of positive cases with a specificity rate of 91 percent (Buchsbaum et al., 1993). Fingerhood (2000) recommends, however, embedding *CAGE* within other assessment devices in light of recent studies where *CAGE* on its own failed to identify heavy or binge drinking among older primary care patients (Adams et al., 1996).

Relatively simple and useful assessment devices have also been recommended to social workers. These include *the WART Assessment, T-ACE,* and *HEAT*. The WART Assessment developed by Ehline and Tighe (1977) stands for "With Alcohol, Repeated Trouble." The assumption put forward here is not to determine how much, when, where, or what an elderly person drinks, but focuses on the trouble (i.e., social, behavioural, familial, etc.) drinking may be causing and the role that drinking plays in the person's life. The *T-ACE* resembles the *CAGE*, but substitutes the question on guilt for one on tolerance (i.e., how many drinks can you hold?) (Sokol et al., 1989). It specifically identifies drinking risk. The *HEAT* is another short-item device that taps a person's history of alcohol use (i.e., How do you use alcohol?; Have you ever thought you used alcohol to excess?; Has anyone else ever thought you used too much?; and Have you ever had any trouble resulting from your use of alcohol?) (Willenbring & Spring, 1990). Either of these quick assessments, or similar ones, could easily become incorporated into a more comprehensive diagnostic assessment protocol. Finally, asking elderly clients how they cope or manage stress is often a diagnostic path to discuss alcohol-related issues. This technique is used by many gerontological social workers.

B. Dispelling Myths

The stereotypical image of an alcoholic as a person who drinks daily, sneaks drinks, drinks in the morning, and drinks only hard liquor is still pervasive among both clinicians and the general population. It may be difficult for a social worker to imagine that a sweet grandma who says she has a glass of sherry to stimulate her appetite before supper may have a serious problem with alcohol dependency. For instance, she does not have delirium tremens, is not dishevelled, drinks less than others in her environment, and is open about her drinking. Thus, she may not fit the image of an alcoholic.

As indicated in Chapter 2 of this text, myths get in the way of identification and can only be dispelled by facts. Further, we concur with the suggestion offered in Chapter 2 that it is the responsibility of social work practitioners to dispel myths whenever they can as this is a way of creating awareness about problems such as alcoholism. In turn, knowledge, skills, and behaviour change of practitioners will come about only when such awareness is fully realized. Although we cited only an example of one myth here to make the point, the field of addictions is prone to myth perpetuation and, as a result, is fertile ground for the promulgation of such fabrications. Some of the more frequent ones that prevail and relate to the elderly are: "She or he is old and will die anyway, so let her or him drink," "Alcohol is needed to aid the digestion" (this is synonymous with "It is only for medicinal purposes"), "If you drink only beer or wine, you can't be an alcoholic," "If a person has never been in trouble with the law or at work, how can you say she or he is an alcoholic?", "She or he is not hurting anyone by their drinking," "Alcohol helps one to sleep," "Studies show it helps the heart and circulatory system," "I don't wish to change my drinking behaviour as any radical change in my habits may result in death," "It helps as a laxative," and "They've worked hard their whole life—they are entitled to drink now that they are old." Krach (1998) pointed out that such myths only serve to impede detection of alcohol abuse and dependence among the elderly.

C. Transference and Counter-transference Issues

Social workers with elderly alcoholic clients need to become aware of a number of transference and counter-transference issues peculiar to this group. Sumberg (1985) defined four such issues. First, even when drinking seems to be one of the remaining pleasures in the life of an elderly person, the worker must be aware of the potentially devastating effects of the addiction for the client and be prepared to enable the client to give up drinking. Second, there is frustration when a client relapses and drinks after much work was completed, and a resultant tendency is to see that client as a "hopeless case." Third, if a worker attempts to help a client work through issues of loss and/or death (prevailing themes with this clientele), and the client uses this as an excuse to drink, the effect on the worker may be frustration. Fourth, elderly clients may be using alcohol to cope with other losses, and it is difficult to ask them to relinquish the "only comfort" they have left, even though it is blocking their normal grieving process (Sumberg, 1985, p. 172–173).

In this regard, self-awareness is critical for the worker so that personal apprehension is not projected into the relationship. For example, a social worker untrained in this specialized field may feel inadequate to deal with alcoholism and is unreasonably pessimistic about it; she or he avoids or minimizes the problem and subsequently her or his feelings become a self-fulfilling prophecy as the treatment fails to help (Weinberg, 1983, p. 204).

Beginning with the first contact with the client through to follow-up, social work practitioners must always be mindful of the impact of self and how personal attitudes and values relate to the therapeutic relationship (Strean, 1993). For instance, personal views on drinking and life experience of the worker may have a detrimental effect on a worker's capacity to recognize and bring to light an elderly person's excessive drinking. Our culture gives us decidedly mixed messages about drinking, both glamorizing and condemning it, making it difficult to clearly know how to evaluate its use and abuse. Further, some practitioners may be uncomfortable about drinking, perhaps because of their own use or because of negative experiences with drinking (Willenbring & Spring, 1990). In turn, such negative experiences may be particularly pertinent to direct practitioners as they constantly interact face to face with their clients. For instance, one study of MSW students found that almost half (49.7 percent) of the sample reported the existence of alcohol abuse as a problem in their families of origin compared to 28.2 percent and 23.1 percent respectively for education and business students (Russel et al., 1993). Thus, awareness, peer support, education, therapy, and supervision are all avenues through which social workers may resolve counter-transference issues should they arise.

D. Using Support Systems

Elderly alcoholics are unlikely to refer themselves for services because of reluctance to use services, lack of experience with social service agencies, and the "denial demon" element that is part of alcoholism. When they are referred for services, the social worker will often be working with others in addition to the identified client. When a referral for an elderly person is made by another professional, the referent may be a resource for the assessment process and be part of an interdisciplinary team that will combine resources to assess the client's problems. Some clients, because of their degree of isolation, will lack a social support network and a social environment will need to be developed (Sisson & Azrin, 1989). Thus, the impact of other professionals with whom the elderly person has had contact may be very significant for these individuals. Outreach services to referred clients by professionals has been identified as an effective way to facilitate the assessment process (Health Canada, 2002).

Graham (1986) explicitly recommended that "those interested in identification should exploit other sources of information (i.e., family, neighbours) concerning drinking patterns of the elderly person" (p. 325). If a worker preliminarily screens a problem (by using The *CAGE* or another type of assessment) and is concerned that the elderly person's memory may not be accurate, that he or she is confused, is denying the existence of a problem, or fears stigmatization, altering the questions for corroborating information from family and friends is probably necessary (Jacobson, 1989).

Further, when elderly alcoholics enter the health or social service system for help, their spouses and adult children often feel guilty, responsible, exasperated, and helpless, as well as angry, fearful, frustrated, and resentful. These feelings seem to be more intensified (particularly the feelings of guilt) when the person drinking is older and the condition is critical and life-threatening (Dunlop, 1990). Further, when the family recognizes that the client's drinking is a problem, but the client does not, the family system may provide useful information about the problem and establish contingencies that require the alcohol abuser to seek help (McCrady, 1986) rather than inadvertently enabling drinking patterns by interfering with the natural consequences of his or her drinking because of mistaken beliefs they are helping. In short, workers must use whatever available supports they can, namely other professionals, families, neighbours, or friends in assisting with this identification process.

Finally, in this regard, one of the best-known and effective supports available is Alcoholics Anonymous (AA). Ehline and Tighe (1977) recommended that social workers working with alcoholics and their families attend an open AA meeting. AA has groups specifically for elderly persons, and attending a meeting may increase an understanding of alcoholism in elderly persons and provide first-hand experience of their rehabilitation needs. Further, classic-style intervention, where many friends and family gather together to confront the alcoholic, has been found to have a profound negative impact on an elderly person's self-worth. A mini-confrontation, with one person and/or a counsellor, presented in a supportive and educational manner emphasizes an elderly person's freedom of choice and enhances his or her dignity or self-respect (Dunlop, 1990). The importance of AA as a proven and beneficial support should not be underestimated, in particular for those elderly who have a limited social support network.

In addition to AA, specialized programs available to seniors with alcohol-related problems do exist. Of the 180 specialized programs for substance abuse in Canada, 13 of these are specific to seniors. Many of these programs offer comprehensive intervention plans sensitive to the needs of older people and their family members.

V. Direct Practice Suggestions

Since social workers are often the gatekeepers to service elderly clients in that their assessments must look beyond the obvious for underlying problems that, when resolved, will enhance a client's functioning. Detection of alcohol abuse, through early, comprehensive assessments, leads to early, prompt intervention. In order to create a therapeutic environment that is conducive to detection of alcohol abuse in elderly clients, there are a number of suggestions workers should be mindful of.

1) Just as there is no typical older person, there is no stereotypical older person who abuses alcohol.
2) All social workers in gerontology need to learn at least the rudiments of alcoholism education (Sumberg, 1985, p. 176).
3) Social workers need to hone their assessment skills so that, with older clients, they are alert and attentive to the possibility that alcohol abuse may be present even when at first appearance it may seem unlikely. In order to accomplish this, general intake tools with elderly clients should include questions that screen for alcohol abuse. Even when alcohol problems are apparent, the focus of the assessment should also consider factors of current medical condition, mental status, domestic situation, financial status, and extent of family or social support (Dunlop, 1990).
4) Alcohol-related concerns may very well not be the presenting problem nor the primary concern of the client. More often they present with health concerns, and assisting clients to recognize the impact of drinking on their physical condition can be a valuable starting point toward helping them to accept that their drinking is problematic (Gulino & Kadin, 1986).

5) Social workers working in this field require knowledge of normal physiological, age-specific changes in order to identify and distinguish symptoms of alcohol abuse.

6) One should acknowledge that drinking patterns differ—for some it has been a life-long pattern and for others it is a problem that begins later in life. Thus, with early-onset drinkers, an assessment may likely focus on losses incurred because of drinking, whereas late-onset drinkers may need to discuss losses that occurred that triggered drinking.

7) Regardless of when the drinking began, in addition to all other losses that an older person faces (a main issue with the elderly), giving up the bottle will be another serious loss issue for such clients.

8) Drinking occurs within different contexts, and although normally most elderly people drink alone and at home, there is an increasing concern that the extent of social drinking occurring in retirement communities is placing retirees at risk for alcoholism (Sumberg, 1985).

9) It is very likely that family members will also need to be supported, educated, and worked with in order to assist the older person to recognize that a problem exists. (A list of recommended reading material and resources for families is given at the end of this chapter.)

10) Other professionals and agencies may be involved in the client's care; this may mean arranging for concrete needs such as Meals-on-Wheels, transportation, or home care services. In the event that a client is referred to another agency, the social worker may be required to make the initial appointment, arrange for someone to meet the client there, or obtain releases for the transfer of information.

11) Continuing to support the alcoholic elder by following up and staying in touch may be essential for a positive outcome for that person (Blazer, 1990). Ensuring that treatment is received and that an older person does not get lost in the system may require a liaison person (Gulino & Kadin, 1986).

12) An awareness of personal values and attitudes regarding not only the elderly in general but also in relation to alcohol abuse is necessary.

13) Finally, social workers require a sincere belief in the client and his or her recovery because: "Above all, treating the elderly alcoholic client requires faith on the part of the

worker that recovery from alcoholism is possible. Such faith can feed the recovery of an alcoholic as nothing else can" (Sumberg, 1985, p. 180).

Note

1. We would like to acknowledge the work of Catherine Schenk, BSW, for her work in the earlier versions of this chapter.

References

Adams, W.L., Barry, K.L., & Fleming, M.F. (1996). Screening for problem drinking in older primary care patients. *Journal of the American Medical Association*, 276(24), 1964–1967.

Addiction Research Foundation. (1991, October/November). Stats · facts: Older. *The Journal*, p. 13.

Aims Media. *Alcohol, drugs, and seniors: Tarnished dreams.* (1990). The Educational Media Producers and Distributors Association of Canada [Aims Media]. Film.

American Psychiatric Association. (1987). *Diagnostic and statistical manual of mental disorders*, 3rd ed., rev. Washington: American Psychiatric Association.

Atkinson, R.M. (1984). Substance use and abuse in later life. In R.M. Atkinson (ed.), *Alcohol and drug abuse in old age*, pp. 2–21. Washington: American Psychiatric Press, Monograph Series, 1-22.

Atkinson, R. & Ganzini, L. (1994). Substance abuse. In C. Coffey & J. Cummings (eds.), *Textbook of geriatric neuropsychiatry*, pp. 298–321. Washington: American Psychiatric Press.

Babor, T.F., de la Fuente, J.R., Saunders, J., & Grant, M. (1992). *The alcohol use disorders identification test (AUDIT): Guidelines for use in primary health care.* Geneva: World Health Organization.

Blazer, D. (1990). *Emotional problems in later life: Intervention strategies for professional caregivers.* New York: Springer.

Blazer, D.C. & Pennybacker, M.R. (1984). Epidemiology of alcoholism in the elderly. In J.T. Hartford & T. Samorajski (eds.), *Alcoholism in the elderly: Social and biomedical issues*, pp. 25–34. New York: Raven Press.

Blow, F.C., Brower, K.J., Schulenberg, J.E., Demo-Dananberg, L.M., Young, J.P., & Beresford, T.P. (1992). The Michigan alcoholism screening test—geriatric version (MAST-G): A new elderly-specific screening instrument. *Alcoholism: Clinical and Experimental Research, 16*, 372.

Blow F.C., Oslin, D.W., & Barry, K.L. (2002). Use and abuse of alcohol, illicit drugs and psychoactive medication among older people. *Generations,* 25(1), 50–54.

Buchsbaum, D.G., Buchanan, R.G., Welsh, J., Centor, R.M., & Schnoll, S.H. (1993). Screening for drinking disorders in the elderly using the CAGE questionnaire. *Journal of the American Geriatric Society,* 40(7), 662–665.

Council on Scientific Affairs. (1996). Alcoholism in the elderly. *JAMA,* 275, 797–801.

Crook, T. & Cohen, G. (1984). Future directions for alcohol research in the elderly. In J.T. Hartford & T. Samorajski (eds.), *Alcoholism in the elderly: Social and biomedical issues,* pp. 277–282. New York: Raven Press.

Deblinger, L. (2000). *Alcohol problems in the elderly: Patient care.* Retrieved from www.findarticles.com on November 18, 2003.

Dunlop, J. (1990). Peer groups support seniors fighting alcohol and drugs. *Aging,* 361, 28–32.

Ehline, D. & Tighe, P.O. (1977). Alcoholism: Early identification and intervention in the social service agency. *Child Welfare,* 56(9), 584–591.

Fingerhood, M. (2000). Substance abuse in older people. *Journal of the American Geriatrics Society,* 48(8), 985–995.

Fink, A., Morton, S.C., Beck, J.C., Hays, R., Spritzer, K., Oishi, S., Tsai, M., & Moore, A.A. (2002). The alcohol-related problems survey: Identifying hazardous and harmful drinking in elderly primary care patients. *Journal of the American Geriatrics Association,* 50(10), 1717–1722

Fink, A., Tsai, M., Hays, R.D., Moore, A.A., Morton, S.C., Spritzer, K., & Beck, J.C. (2002). Comparing the alcohol-related problems survey (ARPS) to traditional alcohol screening instruments in elderly outpatients. *Archives of Gerontology and Geriatrics,* 34, 55–78.

Graham, K. (1986). Identifying and measuring alcohol abuse among the elderly: Serious problems with existing instrumentation. *Journal of Studies on Alcohol,* 47(4), 322–326.

Graham, K. (1993). Interventions with older people who have alcohol or drug problems: Recent developments. Paper presented at a national conference on Misuse of Alcohol and Other Drugs by the Older Person: Community-Based Prevention and Intervention, Toronto, Canada, November 25–26.

Graham, K., Zeidman, A., Flower, M.C., Saunders, S.J., & White-Campbell, M. (1990). A typology of elderly persons who have alcohol problems. Manuscript submitted for publication. The University of Western Ontario and Addiction Research Foundation: Programs and Services Research Department and Community Older Persons Alcohol Project, Toronto, Ontario.

Gulino, C. & Kadin, M. (1986). Aging and reactive alcoholism. *Geriatric Nursing*, 7(3), 148–151.

Health Canada. (2002). *Best Practices: Treatment and rehabilitation for seniors with substance use problems*. Ottawa: Health Canada.

Health and Welfare Canada. (1988). *Guidelines for comprehensive services to elderly persons with psychiatric disorders*. Department of National Health and Welfare.

Holzer, C.E., Robins, L.N., Myers, J.K., Weissman, M.M., Tischler, G.L., Leaf, P.J., Nathony, J., & Bednarski, P.B. (1986). Antecedents and correlates of alcohol abuse and dependence in the elderly. In G. Maddox, L.N. Robins, & N. Rosenberg (eds.), *Nature and extent of alcohol problems among the elderly*, pp. 217–244. New York: Springer.

Jacobson, G.R. (1989). A comprehensive approach to pretreatment evaluation: I. Detection, assessment, and diagnosis of alcoholism. In R.H. Hester & W.R. Miller (eds.), *Handbook of alcoholism treatment approaches*, pp. 17–53. Toronto: Pergamon.

Jayck, W.R., Tabisz, E., Badger, M., & Fuchs, D. (1991). Chemical dependency in the elderly. *Canadian Journal of Aging*, 10(1), 10–17.

Johnson, I. (2000). Alcohol problems in old age: A review of recent epidemiological research. *International Journal of Geriatric Psychiatry*, 15, 575–581.

Krach, P. (1998). Myths and facts: About alcohol abuse in the elderly. *Nursing*, 25.

Liberto, J.G., Oslin, D.W., & Ruskin, P.E. (1992). Alcoholism in older persons: A review of the literature. *Hospital and Community Psychiatry*, 43(10), 975–984.

Marino, S. (1991). Selected problems in counselling the elderly. In M.J. Holosko & M.D. Feit (eds.), *Social work practice with the elderly*, pp. 47–74. Toronto: Canadian Scholars' Press.

McCrady, B.S. (1986). The family in the change process. In W.R. Miller & N. Heather (eds.), *Treating addictive behaviours: Process of change*, pp. 305–329. New York: Plenum Press.

Mellor, M.J., Garcia, A., Kenny, E., Lazerus, J., Conway, J.M., Rivers, L., Viswanathan, N., Zimmerman, J. (1996). Alcohol and aging. *Journal of Gerontological Social Work*, 25(1–2), 71–89.

Menninger, J.A. (2002). Assessment and treatment of alcoholism and substance-related disorders in the elderly. *Bulletin of the Menninger Clinic*, 66(2), 166–184.

Rigler, S. (2000). Alcoholism in the elderly. *American Family Physician*, 61, 1710 1716.

Robertson, N. (1988). *Getting better inside Alcoholics Anonymous*. New York: William Morrow and Company, Inc.

Russel, R., Gill, P., Coyne, A., & Woody, J. (1993). Dysfunction in the family of origin of MSW and other graduate students. *Journal of Social Work Education*, 29(1), 121–129.

Saunders, J.B. & Conigrave, K.M. (1990). Early identification of alcohol problems. *Canadian Medical Association Journal*, 143(10), 1060–1068.

Schonfeld, L. & Dupree, L.W. (1990). Older problem drinkers: Long term and late life onset abusers. *Aging*, 361, 5–8.

Schonfeld, L. & Dupree, L.W. (1991). Antecedents of drinking for early- and late-onset elderly alcohol abusers. *Journal of Studies on Alcohol*, 52(6), 587–591.

Sisson, R.W. & Azrin, N.H. (1989). The community reinforcement approach. In R.H. Hester & W.R. Miller (eds.), *Handbook of alcoholism treatment approaches*, pp. 242–258. Toronto: Pergamon.

Sokol, R.J., Martier, S.S., & Ager, J.W. (1989). The T-ACE questions: Practical prenatal detection of risk-drinking. *American Journal of Obstetrics and Gynecology*, 160, 863–870.

Statistics Canada. (1996–1997). *National population health survey*. Ottawa: Statistics Canada.

Strean, H.S. (1993). *Resolving counterresistances in psychotherapy*. New York: Brunner/Mazel Publishers.

Sumberg, D. (1985). Social work with elderly alcoholics: Some practical considerations. *Journal of Gerontological Social Work*, 8(3/4), 169–180.

U.S. Department of Health and Human Services. (1995). *Late-onset alcoholism: Gaining understanding*. Treatment Improvement Protocol (TOP) Series 17. Rockville: DHHS.

Watt, S. & Soifer, A. (1991). Conducting psycho-social assessments with the elderly. In M.J. Holosko & M.D. Feit (eds.), *Social work practice with the elderly*, pp. 47–74. Toronto: Canadian Scholars' Press.

Weinberg, J. (1983). Counselling recovering alcoholics. In F.J. Turner (ed.), *Differential diagnosis and treatment in social work*, 3rd ed., pp. 193–206. New York: The Free Press. Reprinted from *Social Work*, 1973, 18(4), 84–93.

Wetterling, T., Veltrup, C., Ulrich, J., & Driessen, M. (2002). Late onset alcoholism. *European Psychiatry*, 18, 112–118.

Willenbring, M. & Spring, W.D. (1990). Evaluating alcohol use in elders. *Aging*, 361, 22–72.

Zimberg, S. (1984). Diagnosis and the management of the elderly alcoholic. In R.M. Atkinson (ed.), *Alcohol and drug abuse in old age*, Monograph Series, 23–34. Washington: American Psychiatric Press.

Internet Resources

Alcohol and Seniors
>This site is devoted to alcohol issues particular to seniors and those who work with them.
>http://www.agingincanada.ca/

A Guide to Internet Resources in Social Work
>Links to organizations and agencies that provide information specific to both aging and/or alcoholism.
>http://www.abacon.com/internetguides/social/weblinks.html#6b

Health Canada
>Offers information and resources specific to Canadian seniors and substance abuse. http://www.hc-sc.gc.ca
>http://www.hc-sc.gc.ca/hecs-sesc/cds/publications/

Aging and Addiction: Helping Older Adults Overcome Alcohol or Medication Dependence
>The site provides an on-line text on the issue plus additional resources for support and treatment of alcohol or medication dependence among older adults.
>http://www.agingandaddiction.net/

American Society on Aging
>This site is geared toward disseminating information to those who work with older adults and their families.
>http://www.asaging.org/

Additional Readings

Barry, K., Oslin, D., & Blow, F. (2001). *Alcohol problems in older adults: Prevention and management.* New York: Springer.
>This is a text is a practical guide with information related to assessment, prevention, and intervention with elderly adults at risk for alcohol dependence and abuse.

Beresford, T. & Gomberg, E. (1995). *Alcohol and aging.* New York: Oxford University Press.
>Comprehensive text designed for clinicians dealing with diagnosis, treatment, related cognitive disorders, biology and biochemistry, and special populations.

Blow, F.C. (1998). *Substance abuse among older adults.* Treatment Improvement Protocol (TIP) Series 26, Center for Substance Abuse Treatment, Substance Abuse and Mental Health Services Administration, U.S. Department of Health and Human Services.

This is a useful protocol guidebook for substance abuse treatment providers. It makes specific reference to assessment and treatment of elderly clients with alcohol and prescription drug abuse. Included is an effective treatment protocol model.

Colleran, C. & Jay, D. (2002). *Aging and addiction: Helping older adults overcome alcohol or medication dependence*. Center City: Hazelden Publishing. Written by two noted experts in the field of addiction treatment and intervention, this book provides a useful tool for clinicians who work with older adults on issues related to substance use and abuse. Key topics include: understanding the relationship between aging and addiction, finding help for a loved one, and recognizing the treatment needs of older adults.

Osgood, N., Wood, H., & Parham, I. (1995). *Alcoholism and aging: An annotated bibliography and review*. Westport: Greenwood Press. This is a resource guide especially useful to students in the health care professions. The book maps out the field of chemical dependency by citing articles, books, and empirical studies from the 1940s to the present time.

Videos

It can happen to anyone: Problems with alcohol and medications among older adults. (1996). American Association of Retired Persons and Hazelden film. This video discusses factors related to life changes/transitions, substance use, intervention, and treatment among older adults. Highlighted are the stories of older recovered substance abusers. Available through: American Association of Retired Persons, Social Outreach and Support, 601 E. Street NW, Washington, DC, (202) 434-2277.

Looking forward to tomorrow: Medical aspects of seniors and substances. (1995). FMS Productions. This is a 28-minute awareness video for health professionals, older adults, and their families. A medical expert in the area of addictions follows a young medical resident interacting with older patients dealing with substance use issues. Available through: FMS Productions, P.O. Box 5016, Carpenteria, CA, 93014, (800) 421-4609.

Substance abuse in the elderly. (2001). Films for the Humanities & Sciences, a Dartmouth-Hitchcock Medical Center Production. A 28-minute video that profiles older Americans dealing with the issues of alcohol and prescription drug misuse and shows some innovative programs created specifically for the elderly. Available through: Films for the Humanities & Sciences, P.O. Box 2053, Princeton, NJ 08543-2053, (800) 257-5126.

Additional Reading/Resources for Families and Friends

Beattie, M. (1987). *Codependent no more*. Center City: Hazelden Foundation.

Beechem, E. (2002). *Elderly alcoholism: Intervention Strategies*. Springfield: Charles Thomas Publisher.

Beresford, T.P. & Gomberg, E. (eds.). (1995). *Alcohol and aging*. New York: Oxford University Press.

Black, C. (1982). *It will never happen to me*. Denver: MAC Publishing.

Colleran, C. & Jay, D. (2002). *Aging and addiction: Helping older adults overcome alcohol or medication dependence*. Minneapolis: Hazelden Press.

Gurnack, A.M., Atkinson, R., & Osgood, N. (2001). *Treating alcohol and drug use in the elderly*. New York: Springer.

Johnson, V. (1980). *I'll quit tomorrow*. Scranton: Harper & Row.

Marlin, E. (1987). *Hope: New choices and recovery strategies for adult children of alcoholics*. New York: Harper & Row.

Woititz, J. (1983). *Adult children of alcoholics*. Deerfield Beach: Health Communications.

Self-help groups are available in your community, such as Al-Anon for adult family members and friends of alcoholics, Adult Children of Alcoholics (ACOA), of Alafam for alcoholic families.

Contact the local AA group for information or assistance; there are some localities that have groups specifically for older adults. AA also has publications available, including information regarding older alcoholics, that can be ordered from the General Service Office of Alcoholics Anonymous, Box 459, Grand Central Station, New York, NY 10163.

Canadian Centre on Substance Abuse

The CCSA has been in operation since 1988 and is considered Canada's only national addiction agency. Their website provides information on various aspects related to substance abuse, research, prevention, assessment, and treatment.

http://www.ccsa.ca/default.htm

Centre for Addiction and Mental Health

This is Canada's largest health sciences centre and focuses specifically on mental illness and addiction. It provides clinical services, conducts research, and engages in educational initiatives and health promotion mandates.

http://www.camh.net

National Institute on Alcohol Abuse and Alcoholism

An American organization whose efforts aim to reduce alcohol related problems. Their website provides comprehensive information ranging

from diagnosis to treatment to prevention. Information pertaining to elderly is included.
http://www.niaaa.nih.gov/

CHAPTER 8

CASE MANAGEMENT PRACTICE WITH THE ELDERLY

CAROLE D. AUSTIN AND

ROBERT W. MCCLELLAND

By using the frail elderly as an example, this chapter presents a comprehensive overview of the state-of-the-art of case management. Discussion about case management centres around its origins, definition, various components, goals, role conflicts, models, client-centred issues, caregiving, and ethical issues. Given the demographic realities of the elderly population and their demands for increased and cost-effective services, quality case management seems inevitable for social workers practising in this field.

I.   Introduction

The growth of the older population has stimulated more attention to their functional disabilities and to their capacity to live independently in the community. As indicated in Chapter 1 of this text, it is the increase of the oldest old, those over the age of 85, that most dramatically demonstrates the need for health and social services that can assist frail elders to continue to remain independent. Since the early 1970s, public policy-makers have become more aware of future population shifts and developed a variety of responses for a range of complex and critical issues. These concerns illustrate the profound social changes that will be present in an aging society and demonstrate the far-reaching effects of public policy on the daily lives of the elderly and their families.

A number of questions/concerns emanate from these changes. Who will care for the large and growing number of elders who are no longer able to care for themselves? When, if at all, should publicly funded services replace or substitute for the care that family members might provide? Should public policy encourage the use of nursing homes to serve the larger numbers of frail elders who can no longer live independently in the community? Institutional care is costly—how much of it should be provided and to whom? Can community-based services provide enough to support frail elders and enable them to remain in the community? What kinds of services should be available and who should authorize their provision? How will these policy directions affect the lives of elders, their autonomy, their integrity, and the quality of their lives?

As public policy-makers have designed programs, funding strategies, and delivery systems, case management has been a consistent and central component. Over the last two decades, a massive investment has been made in North America on the development of community-based services and delivery systems with the aim of helping frail elders remain in their own homes or in the community. In this regard, case management has become ubiquitous in community-based, long-term care programs for the elderly. Although it is frequently given another name (i.e., case coordination, care management) the case management role and function are virtually universally present. Case management continues to be an important part of social work practice with frail elders and their families.

II.   Origins

Case management has been hailed as a cure for the ills of any type of long-term care service delivery. Although it has enjoyed considerable popularity recently, it is not new. Its origins are found in the early 1900s and the beginnings of North American social work practice. It is rooted in early social work activities designed to arrange and coordinate care for clients. Case management activities were identified in both the early settlement house movement and in the operations of the charity organization societies. As such, case management is closely related to social casework, a basic social work practice method.

Early caseworkers adopted what is now known as the "person-in-environment" perspective, directly working with and indirectly working on behalf of their clients.

The concern to provide carefully coordinated services for clients ... and to account for service provision and the use of resources has its roots in the record keeping methods developed in these early movements .... Through its history, case management has had a dual sets of goals—one set related to service quality, effectiveness and service coordination, and the other set related to goals of accountability and cost effective use of resources. (Karls et al., 1985, p. 153)

Contemporary case management practice rests on these roots and is based on a commitment to address both client and system issues.

This dual emphasis is also apparent in the current delivery of case management in community-based, long-term care programs. A wide range of goals has been associated with case management, those regarding direct service, system developmen, and cost containment. Direct service goals are primarily focused on clients, caregivers, and family members, with attention to improving service coordination, access, quality, and efficiency. In the area of system development, case managers assess the local delivery system to identify, develop, and expand needed services. Case managers also function as resource allocators, service authorizers, and system gatekeepers in pursuit of cost containment goals. This is an extremely complex role that requires extensive expertise, diverse skills, and comprehensive knowledge.

III. What Is Case Management?

Various definitions have been advanced (Applebaum & Austin, 1990; Berstein et al., 1986; Carter & Steinberg, 1983; Cline, 1990; Grisham et al., 1983; National Association of Social Workers, 1992; Quinn, 1993). Indeed, the question "What is case management?" has been hotly debated. Although the discussion has abated recently, there remains considerable variation in how case management is defined and implemented. It is not safe to assume that all participants share the same definition, philosophy, or approach. Over time, however, substantial consensus has developed regarding the core components of the case management role and function.

Perhaps the most comprehensive definition is included in the National Association of Social Workers' standards for social work case management: "Social work case management is a method of providing services whereby a professional social worker assesses the needs of the client and the client's family, when appropriate and arranges, coordinates, monitors, evaluates and advocates for a package of multiple services to meet specific client's complex needs" (National Association of Social Workers, 1992, p. 5).

IV. Components of Case Management

Case management is recognized as having a common set of core components: (1) outreach, (2) screening, (3) formalized assessment, (4) care planning, (5) service arrangement, (6) monitoring, and (7) formalized reassessment. In the following discussion, the target population for case management services will be frail elderly, specifically individuals who require a nursing home level of care, as it is this group who may be diverted from nursing home placement. This is only one of several possible target populations served by community-based, long-term care programs that provide case management.

A. Outreach

Outreach activities include efforts to publicize the services offered by an agency and to identify persons likely to qualify for and need case management and supportive services. "Case finding" and "locating the target population" are other terms for outreach. Older persons experiencing high levels of disability may have the most difficulty gaining access to services. Outreach efforts help to locate these persons and connect them with appropriate services. Outreach mechanisms may include listing the program with an informal referral agency and negotiating agreements with provider agencies to make accurate referrals and public information campaigns.

Outreach activities represent the first step toward reaching the program's target population in locations where screening is required before nursing home admission. These case finding efforts are designed to ensure that only individuals who clearly meet eligibility criteria are served. Others are referred to more appropriate programs. Caseloads will be more heterogeneous than desired since outreach, screening, and targeting efforts are not foolproof. In fact, providers have come to understand that "not all consumers require full levels of case management, and not all consumers desire it ... self-directed or reduced case management [may be more appropriate] for consumers who may need no or minimal case management" (Connecticut Continuing Care Inc., 1994, p. ii).

B. Screening

Screening is a preliminary assessment of clients' circumstances and resources in order to determine presumptive eligibility. In many community-based, long-term care programs screening criteria are designed to target those clients at risk for institutionalization. Screening criteria are applied to determine whether the clients' needs and circumstances match the target population definition(s) in the program. A standard instrument, considerably shorter than one used for a comprehensive assessment, is generally used to screen potential clients.

It is critical that screening procedures accurately identify appropriate clients. This is particularly important since once a client is screened into a program, s/he will receive a comprehensive assessment. The comprehensive assessment process is time consuming, labour intensive, and costly. Comprehensive assessment is an expensive service that should not be provided to individuals who do not meet a program's target criteria. Effective outreach and screening are necessary for efficient program operations and management. If individuals who do not meet target population criteria are accepted, the program will experience difficulty in meeting its goals and managing its operations. Outreach and screening are critical gatekeeping tasks.

C. Comprehensive Assessment

Comprehensive assessment is "a method of collecting in-depth information about a person's social situation and physical, mental and psychological functioning which allows identification of the person's problems and care needs in the major functional areas" (Schneider & Weiss, 1982, p. 12). The areas commonly evaluated in the comprehensive assessment include physical health, mental functioning (both cognitive and affective), ability to perform activities of daily living, social supports, physical environment of the home, and financial resources. Because frail elderly usually have multiple health problems, functional disabilities, and social losses, a comprehensive multi-dimensional assessment is required for effective care planning and service arrangement.

Comprehensive assessments are conducted for every client who is screened into a program, and optimally the assessment interview is conducted in the client's home. The benefit of an in-home assessment is having the opportunity to observe the client and her caregivers in their own environment. Assessments can also be conducted in hospitals and nursing homes, although these are limited by the lack of information regarding the home environment. Family members are typically interviewed as well to assess the state of the client's support system and the family's interest and capacity to provide care to the client. In many cases, caregivers have overextended themselves and are physically and emotionally spent. Here the assessment becomes even more comprehensive, including the caregiver [more directly] as a client. Thus, assessments must attend to the caregivers' capacity to effectively continue in that role in light of her physical and emotional status.

Many provinces and states have developed their own standardized assessment instruments, protocols, and formats used throughout their jurisdictions. These instruments are normally comprehensive in nature, including extensive health and social history data. Most programs have adapted standardized multi-dimensional instruments based on the long-term care minimum data set. These instruments have been rigorously developed and validated on large numbers of clients. Risk assessment tools are also being used by some programs in the assessment process to determine a client's risk of being institutionalized. Less comprehensive tools may be used to assess specific domains. For example, *The Mental Status Questionnaire (MSQ)* measures cognitive functioning and *The Beck Depression Inventory* provides a measure of affective functioning.

Comprehensive assessment is characterized by consumer involvement and input. As a result, it should focus on strengths not solely on disabilities and deficits. The assessment is designed to identify and support the client's ability to live independently. Thus, in collecting assessment data, a case manager obtains consumer permission to request information from other sources (i.e., health providers, family members, neighbours). The quality of relationship established during assessment often influences the nature of contact between the client and case manager in the later stages of the relationship. One common observation is that these instruments are lengthy and demand considerable attention and energy from frail elderly. Often it is necessary to make more than one home visit to complete the assessment. Thus, case managers must remain sensitive to client fatigue and its impact on the quality of assessment data.

Quality assessment services demand that case managers possess broad knowledge and well-honed skills. The knowledge base is so comprehensive that interdisciplinary teams and consultation models have been developed and implemented. Nelson (1987) observed that quality assessments require expertise in technical competence, interpersonal competence, and the amenities of service encounters with older persons (i.e., privacy, confidentiality, and dignity).

D. Care Planning

Information gathered during a comprehensive assessment is used by the case manager in developing a care plan. Care planning is perhaps the most demanding case management activity. It requires clinical judgment, creativity, and sensitivity as well as knowledge of community services and the ability to create a care plan within the fiscal limits imposed by budget requirements.

Schneider (1988) has identified components that she asserts should be present in all care plans. These are:

> A comprehensive list of problems; a desired outcome for each problem; the types of help needed to achieve each desired outcome; a list of the services and providers that will be supplying help; an indication of the amount of each service to be provided; a calculation of the costs of providing the listed services for a specific periods of time and an indication of the sources of payment; an indication of agreement by the client and, when appropriate, the informal caregiver. (pp. 16–17)

Care plan development takes into account the willingness and availability of informal caregivers to provide care. Most care plans include a combination of formal services and informal care. It is the mix of formal and informal that is often a central issue in the care planning process. The significance of available and able caregivers cannot be overestimated.

The case manager can assist in stimulating and enhancing their clients' independent functioning and providing support to clients' caregivers. Caregiver support services may become a significant component of the care plan. Thus, the case manager may be able to identify new sources of informal support and strengthen existing sources by expanding the existing support network. Case managers often find that clients are referred when their caregivers have reached the point of burnout. In these cases, the case manager's client is both the older person and her primary caregiver.

Elders lacking a support system in the community are more likely to be admitted to institutional care. The balance between formal and informal service provision continues to be a central public policy issue. Two key questions emerge: what should families be expected to provide and what kinds of support should be available to assist caregivers in this key role?

A guiding principle in the development of care plans is the direct involvement of the client and her caregivers. The NASW *Standard for Social Work Case Management* states that "the social worker shall ensure that clients are involved in all phases of case management practice to the greatest extent possible" (National Association of Social Workers, 1992, p. 10). Involvement and participation are essential, and client autonomy and independence must be enhanced and protected. Clients and caregivers are critical care plan decision-makers as without their participation, case managers will not likely develop care plans that can be successfully implemented. Client self-determination remains a core social work practice requirement, and is a commitment that is honoured in care plan decision-making.

Finally, through care planning, the case manager performs an important resource allocation function. The care plan is a service prescription that identifies what services are to be delivered, by which providers, and with what frequency. Thus, care plans can specify the costs of individual services and the total cost of the entire service package.

E. *Service Arrangement*

The service arrangement function is a process of contacting both formal and informal providers to arrange for services identified in the care plan. Service arrangement is really care plan implementation and it involves negotiating with providers for services when the case manager makes referrals to other agencies. It also involves ordering services from providers when the case manager has the authority to directly purchase services on behalf of their clients. The process of arranging for care plan implementation serves the function of distributing resources to the various formal providers in the delivery system. This is clearly the case when the case manager can directly purchase services on behalf of her clients.

A key aspect of service arrangement involves sharing client assessment and care plan information with relevant family members and formal providers. Although families provide the majority of services, family members may not be adequately informed about what formal services are to be provided or what they are expected to do as part of the overall care plan. Accurate and clear communication are essential for the successful implementation of care plans, and persons involved in care plan decision-making must be adequately informed.

The process of implementing care plans provides important information about the capacity of the local delivery system to meet service demands. Case managers can identify service gaps and services that are in short supply, and this information is necessary for case managers to pursue their system-level activities.

F. Monitoring

Monitoring is a critical case management task that enables the case manager to respond quickly to changes in the client's situation and increase, decrease, terminate, or maintain services as required. The frequency of monitoring varies depending on the intensity of client needs and the types of services being delivered. For example, a client who has been discharged from a hospital after an acute illness and is temporarily receiving home health care from two shifts of in-home workers may need substantial monitoring. Occasional case monitoring may be all that is required by a client who is stable and whose care plan has not changed. Indeed, careful attention to changes in client needs can have significant effects on service costs. Clients may experience changes in their functional capacity, in their living arrangements, in the availability of caregivers, and/or in their health status. Systematic monitoring allows the case manager to identify such changes and to alter care plans to more adequately meet clients' current needs. Ongoing monitoring combined with appropriate changes in care plans increase confidence that program expenditures reflect current client needs and are not based on out-of-date assessment data.

G. Reassessment

Reassessment can be routinely scheduled or precipitated by specific events. In either case, it involves a systematic examination of the client's current situation and functioning. The goal here is to identify whether changes have occurred since the initial or most recent assessment and to determine how much progress has been accomplished toward the outcomes specified in the care plan. Reassessment often takes the form of a partial re-evaluation of the most significant client problems. In some programs, reassessment is a modified form of the original assessment, focused primarily on changes since the last reassessment.

Dates for routine reassessments can be written into the care plan and are often based upon a case manager's judgment of an appropriate time frame. Other programs require reassessments at specific intervals (i.e., six months, annually). Major events in a client's life can trigger a reassessment such as: loss of a major caregiver through death or relocation; death of the client's spouse or member of the household; acute medical crisis; major deterioration in physical or mental status; placement in a hospital, lodge, or nursing home; and forced relocation of the client. Reassessment can also be triggered when the initial problem has been resolved, alleviated, or redefined; when a planned service is terminated by the client or service provider; or when there is the need to prepare clients for a planned withdrawal of services. Often reassessments are conducted when the client is terminated from the program and when a new worker is assigned.

This final task creates a feedback loop back to the overall care planning process. As a result, case management becomes an ongoing process. Reassessment can result in substantial changes in care plans, which can have a substantial impact on program costs. Finally, reassessment provides an important opportunity to ensure that the most appropriate clients are being served by the program and that their care plans reflect their current status and situations. In this respect, reassessment is a major gatekeeping function.

V.   Case Management Goals

Although there is considerable consensus on the core components that constitute case management, there appear to be multiple goals or expectations concerning these core activities (Applebaum & Austin, 1990; Carter & Steinberg, 1983; Kane, 1988; Karls et. al., 1985; Quinn, 1993; Radol-Raiff & Shore, 1993). An examination of goals that have been associated with case management practice reveals role conflicts — conflicts that make case management simultaneously challenging and frustrating. Case management goals fall into two categories, those that are primarily client focused and those that are aimed at potential change in delivery systems (Applebaum & Austin, 1990). Although these goals are discussed separately, they are interdependent.

Goals That Are Primarily Client Oriented
1.   To assure that services are appropriate to the needs of a particular client.

2. To monitor the client's condition in order to guarantee the appropriateness of services.
3. To improve client access to the continuum of long-term care services.
4. To support the client's caregivers.
5. To serve as bridges between institutional and community-based care systems. (Applebaum & Austin, 1990, p. 7)

The needs and circumstances of each client are individualized in the case management process. This emphasis is present throughout from assessment to care planning and reassessment. Care plans are really individualized service prescriptions, unique to each client. Monitoring allows the case manager to identify changes in a client's circumstances and to change the care plan to more accurately reflect currently assessed needs.

Case managers are responsible for enhancing access for individual clients to the continuum of long-term care services. The sheer complexity of programs and agencies, coupled with bureaucratic procedures, are daunting barriers for clients seeking service. This is particularly the case for the most impaired whose needs are substantial and who often experience the most difficulty accessing the system. Case managers function as the single contact point for clients, have knowledge of community services and resources, and are responsible for making the delivery system(s) more responsive to the clients' needs.

The presence, willingness, and capacity of informal caregivers are among the most critical considerations in the development of care plans. Indeed, the quality and strength of a client's support system can be the difference between remaining in the community and being institutionalized. In some instances, caregivers also become clients as they become more vulnerable themselves when faced by the continuing demands of continuing to provide care. A case manager's intervention on behalf of the caregiver, with additional services and respite, can be crucial for those families whose resources have been depleted.

Continuity is critical in the provision of case management services. Ideally, a client will work with the same case manager regardless of at what point in the delivery system they may be residing. This means that the same case manager follows the client from home care, to community services, to acute care, to nursing home care, and back to home. The involvement of multiple case managers, each assigned at different points in the delivery system and by various service providers, is neither effective from the client perspective nor efficient from a delivery system perspective. Case management will not be as client centred as it should be if multiple case managers are involved with the client.

Goals That Are Primarily System Oriented
1.   To facilitate the development of a broader array of non-institutional services.
2.   To promote quality and efficiency in the delivery of long-term care services.
3.   To enhance the coordination of long-term care service delivery.
4.   To target individuals most at risk of nursing home placement in order to prevent inappropriate institutionalization.
5.   To contain costs by controlling client access to services, especially high cost services. (Applebaum & Austin, 1990, p. 7)

In the development of care plans, case managers make decisions about how much of which services will be provided to the client by which provider. In the care planning process, the case manager can identify service gaps in the community, facilitate the development of new services, and may discover the presence of costly duplications. Case managers are also in the position to foster coordination among providers in the local delivery system. *The NASW Standard for Social Work Case Management #6* states: "the social work case manager shall intervene at the service system level to support existing case management services and to expand the supply of and improve access to needed services" (National Association of Social Workers, 1992, p. 15).

In many communities, the direction of system development is toward the expansion of the scope and volume of community-based services that are present. Such delivery system expansion provides a significant opportunity for case managers to influence the quality and efficiency of newly developed as well as existing services. "By working with providers and monitoring services that clients receive, case managers are able to evaluate the quality of providers' care. In the care planning process, case managers can also offer incentives to providers by directing the flow of referrals, thereby promoting quality and efficiency" (Applebaum & Austin, 1990, p. 9). Case managers also have major responsibility for coordinating services to clients, a responsibility that can be particularly challenging when the client is receiving multiple services from different provider agencies.

The combination of case management and community-based services has been advanced as the programmatic strategy for preventing or delaying premature or unnecessary admission to nursing homes. One of the goals of this approach is to divert clients from institutional placement. From a systems perspective, it has been asserted that effective and efficient targeting and close attention to cost in the care planning are necessary for case managers to fulfill their responsibilities regarding cost containment. "Case management, whatever setting in which it is applied, should be accountable so that costs are as streamlined as possible and that public and private financing of case management is spent in a way that protects consumers, payers of case management and direct services and the general public" (Connecticut Continuing Care Inc., 1994, p. 69).

VI. Role Conflict

These goals create a major dilemma. For instance can case managers function as client advocates and agents of the system simultaneously? Are the goals of clients and the delivery system consistent? A single service delivery role that can actually address such a broad range of goals is attractive but may be limited by insufficient authority. Most often, the major focus in the delivery of case management services has been on clients. This suggests that the basic service delivery problem is a lack of information on the part of clients. That is, if only clients had sufficient accurate information about how services were organized and where to access the system, entry into the system and receipt of services would follow smoothly. Access to community services, from the perspective of adequate information about client services, becomes the primary concern of case management services.

Another view is "... case management has enjoyed such widespread acceptance because it has not been viewed as a systemic reform, but as a function that can be incorporated into ongoing delivery systems without changing structural relationships among providers" (Austin, 1983, p. 17). Over the last 30 years there has been growing recognition that a key to the effectiveness of case management, in terms of systems development and cost containment, is the extent to which case managers have authority to directly purchase services in the implementation of care plans. The nature of the resource allocation authority dramatically shapes case management activity. The mix of client-centred and system-oriented activity In the practice of case management reflects the way it is defined and operationalized in a given program.

VII. Models of Case Management

Case management has evolved across time, organizational settings, programmatic fiscal limitations, and public policy directions. What is clear is that past, present, and future methods of organizing and financing long-term care services include some form of case management. Numerous models of case management have been offered. Cline (1990) identified three case management practice models: medical care case management (hospital-based), catastrophic care case management (insurance company-based), and long-term care case management (community-based). The central defining feature in these models is the primary location from which the case management services are provided.

Another critical variable in the specification of case management models is tied to the nature of a program's funding. As indicated, fiscal considerations become more critical in case management practice. Three case management models have been identified, each of which can be specified by the extent to which case managers possess direct authority to purchase service in the care plan development process.

First, case managers function as *brokers* when they do not have service dollars to spend on behalf of their clients. Brokers develop care plans and make referrals to providers. Brokers cannot guarantee the provision of service and frequently clients will end up on waiting lists, waiting for services to be delivered by the provider agency. In this situation, the case manager has minimal leverage with the provider agency and cannot ensure that services will be provided. Here the case manager is primarily passive, following up with the client and provider once a referral has been made, attempting to influence the provider to serve the client quickly through personal persuasion and influence. Brokers cannot directly purchase services since they do not have specific service funds, which are used to buy services prescribed in the care plan [much of this activity is conducted on the telephone]. Clearly, when time is a critical issue, brokers cannot be very responsive to client need since service provision cannot be assured. Brokered case management is weak in that it is not optimally responsive to clients' assessed needs and will not produce changes at the delivery system level. Since they are not spending their own program funding, brokers do not systematically calculate the cost of their care plans. Normally, they are not aware of the cost of their care plans, reflecting the program's limited attention to tracking costs.

The source of program funding typically determines the extent to which case managers are fiscally responsible. The power to authorize services is the critical feature of the *service management* model. Here, a case managers' care planning activities are limited by the kinds and amounts of services available in the local delivery system and by budget caps placed on the costs of individual care plans. Once the care plan has been developed, the case manager's functioning in the service management mode determines which providers to contact and then orders specific services to be delivered at a defined frequency. In this model, the case manager develops care plans within predetermined cost caps, frequently within a specified percentage of the cost of nursing home care. Service management case managers can affect the shape of the local delivery since they develop care plans and decide which providers to contact in order to arrange for services. In turn, these resource allocation patterns can influence unit costs, service quality, and the supply of services in the local delivery system.

The third model, called *managed care*, has emerged most recently. It has developed directly from service management and adds another critical dimension, prospective financing. Here, case managers develop care plans within a fiscal environment where the case management agency receives a specified amount of funding for each client served. This is often called capitation. Prospective payment or capitation creates a so-called "provider risk," where financial responsibility and liability for expenditures are shifted to the provider agency. Thus, provider agencies must keep costs below the aggregate capitation payment or they are at financial risk for expenses exceeding the prepaid amount. Thus, prospective payment puts additional emphasis on the care planning process, creating pressure on case managers to control total costs, provide and promote prevention-oriented services, and substitute lower cost services without sacrificing quality or underserving clients. Loomis (1988) noted:

> If case managers control the funds for care provided in all settings, then case managers exert significant influence when service providers decide if clients should be treated in a hospital, a nursing home, or under hospice or home care. Case managers can decide what additional services, in what amount, are necessary or unnecessary to care adequately for the client. (p. 164)

A central feature of managed care case management involves contract negotiations with providers. These negotiations centre on service costs and agreement on the volume of referrals a provider can expect to receive. At the system level, cost containment is the driving force here. In the context of provider risk, the questions are: Should certain services be provided internally and not contracted out? If so, which ones? From a systems perspective, the managed care approach most dramatically provides incentives to keep clients at the least costly level of care, which appropriately meets clients' assessed needs and assures quality. In managed care, the case manager may be conflicted in terms of the juxtaposition of client-centred and system-oriented goals. The danger here is to underserve clients in the name of fiscal management and/or cost containment. Thus far, the evolution of case management indicates the overall trend is away from brokering, more into service management and recently into managed care. This suggests that case managers will continue to function with more authority and fiscal responsibility for care plan development and implementation.

VIII. Client-Centred Issues

Much of case management practice involves direct work with elders, their families, and caregivers. Case managers will perform tasks for, collaborate with, and/or facilitate services at various times for clients. A familiar criticism has been that clients are not cases and do not need to be managed. As in other social work practice settings, there is the danger of objectifying clients, particularly when caseloads are high and service supply is inadequate. Relationship is a core concept in case management as it is in the more generalized practice of social work. As well, theory and practice may diverge in case management as it does in social work.

Burack-Weiss (1988) suggested several ways that the theory and practice of case management are discrepant. Case management practice is frequently discussed in a sequential, linear fashion. Ideally, one task follows the previous one smoothly, apparently without a hitch. Yet practice experience indicates that "smooth" is sometimes the least accurate adjective to describe case management interactions with clients, the families, and caregivers. Indeed, many clients are "non-compliant," and they may not cooperate even if they have been involved in the development of their care plans. However participatory, clients may perceive the case management process as directive—i.e., "telling them what to do." Further, clients may want services that are not available because of inadequate service supply, excessive costs, or unrealistic expectations. As well, they may only be willing to accept part of the care plan, rejecting other services. Similarly, as one may surmise, families are not always facilitative. In short, some are willing but not capable of caring for their relatives, while others are capable but not willing.

There is also a tendency to view elders as homogeneous when in fact this age group is just as much if not more heterogeneous than others (see Chapter 1). This is a reflection of ageism, where elders are viewed as the same, except for their various functional disabilities and needs for supportive service. One manifestation of ageism is stereotyping of all members of a group as the same, ignoring cultural, social class, educational, ethnic, and economic influences (see Chapter 2 for more elaboration on ageism). Individualizing case management practice is a core practice commitment. Unfortunately, overworked case managers who are asked to manage unmanageably large caseloads may be in danger of treating clients as "treatment labels" or stereotypes. Here agency pressures can adversely affect the quality of service provision. In turn, client self-determination and individualized care plans can be sacrificed in programs that are not committed to quality service delivery.

The theory of case management is frequently articulated in technical terms, while in practice it is often emotional. Case management terminology includes comprehensive assessment, providers, care plans, budget caps, care planning, systems, networks, and monitoring, among others. The language of practitioners is affective, not abstract, including anxiety and depression. This is another reflection on the dual focus of case management. Case management theory is not client centred in the counselling sense and care planning is individualized within the larger context of program, costs, and delivery system. In an effort to move away from a psychotherapeutic orientation, case management theory has obscured the relationship focus in the role. More specifically, the reciprocal relationships among the elderly, the family, and the case manager over time are also significant features of case management service.

Burack-Weiss (1988) astutely noted that "with the advent of case management, practice with the aged has inexorably moved from looking at the person-in-situation to looking for the situation in the person" (p. 24). The danger here is that assessment and care planning will dwell on "where the client fits into the system" rather than on her individual needs and the development of a tailored care plan. Even when care plans are developed from a client-centred rather than a system-focused perspective, clients may not follow through, perhaps reflecting an underdeveloped relationship between the case manager and the client. Since assessment is ongoing, case managers and clients determine those interventions that are most appropriate given the client's functional ability over time.

Mainstream case management for the elderly has not emphasized clinical mental health aspects. It is interesting to note that recent books on case management practice have devoted little attention to clinical mental health issues (Applebaum & Austin, 1990; Quinn, 1993). Their focus has been on pragmatic problem-solving and coordination within the context of community-based care planning. Indeed, clinical case management is more relationship and psychotherapeutically oriented. Clinical case management has a two-pronged thrust: it is more focused on the changes, options, and pacing of relationships other than "broker" models and it weaves clinical understandings throughout the process of dispositions planning, service referral, advocacy, and follow-up (Radol-Raiff & Shore, 1993, p. 85).

Mental health concerns normally have been addressed as part of the case management process, a process that is not particularly clinically oriented. It should be noted, however, that the increasing prevalence of Alzheimer's disease and other dementias has affected care planning dramatically. In these cases, the focus of care planning is often the caregiver and her or his needs for support and respite. Thus, the focus here is not psychotherapeutic in nature.

Case management is not an orderly sequence of tasks that unfolds effortlessly. It inevitably gets caught up in clients' feelings and reactions, responses that well-organized care plans may not adequately address. If clinical aspects of case management are not adequately addressed, there is the risk that the client will be lost within the larger delivery system when in fact the client is its centre. The risk is major goal displacement, a risk that creates additional vulnerability for the client and significant ethical problems for social workers.

IX. Caregiving

A further note on caregiving is necessary at this point. Case managers know that the presence, strength, and capacity of the informal caregivers is a critical component in the development of a care plan. Consistently, programs have stated that a primary goal is to support, not supplant, the care provided by family, friends, neighbours, volunteers, church members, and other community contacts. Some elderly are fortunate to have a network of support, which might include an adult daughter, a neighbour, a local friend, and friends or relatives who are in touch by telephone. Others are more isolated, lacking in support from any of these sources. Informal caregivers can provide assistance with a wide range of activities, including meal preparation, errands and shopping, transportation, medication management, home maintenance, house cleaning, financial management, financial contributions, laundry, personal care, emotional support and companionship, and advocating for services and benefits (Scharlach, 1988; Sterthous, 1986). In the absence of caregivers to provide these services, more formally delivered care will be necessary and more public funding will be required to address the needs of isolated elders.

A significant assumption in public policy regarding community-based, long-term care is that families and other informal caregivers are present, willing, and able to perform this critical role. In fact, some elderly do not have caregivers and others have potential caregivers who are neither willing nor able. Family care is not always the best choice. Some families are abusive, while others are not interested. Here the case manager may be caught between the assessed capacity of the informal network and program policies regarding the involvement of caregivers. In fact, in some programs the presence of a caregiver may be the basis upon which services are denied.

X.   Ethical Issues

In a study of 251 case managers, Kane, Kivnick, and Penrod (1994) asked respondents to identify ethical issues they had experienced in their practice. Forty-nine percent of respondents [the largest group] reported that conflicts between the family and the client or case manager regarding nursing home placement was the ethical issue they encountered most frequently. The second most frequently encountered (37 percent) was family and client with differing views, excluding the issue of nursing home placement. The most frequent solution reported by the case managers was providing support for client preferences if the client was competent. This study also included ethical problems that emerged as a result of a discrepancy between client needs and wants. Here, case managers reported two issues that were familiar as conflicts with so-called "non-compliant" clients. "The most frequently (32 percent) mentioned ethical issues in this category were: 1) the client wants an unsafe or unhealthy lifestyle; and 2) client conflict (for 28 percent of the sample)" related to the client needing home care and does not want it (p. 7).

While the universal value of participation in care planning decisions is asserted, it is also necessary to recognize that preferences differ regarding involvement of families and clients in decision-making and the nature of decisions being made. The question here becomes *who is the client?* All family members are not necessarily involved in decision-making and planning for a vulnerable relative. Knowledge of family history is critical for determining which family members are in the best position to constructively participate in such decision-making.

Protecting client autonomy includes two basic steps. First, the client expresses her or his wishes. Second, those wishes are carried out. Even though a client has articulated her choices, there is real cause for concern that those preferences will actually be carried out. Case managers need to be knowledgeable about the variety of advanced directives (i.e., living wills, power of attorney for health care, etc.) that may prove useful and how to skillfully plan for their timely and successful implementation.

Social workers and other human service professionals are ethically bound to provide quality services. Indeed, in recent years the discussion has shifted from what is case management to what is quality case management (Applebaum & McGinnis, 1992; Kane, 1988; Kane & Kane, 1987; National Association of Social Workers, 1992; National Institute on Community-Based Long-Term Care, 1988). Increasing attention is being paid to the design and implementation of quality assurance systems in case management programs. This represents a significant challenge since there are at least two layers of activity that require qualitative review and assessment. First is case management itself. As a distinct service, case management must meet criteria to demonstrate the quality of its service delivery. As well, case management itself functions as a case management mechanism, focused on improving the quality and suitability of community-based, long-term care services.

A comprehensive quality assurance program is based on consensus regarding desired outcomes of case management services at both the client and community levels. Quality goals include attention to multicultural realities and demonstrate a commitment to comprehensive quality outcomes in the agency's functions and activities. Consumer empowerment, through direct participation in care planning as well as feedback through client satisfaction surveys, is a crucial element of quality. Case managers' competencies and clinical skills should also be routinely assessed in order to determine how well they are performing core case management tasks.

Quality case management service delivery is one of several ethical considerations. Another fundamental concern is client self-determination. "Intrinsic to case management practice is the principle that consumers have the right to self-determination and autonomy. Case management strives to promote the highest level of independence consistent with the consumer's capacity and preferences for care, allowing consumers to maximize self-directed care to the extent possible" (Connecticut Continuing Care Inc., 1994, p. 6). This is a commitment at the core of professional social work practice. The enhancement and protection of client self-determination are significant challenges for clients in this population.

XI. Context: The Definitive Issue

It is necessary to contextualize case management, to understand how it is delivered in diverse service settings and that this affects how case management is practised in any specific setting. Case management provided to a defined target population is embedded in a particular policy context, history, culture, community, organization, and advocacy experience reflecting a client's social status. The observed variability in the way case management is delivered in different North American programs and organizations is a product of the specific context of each setting. Although the context of case management profoundly influences service delivery, its impact can be overlooked given the pressures of day-to-day practice.

There are several levels of context: policy, system, community, and organization.

National values and culture are powerful determinants of public *policy* that directly affect service delivery. The presence of case management in human service programs, as well as expectations regarding its effectiveness and efficiency, are products of specific national, public policies. While case management is national policy and is mandated in federal legislation in Australia and the United States, in Canada provinces authorize the provision of case management in community-based long-term care programs. In Canada, case management is not embedded in the current national policy framework.

Thus, ambiguous public policy is the source of conflicting messages and contradictions that surround case management. Case managers are expected to simultaneously control expenditures and improve quality, to view the client as "a customer" with limited choice, to efficiently manage unmanageable workloads, and provide client-centred services. Case managers experience role conflict as they attempt to be both a client advocate and an agent for the delivery system.

The *system* context reflects various structural characteristics of delivery systems. Case management does not exist in a vacuum (Applebaum & Austin, 1990; Austin, 1993). It is at the centre of complex delivery systems that routinely include conflicting elements and pressures. What kinds of relationships exist among providers? The presence of collaborative and/or consortia arrangements, the integration of programs and agencies into multi-provider systems, for example, influence the programmatic configuration of case management. How have providers traditionally related to each other? How does the implementation of case management alter these existing relationships? Are there conflicts in the delivery system? Are multiple models of case management operating? What resource problems exist? Case management is particularly sensitive to inadequacy of resources in basic community domains, including housing, mental health, and health care.

Case managed services are provided in specific *community* contexts. Communities vary in terms of their resources, strengths, and capacities. It is necessary to assess the strengths and limitations of specific communities through the development of resource inventories, needs assessments, strength assessments, and environmental scans. To what extent can mediating community organizations (i.e., churches, community associations, clubs) provide informal supports as case managers and their clients develop care plans? "A case management program in the context of a weak community support system can be overwhelmed by the sheer number of clients requiring service" (Moxley, 1997, p. 70). Case managers can mobilize community resources using community development strategies. A significant, frequently untapped resource are healthy, active older adults, individuals who will be seeking ways to be vitally involved in their neighbourhoods and communities [see Chapter 14].

Case management is delivered through provider *organizations* that have specific cultures and contexts. The host organization's mission, values, culture, history, disciplinary orientation, funding, and staffing patterns will have direct impact on case management program development and service delivery. For example, it can be anticipated that case management delivered by the health care system will substantially differ from case management provided by a community social agency.

A Canadian study (Desai et al., 2000) provided an instructive example of how organizational contexts can affect the provision of case management services. Experienced nurse case managers identified decision criteria for selecting the most appropriate case management approach. The case managers were then asked to use these criteria in deciding the most appropriate case management approach for clients randomly selected from their caseloads. With caseloads ranging between 120 and 200 clients, case managers were physically removed from their clients in middle management positions and had inadequate knowledge of their clients to make evidence-based, client-centred decisions about care management needs. Since these case managers had limited direct client contact, their decisions about the most appropriate case management model was based on information immediately accessible in case records: medical diagnoses, level of education, and level of informal support. In this study, caseload size, an organizational variable, had significantly more influence on care plan decision-making than direct contact that provided specific knowledge of clients. The authors concluded that "service administrators may experience pressure to increase caseloads of case managers to attain further budgetary savings, thereby only adding to the challenge of optimizing sound professional judgement by case managers" (p. 43). Here the fiscal constraints experienced in the agency meant that case managers carried large caseloads. In short, the size of the case manager's caseloads proved to be more significant than client characteristics in determining what kind of case management the client would receive.

Although there is consensus on the core components that constitute case management, the actual delivery of case management can vary considerably. The policy, system, community, agency, and programmatic contexts profoundly affect case management practice. These complex, layered service delivery contexts will determine the relative emphasis on client versus system goals; which and how much service clients actually receive; which models of case management are dominant; how caregivers are viewed in the care planning process; what ethical dilemmas case managers may face; what standards guide case management practice; whether a quality assurance mechanism for case management exists; and the extent to which social workers are employed as case managers. Context is truly the definitive issue and profoundly affects the practice of case management.

XII. Concluding Remarks

There can be little doubt that case management will continue to be a central function and service in the provision of community-based, long-term care services in North America. The intrinsic stress between the client-oriented and system-focused responsibilities will not disappear. Social work involvement in case management will vary from one location to another depending on how the role is defined and the presence of other professional groups competing for the designation. Wherever social workers provide case management services, it is necessary to demonstrate three core competencies: psychosocial assessment, skilled intervention, as well as professional accountability within the context of program and policy commitments. All are characteristic and central to social work practice and are built upon extensive professional experience. Social workers choosing to become case managers will be challenged to learn and continue to be current about a broad range of knowledge and specialized skills. A larger and older population is the demographic reality in North America, and case management in community-based, long-term care programs is a predictable component of future service delivery. Social work's work in this area has just begun!

References

Alberta Health and Wellness. (2002). *The Alberta continuing care minimum data set initiative. Final report*. Edmonton: Alberta Health and Wellness.

Applebaum, R. & Austin, C. (1990). *Long-term care case management: Design and evaluation*. New York: Springer

Applebaum, R. & McGinnis, R. (1992). What price quality? Assuring the quality of case-managed in-home care. *Journal of Case Management*, 1(1), 9–13.

Austin, C. (1983). Case management in long-term care: Options and opportunities. *Health and Social Work*, 8(1), 16–30.

Austin, C. (1993). Case management: a systems perspective. *Families in Society*, 74(8), 451–459.

Austin, C. (2002). Case management: Who needs it? Does it work? *Journal of Case Management* 3(4), 178–184.

Beck, A., Erbaugh, J., Mendelson, M., Mock, J., & Ward, C. (1961). An inventory for measuring depression. *Archives of General Psychiatry, 4,* 53–63.

Bergner, M., Bobbit, R., Gilson, B.S., & Pollard, W. (1976). The sickness impact profile: Conceptual formulation and methodology for the development of a health status measure. *International Journal of Health Services, 6,* 393–415.

Berstein, J., Capitman, J., & Haskins, B. (1986). Case management approaches in coordinated community-oriented long-term care demonstrations. *The Gerontologist, 26,* 398–404.

Burack-Weiss, A. (1988). Clinical aspects of case management. *Generations,* 12(5), 23–25.

Carter, G. & Steinberg, R. (1983). *Case management and the elderly.* Toronto: Lexington Books.

Cline, B. (1990). Case management: Organizational models and administrative methods. *Caring,* 9(7), 14–18.

Compton, A. & Ashwin, M. (eds). (2000). *Community care for health professionals.* Oxford: Butterworth-Heinemann.

Connecticut Continuing Care, Inc. (1994). Guidelines for long-term care case management practice. A report of the national advisory committee on long term care case management. Bristol, CT.

Desai, K., Galajda, J., McWilliam, C., Stewart, M., & Wade, T. (2000). Case management approaches for in-home care. *Health Care Management Forum,* 13(3), 37–44.

Dill, A. (2001). *Managing to care: Case management and service system reform.* New York: Aldine de Gruyter.

Duke University Center for the Study of Aging and Adult Development. (1978). *Multidimensional functional assessment: The OARS methodology.* Durham: Duke University.

Gray, L. (2000). Care management: The care planning process and international perspectives. In A.L. Compton & M. Ashwin (eds.), *Community Care for Health Professionals,* pp. 88–99. Oxford: Butterworth-Heineman.

Grisham, M., Miller, L., & White, M. (1983). Case management as a problem solving strategy. *Pride Institute Journal of Long Term Health Care,* 2(4), 21–28.

Gursansky, D., Harvey, J., & Kennedy, R. (2003). *Case management: Policy, practice and professional business.* Crows Nest: Allen & Unwin.

Gwyther, L. (1988). Assessment: Content, purpose and outcomes. *Generations,* 12(5), 11–15.

Huber, D.L. (2000). The diversity of case management models. *Lippincott's Case Management* 5(6), 248–255.

Kane, R. (1988). Introduction. *Generations,* 12(5), 5–6.

Kane, R. & Kane, R. (1987). *Long-term care: Principles, programs and policies.* New York: Springer.

Kane, R., Kivnick, H., & Penrod, J.D. (1994). Case managers discuss ethics. *Journal of Case Management,* 3(1), 3–12.

Karls, J., Weil, M., & Associates. (1985). *Case management in human service practice.* San Francisco: Jossey Bass.

Loomis, J. (1988). Case management in health care. *Health and Social Work,* 13, 219–225.

Moxley, D. (1997). *Case management by design: Reflections on principles and practices.* Chicago: Nelson Hall.

National Association of Social Workers. (1992). *NASW standards for social work case management.* Washington: National Association of Social Workers.

National Institute on Community-Based Long-Term Care, affiliate to the National Council on the Aging, Inc. (1988). *Care management standards: Guidelines for practice.* Washington: National Institute on Community-Based Long-Term Care.

Nelson, G. (1987). *Effective social work practice and management in adult services.* Chapel Hill: School of Social Work, University of North Carolina at Chapel Hill.

Ontario Case Managers Association & Ontario Community Support Association. (2000). *Provincial standards and guidelines for case management.* Newmarket: Ontario Case Managers Association & Ontario Community Support Association.

Pfeiffer, F. (1975). A short portable mental status questionnaire for the assessment of organic brain deficit in elderly patients. *Journal of the American Geriatrics Society,* 23, 433–441.

Quinn, J. (1993). *Successful case management in long-term care.* New York: Springer.

Radol-Raiff, N. & Shore, B. (1993). *Advanced case management.* Newbury Park: Sage.

Regina Qu'Appelle Health Region. (2001). *The Regina risk of institutionalization tool.* Regina: Regina Qu'Appelle Health Region.

Regina Qu'Appelle Health Region. (2003). *Guidelines for case coordination of community elderly.* Regina: Regina Qu'Appelle Health Region.

Scharlach, A. (1988). *Survey of caregiving employees.* Los Angeles: TransAmerica Life Companies.

Schneider, B. (1988). Care planning. The core of case management. *Generations,* 12(5), 16–19.

Schneider, B. & Weiss, L. (1982). *The channeling case management manual.* Prepared for the national long-term care channeling demonstration program. Philadelphia: Temple University Institute on Aging.

Sterthous, L. (1986). *Informal services and supports in the national long-term care channeling demonstration: A collection of practice oriented papers.* Philadelphia: Temple University Institute on Aging.

Internet Resources

American Case Management Association
    The Professional Association that offers solutions to support the evolving collaborative practice of Hospital/Health System Case Management.
    http://www.acmaweb.org

Case Management Resource Guide
    A searchable database of over 160,000 specialty health care services, facilities, businesses, and organizations.
    http://www.cmrg.com/

Case Management Society of America
    Goal is to promote the growth and value of case management and to support the evolving needs of the case management professional.
    http://www.cmsa.org

National Association of Professional Geriatric Case Managers
    A non-profit, professional organization of practitioners whose goal is the advancement of dignified care for the elderly and their families.
    http://www.caremanager.org

Additional Readings

Applebaum, R. & White, M. (2000). *Key issues in case management around the globe.* San Francisco: American Society on Aging.

Chapin, R. & Fast, B. (2000). *Strengths-based care management for older adults.* Baltimore: Health Professions Press.

Frankel, A. & Gelman, S. (1998). *Case management: An introduction to concepts and skills.* Chicago: Lyceum.

Holt, B. (2000). *The practice of generalist case management.* Boston: Allyn & Bacon.

Summers, N. (2001). *Fundamentals of case management practice.* Belmont: Brooks Cole.

CHAPTER 9

SOCIAL WORK PRACTICE WITH SENSORY IMPAIRMENTS: HEARING, TASTE, TOUCH, SMELL, AND VISION LOSS

DONALD R. LESLIE AND

M. KAYE LESLIE

This chapter reviews the changing demographics of the elderly, highlighting the projected increase of numbers experiencing one or more sensory impairments. The underlying causes of sensory impairments are explored in order to promote understanding required for social work practice. Significant impacts of these impairments upon individual and interpersonal/ relationship functioning are outlined. This increased understanding of potential impacts forms the basis for delineating the implications for social work practice with an elderly population. Sensitivity to and awareness of these impacts and implications are seen as necessary, but insufficient for sound social work practice. The need to assess each individual within his or her particular person-problem-environment situation remains as the core practice component.

The changing demographics indicating a significant increase in the proportion of the North American population over age 65 means that a disproportionate number of these individuals will face their elder years with one or more disabilities. Estimates range from 60 percent to 100 percent of the population having more than one disability with the likelihood of multiple impairments increasing directly with chronological age. This is true particularly in the areas of sensory impairment. These factors imply that a major area of social work practice is now, and will be even more so in the future, providing services to elderly individuals learning to cope with these impairments. The sensory impairments discussed in this chapter include hearing loss, reduction in taste, touch, and smell, and vision loss.

For each of these impairments, a discussion will include an overview of research findings, impact on the individual, impact on interpersonal/family relationships, and implications for practice. Interspersed throughout are a social worker's observations of case studies made working directly with this population.

I.   Hearing Loss

This pervasive loss impacts on social functioning, self-esteem, interpersonal communication, health, safety, intimacy, and interpersonal relationships. Its significance cannot be minimized, since 50 percent of the population over the age of 65 experiences hearing loss, and 95 percent of elders who have been institutionalized [for whatever reason] have significant hearing loss. Hearing loss is one of the four leading chronic conditions experienced by elderly persons (U.S. Department of Health and Human Services, 1991). Census figures for 1989 reported the rate of hearing loss among people age 45 to 64 to be approximately 13 percent, age 65 to 74 to be 24 percent, and age 75+ to be 36 percent (National Center for Health Statistics, 1990). Other researchers have found the prevalence to be much higher than that suggested by the census, with estimates ranging from 50 percent to 74 percent (DiPietro & Wax, 1984).

While aging may be the primary cause of hearing loss, others include medication, surgery, neurological disease (e.g., Alzheimer's and Parkinson's), epilepsy, head trauma, exposure to toxins, smoking, and viral conditions. It is important to note that the average person acquires this loss gradually, and deterioration associated with degenerative change is thought to progress at such a slow rate that an individual usually is unaware of the loss or the extent of its effects (Bienenfeld & Stein, 1992). After noticing the onset of hearing loss, most elderly take from 5 to 7 years to seek assistance. This is partly due to both its gradual onset and the negative social attitudes toward aging and disability.

Because hearing loss is a so-called "invisible" disability and is so pervasive (Wright, 1983), other persons may not deem it to be a true disability per se. For instance, Butler and Lewis (1977) reported that due to its invisible nature, deaf elderly are generally given less consideration than blind elderly. As such, it may in turn lead to greater social isolation because verbal communication is so crucial in social interactions.

A.   A Social Worker's Observation

This brings to mind a complaint disclosed by one of my elderly hard-of-hearing clients. Due to her hearing loss, she noticed a change in the behaviour of the tellers that served her on a regular basis at her bank. She took great pride in being financially astute, and found it very distressing when these tellers condescendingly spoke more loudly and slowly, as though she also had a cognitive impairment. She also expressed sadness about the fact that when her daughter called her on the phone, she was unable to hear the tone of her grandchildren's voices and, therefore, made excuses not to speak to them. In social situations, she found herself laughing when others laughed, although she did not hear the comment or the joke, just to feel included. On a brighter note, she expressed great joy the first time that she attended live theatre and was able to hear the performers through the use of an infrared system—a headset connected to her seat. [Some theatres and churches now have such systems in place].

In order to understand the impact of a hearing impairment, one must first consider the functions of normal hearing. Ramsdell (1978) outlined three psychological levels of hearing: primitive, signs or warnings, and symbolic.

The *primitive level* involves an unconscious awareness of one's own body noises (i.e., breathing, body movements) and of background sounds (i.e., ticking clock, creaking chair) that provide individuals with a sense of self and of being a part of their environment. Without this level of hearing, a person may feel detached from himself or herself and the world. Such detachment can result in a profound experience of isolation, and/or "deadness" that affects individuals in a pervasive and constant manner often being associated with depression (Luey, 1980; Ramsdell, 1978).

The *signs or warnings* level involves a conscious awareness of the environment that is outside the visual field (Ramsdell, 1978). At this level, sound is used as a signal of events about to happen (e.g., approaching footsteps, car brakes squealing). Awareness at this level serves to alert the individual not only to the presence of environmental events, but also to the direction and nature of these events. Such awareness enables the individual to make decisions regarding environmental threats and to take protective action. Without the signs or warning levels, persons may feel a sense of disorientation and vulnerability, creating ongoing apprehension or stress (Brinson, 1983; Hull, 1977; Luey, 1980). Elderly persons with hearing impairment often mistake environmental noises (e.g., thunder is thought to be a knock on the door) (Granick et al., 1976). Misunderstanding environmental noises, especially when coupled with communication difficulties with others, lead generally to embarrassment, fear, anxiety, and some form of withdrawal and/or unusual behaviours (Hull, 1977).

Finally, at the signs or warnings level, sound also contributes to aesthetic experiences in life (e.g., music, running water, or the sound of birds). Without this level of hearing, persons may lose a sense of enjoyment that they previously experienced (Williams, 1984). Because they may no longer be able to hear the sounds of leaves rustling, birds singing, rain on the roof or music, they may feel particularly disconnected with their environment. They may also lose the ability to use various relaxation techniques (e.g., tapes or natural experiences) available to others to reduce stress and anxiety.

The *symbolic level* involves communication with others, and is the level that most people associate with definite hearing loss (Ramsdell, 1978). Because older adults' language skills have already been developed prior to such loss (Delk & Schein, 1974), the hearing impairment should have a limited effect upon speech. Some difficulties, however, may occur because hearing loss affects the ability to appropriately assess one's own volume/loudness and more audible speech sounds such as *sh*, *f*, and *s*. These may become louder or softer than required of the situation or somewhat distorted. For instance, distorted speech and speech comprehension is more typical of an individual who has had a hearing loss for quite some time (Calvert & Silverman, 1978). Decreased speech comprehension ultimately affects the ability to understand and communicate fully with others. High tonal frequency loss affects the ability to hear consonants, and because consonants are important elements of speech, such loss can cause difficulty in understanding spoken conversation, especially when background noise exists (Carlsson et al., 1992). Therefore, loss of hearing at the symbolic level can have a devastating impact on an individual's social-emotional life (Brinson, 1983; Kampfe & Smith, 1997, 1998). Individuals may also tend to stay in the denial stage for long periods of time. Significant isolation, frequent miscommunication, and decreased contact with friends and family may occur. These might be accompanied by feelings of frustration, anger, resentment, and helplessness (Kampfe & Smith, 1998; Luey, 1980; Orlans, 1987).

B. The Impact on the Individual

The functional impact on older individuals may be substantial. Because the richness and complexity of conversations are reduced (Brinson, 1983; Luey, 1980; Oyer & Oyer, 1985), information about physical diagnoses, surgeries, medications, investments, or banking may not be available, resulting in a lack of ability to make truly informed medical or financial decisions (Kampfe & Smith, 1997, 1998). Information about philosophical issues, news items, or family concerns may go unheard, resulting in the inability to engage in meaningful conversations or family decisions. For example, an older person who has always been informed, sympathetic, or is a complex thinker may find him or herself operating in a world of simplistic concrete communications about basic life needs or logistics. If there is in addition a vision loss, the comfort and intellectual benefits gained through reading may be reduced (Kampfe & Smith, 1997).

For individuals having both vision and hearing loss, the impact of the hearing is accentuated because s/he cannot compensate by seeing facial expressions or lip reading. Thus, sensitivity to sound, understanding of speech, and maintenance of equilibrium are all affected.

Two frequently occurring problems associated with hearing loss are vertigo and tinnitus (Agnew, 1986; David & Trehub, 1989; Thomas, 1984). Vertigo is a disturbance in balance that ranges from mild to severe (Rakel, 1994). Tinnitus is a sensation of noise in one or both ears or in the head itself that also has a broad range of severity and concomitant complications (Erlandsson & Hallberg, 1993). Both tinnitus and vertigo can be extremely debilitating in that they may affect mobility, appetite, perception, sleep, and social activities (Agnew, 1986; Gant & Kampfe, 1997; Rakel, 1994).

In addition to difficulty in actual hearing, persons with hearing loss will experience distortions in what they actually do hear. As a result, even when they hear speech, they may not be able to understand it or they may misunderstand it (Cox & McFarland, 1985). Further, external sounds may be misinterpreted, resulting in misconceptions of environmental cues (Hull, 1977; Luey, 1980; Ramsdell, 1978). These compounding problems result in differential hearing (i.e., seeming to hear sometimes and not other times).

When effects of hearing loss are combined with general aging, less energy is available (Smith, 1986). With the addition of other stressors, such as the emotional reactions to several losses and coping with reactions of family and friends, a great deal of energy may be required. Older persons in such situations may become exhausted quickly, and may give up or refuse to try because the energy demands are so great and their resources are so depleted (Thomas, 1984). Thus, in general, older persons with hearing loss may be less active than before. Energy depletion for a specific individual may, of course, vary with a wide range of factors.

C. Impact on Interpersonal/Family Relationships

Because of the prevalence of hearing loss among older persons and because of its pervasive effects, family members, service providers, and older persons themselves can benefit from understanding the potential effects and implications of such loss on interpersonal/family relationships. These effects can be significant, and many older persons with hearing loss experience pronounced modifications in relationships and interpersonal functioning. These may include energy depletion/ fatigue; isolation; decreased recreational outlets; anxiety/fear/distrust; presumption by others that the older person is experiencing cognitive deterioration; changes in family dynamics and roles; depression; loss of independence; and limitations in living environment options (Kampfe & Smith, 1997).

Family members, care providers, medical personnel, and older persons themselves are often unaware of the implications of hearing loss on interpersonal relationships (Butler & Lewis, 1977). Hearing loss may result in a sense of isolation, and almost every human relationship can be affected (Luey, 1980; Oyer & Oyer, 1985; Thomas, 1984). Messages may be misunderstood (Hull, 1977; Luey, 1980), the ability to interact freely with significant others may be stifled (Luey, 1980; Oyer & Oyer, 1985), and intimacy may be difficult to achieve (Hull, 1977). As a result, old friends may avoid the person with a newly acquired hearing impairment (Luey, 1980). Family relationships may be substantially affected by changes associated with late deafness/hearing loss (Alberti, 1987). Both the family and the older person with hearing impairment may become impatient and weary when attempting to communicate (Orlans, 1987). A common misconception is that the older person with a hearing loss hears what or when s/he wants to hear (Christensen et al., 1978). This may lead to resentment because significant others may not understand how to interpret the loss, and may conclude that the loss is deliberate. They may further attribute various motives to the behaviour such as: "He doesn't listen when he wants to make me angry," or "She always tries to get attention from Harry by getting him to repeat everything."

Another common misconception of family members is that wearing a hearing aid should result in good speech discrimination. Family members may not be educated about the disadvantages of hearing aids (Butler & Lewis, 1977). Family members and other hearing people may respond to the deaf person by becoming impatient or angry (Luey, 1980; Orlans, 1987). They may exclude the person from discussions and decision-making (Luey, 1980), or talk about them in their presence (Luey, 1980; Hausman & Rezen, 1985). They may also withhold information, neglect to make accommodations for the hearing loss (Luey, 1980; Orlans, 1987), or take over responsibilities that the individual is capable of handling (Hausman & Rezen, 1985).

The resulting anger felt by the elder may affect his or her relationships with others (Orlans, 1987). Family and friends may not understand the source of the anger or may be offended by it, creating permanent rifts in relationships. Irritability and/or non-responsiveness of the older family member may be perceived as rejection, causing family members to respond negatively in return.

Just as differences in environmental conditions may result in variability in hearing (Birren & Schaie, 1985), changes in characteristics of speakers may result in fluctuations in one's general ability to understand (Kampfe, 1990, 1994; Orlans, 1987). Similarly, the elder person may prefer to communicate with a family member who faces them, speaks clearly, does not have a beard, or smoke or chew gum while speaking. The older person may be more comfortable with a relative who lives in a quiet home and does not tend to go out to noisy restaurants for dinner. This may result in a false perception of favouritism and additional feelings of resentment. After having experienced numerous embarrassing, frustrating, or tiring experiences while attempting to socialize, the person with a hearing loss may begin to withdraw from social activities (Orlans, 1987; Thomas, 1984). Family and friends often fail to inform the older person of upcoming or significant events. In turn, the older person may respond with feelings of distrust.

D. A Social Worker's Observation

An elder spouse, with hearing loss, described her feelings of distrust toward her husband. Because he thought that she could not hear the answering machine clearly, he would erase her phone messages and relay his own version of the messages to her later. On one occasion, he omitted to tell her that her brother had called and had been admitted to hospital. She found out a day later. This event undermined permanently her confidence and trust in her marital relationship.

Thus, it can be seen that hearing loss can affect interpersonal relationships in a variety of ways. Levels of ability to communicate and maintain relationships may change, requiring the development of various coping mechanisms. However, there is no reason why elders with hearing loss should not lead active, happy, and productive lives. Through understanding and knowledge, the individual, their family members, and friends can reach a level of open communication where they feel comfortable expressing their needs, while maintaining respectful interactions.

E. Implications for Practice

There are a number of techniques and/or courtesies relating to communication that should be considered in working with hearing impaired elderly. These include:

- Be aware of the communication process from the perspective of difficulties arising in the interaction that are attributable to the hearing loss.
- Touch the individual to ensure that you have his or her attention before you begin speaking.
- Make sure that the individual is facing you when you speak.
- Ensure that you are not chewing gum, smoking, or have any objects in front of your mouth when you are speaking.
- If a deaf person is using the aid of a sign language interpreter, address your questions and comments to the deaf person and not to the interpreter.
- If the individual is unable to understand what you are saying, do not raise your voice. Rephrase the statement or write it down.
- Because of the compounded problems including loss of balance, practitioners may offer to provide an arm for support or suggest the use of a cane or a walker to avoid falls.
- It may be necessary to have a friend or relative accompany the hearing impaired elderly person to medical appointments to ensure that accurate information is being

conveyed, but do not allow this to preclude direct interaction with the client.

- Ensure a quiet, private space for interviewing that limits background noise and confusion.
- Workers should develop knowledge of the range of assistant devices along with an understanding of their strengths and weaknesses.
- If the elderly person uses assistant devices, ensure that these are available for the interview.
- Given the isolation that can develop subsequent to this impairment, it is essential for workers to explore sensitively the elder's openness to participation in support/self-help groups. This can be important not only to overcome isolation, but also to establish a sense of connection to and affiliation with individuals experiencing similar conditions.

While a number of assistant devices can be helpful, many elderly do not readily embrace technology. In addition, amplification and hearing aids do have limitations, and in fact, may cause additional stress and anxiety for the user. As with any sensory loss, the adjustment takes time.

The Canadian Hearing Society runs support groups across the country for elders, and has an excellent technology department that features adaptive technology. Items such as vibrating alarm clocks, pagers, TTY phones (that convert speech into print), and other devices are available. There is also a service called Bell Relay that individuals may use in order to communicate by phone. The operator types your spoken word and the deaf individual reads it on the TTY machine. Telephones with amplified receivers and smoke detectors that light up when activated are also available. However, social workers must be sensitive to the fact that individuals accept or reject the use of assistant devices and/or participation in groups for a variety of emotional, practical, attitudinal, and cultural reasons.

Finally, in this regard, their right to self-determination must be respected. Further:

- Ensure that all relationships and social activity difficulties are assessed for the possible influence of hearing impairment.
- Explore all unusual behaviours/interpersonal dynamics for meanings or functions attributable to the impacts of hearing loss.

- It may be necessary to provide education for family, friends, and/or caregivers to increase awareness and avoid or overcome misunderstandings arising from the impact of the hearing loss.

II.   Taste, Touch, and Smell (TTS)

This subsection is perhaps one of the most important, yet neglected, in the study of sensory loss because unlike hearing or vision loss, elders and others may not be aware of TTS. Statistics reveal that over one half of individuals over the age of 65 experience diminished ability to smell and taste. The consequences and impact of these losses can be serious, and in some cases even fatal. This loss may be manifested in weight loss or malnutrition, overeating, or can contribute to hypertension and stroke. It is important to note also that loss of smell and taste can be indicators of neurological disorders such as Alzheimer's or Parkinson's disease. At a time of life when other forms of gratification are being reduced, the ability to enjoy food is important in preserving an elderly person's physical and psychological well-being. For instance, when flavour falls flat, the problem may lie not in the food itself, but in a waning ability to taste and smell (Rutherford, 1999).

As many as half of the population over the age of 65 have experienced some loss of smell, often as a result of diseases that become more commonplace later in life (Gillyatt, 1997). It is important to note that hundreds of medications affect one's sense of taste (Rutherford, 1999). Medical research has also identified smoking as a contributing factor to the loss of taste and smell. According to the American Medical Association, taste and smell loss can be caused by medications, certain diseases, viral infections, chronic exposure to environmental toxins, and head injury (Schiffman, 1997).

In a study conducted by Doty (1997) at the University of Pennsylvania's Smell and Taste Centre, 68 percent of 750 consecutive patients with primarily olfactory problems reported that their dysfunction significantly altered their quality of life. Forty-six percent indicated that the disorder changed either their appetite or body weight, and 56 percent complained that it influenced their activities of daily living and/or psychological well-being.

Overall, decreased neuronal density and nerve conduction in the central nervous system causes decreased tactile sensation, decreased response to pain, decreased motor readiness, loss of fine control of response timing, impaired balance, and decreased coordination of fine motor movement. The ability to perceive and adjust to temperature, particularly in patients older than 75 years of age, is affected due to slowed blood circulation, structural and functional changes in the skin, and decreased heat-producing activities (Hazen et al., 1997).

It is important for social workers to identify TTS possible impairments, and ensure that individuals bring them to the attention of their physicians and other caregivers since they not only affect one's quality of life, but also may have significant health and safety implications.

A. Impact on the Individual

It is important to realize that when the senses of taste and smell (which together enable us to savour food) are compromised, there can be safety and health issues over and above the impact on quality of life. The loss of these senses can lead to serious health concerns including undereating, overeating, food or gas poisoning, depression, and death (Rutherford, 1999). Individuals experiencing the loss of taste or olfactory sensitivity may be unaware of their condition, and tend to blame the food since smell supplies all the nuances of flavour. Research has shown that the nose can recognize about 10,000 scents, ranging from the very subtle aromas to strong and pungent, whereas the tongue lumps everything into four crude categories — salty, sour, bitter, or sweet. These losses are significant, as they affect over three-quarters of the elderly over the age of 80 (Schiffman, 1997).

One of the dangers resulting from these sensory losses is the desire to add sugar, salt, or spices to foods in order to enhance their flavour. Adding salt to foods may have an adverse affect on individuals who are prone to hypertension. Likewise, adding excess sugar to food may cause serious problems for diabetics or contribute to its onset.

"Some people undereat because food is so unpalatable that they've lost the desire," says Arlene Spark, coordinator of Public Health Nutrition at Hunter College (Rutherford, 1999). "Others overeat because they're looking for something that tastes good." Still others omit important food groups, like vegetables, which to smell-impaired people can taste bitter (Rutherford, 1999). Further, a loss of smell can lead to increased disease susceptibility. Sensory stimulation derived from food is especially important in old age when other sources of gratification may be less frequent (Schiffman, 1997). The loss of smell may result in additional complications, as the individual may not be able to detect spoiled food and become a victim of food poisoning.

B. A Social Worker's Observation

The effects of the loss of taste and smell became apparent in the case of an 85-year-old female client. She suddenly began to make her instant coffee with two teaspoons of coffee instead of one. At the same time, she knew that it was important to eat broccoli for her calcium intake, but reported that it tasted like medicine. Her weight dropped from 105 pounds to 98 pounds and when urged to eat, she would reply that she simply had no appetite. Oddly enough, she had never been fond of sweets or desserts in her earlier life. However, upon entering her 80s, she developed a real sweet tooth and would eat half a box of chocolates at one sitting.

C. Impact on Interpersonal/Family Relationships

Unfortunately, changes in behaviour resulting from TTS impairments may lead to misunderstandings within family or caregiver relationships. For one, many caregivers may assume that little can be done to assist the individual with TTS, and may miss opportunities to explore health, safety, or quality of life adaptations.

Individuals may also lose interest in going out for dinner as a result of lack of appetite, whereas these social outings were much enjoyed in the past. Family members and caregivers may consider this change in behaviour to be a result of disinterest or laziness when in fact the individual may feel awkward about the inability to eat, and may even feel guilty about what he or she perceives to be wasting food and/or money.

Elderly individuals with decreased senses of taste may complain about the cooking at the nursing home or by family members, and be labeled as "chronic complainers." They may comment that everything needs salt, or that the vegetables "all taste bitter." These individuals may feel that family members are imposing their own habits or values on them by throwing out milk or spoiled bacon, and may simply view this as being fussy, or making an assumption that everything in the fridge must be beyond the "best before date." All of these activities and behaviours on the part of family members may be interpreted as being burdensome or patronizing rather than helpful to the elder person.

Elders experiencing TTS may not be as aware of hygiene problems and may be shunned by caregivers or family members. They also may not notice smells in their home that indicate a need to clean more frequently. These may include changing the garbage, cleaning the bathroom, or airing the house, especially if the individual is a smoker. Elders with limited ability to smell may think that family members are being overly protective by installing additional smoke detectors or carbon-monoxide detectors when in fact these items are necessary to ensure their safety.

Elderly persons with a decreased sense of touch have less ability to adapt to changes in temperature or to tolerate cooler temperatures. This can cause family members or friends to be reluctant to visit the person in his or her own home since they may find it uncomfortably warm. This can be a particular area of conflict where these elderly are sharing a residence with other family members. Often open hostilities can exist revolving around who adjusted the thermostat last. Younger family members may find themselves in conflict with one another over how far to go in accommodating the needs of the elderly co-habitant.

In general, TTS impairments can significantly impact the elderly person's ability to enjoy his or her quality of life. This lack of enjoyment can lead to a generalized change in personality, resulting in friends and family members finding the individual more irritable and less approachable.

D. A Social Worker's Observation

An 83-year-old lady, living in a large city near her family, took great pride in baking cookies for the enjoyment of her grandchildren and company. When her son noticed the distinct absence of cookies in the house, he inquired why she had not been baking. She replied that her cookies did not taste right anymore, that she had obviously lost her knack for baking. Unfortunately, friends and family members had interpreted this change in behaviour as her not wanting to have company and a lack of a desire to socialize anymore.

E. Implications for Social Work Practice

Because these sensory losses often go undetected, social work practitioners should persuade elderly clients to be tested regularly. Upon identification of impairment, the following safety considerations can be implemented:

- additional smoke detectors,
- the use of electrical appliances rather than gas,

- pre-measured amounts of salt for cooking, and
- regular monitoring of perishable foods.

Care providers may find it helpful to offer an arm for support when guiding an elder with diabetes whose circulation problems have affected his or her touch sensation in the feet and hands since neuropathy may have affected this person's sense of balance. In addition to the precautions outlined above, Rutherford (1999) suggested several techniques that can be used to enhance the pleasure of eating, and provide tactile and visual cues to supplement the weakened perception of taste and odour. These include:

- Ensure that meals are varied in texture, temperature, and colour.
- Be aware that smaller portions of food and a pleasing visual presentation may make a genuine difference in the desire to eat.
- Be aware that dining with others often results in an increase in appetite and in quantity of food consumed.
- As memory plays an important role in the enjoyment of food, the practitioner may find out what foods are associated with special occasions and happy family traditions.
- Sauces and additional flavouring can be used to enhance the taste of foods, e.g., lemon zest or chicken broth.
- Frozen dinners can be convenient and easy for an elderly person to use and help to ensure adequate nutrition.
- Elderly with multiple sensory losses will need to be particularly cautious. For example, someone with vision loss may have a more difficult time identifying spoiled food. Likewise, an elder affected by Alzheimer's will need to have food date-stamped and monitored. Through increased understanding, practitioners can help to enhance the quality of life of individuals experiencing TTS sensory losses. It is important to remember that medical treatment and practical solutions can help alleviate the negative consequences of these losses. Finally, the following suggestions should be considered in working with elders, families, and caregivers.
- Provide a safe and comfortable environment.
- Practitioners should ensure that they have access to warm clothing, extra blankets, and a supportive arm when walking.

- Be aware that for elderly persons who may not readily respond to heat sensations, the use of a microwave oven may be a better alternative than the stove.
- It is important to remember that TTS losses seldom occur in isolation.
- Be cognizant of the effects smoking and medications can have on these senses.
- There is a need to watch for changes in weight, as a weight loss or weight gain may be indicators of loss of taste and smell.
- It may be necessary to provide education for family, friends, and/or caregivers to enhance the quality of life and avoid unsafe situations.
- Consider pre-measuring salt in the case of hypertension, and sugar in the case of diabetes.
- Ensure that the individual has regular appointments with a physician in order to monitor nutrition and weight.
- In addition to the safety implications, the social worker should also consider the need to examine the social and psychological impact of TTS loss. Because they often go undetected and are not treated with the same degree of importance as other sensory losses, social workers may become the primary identifiers of this condition.

III.   Vision Loss

As our population ages, there will be a large demand for services for the elderly blind. It is estimated that 209,495 Canadians will have low vision or blindness by 2016. In 1996, 56.5 percent of Canadians who had severe visual impairment were aged 75 and over. By 2016, 64.8 percent of the total blind population will be aged 75 and older (Robinson, 1999). The baby boomers' impact on the incidence of vision loss has commenced, since onset occurs as they enter their 50s when the first signs of vision loss become apparent.

One out of six elders experience vision loss to the extent that they are not able to read the newspaper, and it is projected that the population aged 65 and older will increase by 100 percent between 1980 and 2020, thus doubling the population potentially in need of specialized services (United States Census Bureau, 1994–1995). There are currently 35,000 legally blind persons in Canada. Almost half of these are over 65 years of age, making the visually impaired the second largest group of disabled people in the United States and Canada. As indicated by Dr. Graham Strong, the four major eye conditions associated with aging are macular degeneration, cataracts, glaucoma, and diabetic retinopathy (U.S. House of Representatives, 1985).

When one thinks of blindness, it is often assumed that it means a total loss of sight. In actual fact, only one in ten legally blind individuals is totally sightless. The degree of residual vision varies from person to person according to his or her eye condition (Goodman, 1985). For example, someone with macular degeneration will have difficulty recognizing faces and reading because the macula, which is responsible for detail vision, has deteriorated. A common regret stated by elderly people with this condition is that they are unable to see their grandchildren's faces. Glaucoma, on the other hand, permits a person to see clearly straight ahead; however, their peripheral vision is limited, resulting in tunnel vision. Two cases illustrate examples of these issues and conditions as follows.

A. A Social Worker's Observation

i) One of the frustrations voiced by an elderly gentleman, with glaucoma, living in rural Canada was that he could still see well enough to build beautiful furniture; however, he would often misplace his tools if he set them down, as they would be out of his limited field of vision.

ii) During a client visit with a 76-year-old woman with diabetic retinopathy, it was discovered that she was not adjusting to her vision loss, and in fact had become increasingly depressed. During a home visit and conversation, she revealed that her difficulty was not so much adjusting to her vision loss but rather to the fact that her vision was not stable. On a good day, she was able to see television fairly well, read a large-print Reader's Digest, and even sew a little. This optimism would then be dashed the following day when a haemorrhage behind the eye would obstruct her vision, leaving her with only light and shadow perception. This may indicate that it is more difficult emotionally to adjust to vision that continually fluctuates.

The Canadian National Institute for the Blind (CNIB) defines a blind person as one whose visual acuity is 20/200 or less, or who has a field restriction of 20 degrees or less with corrective lenses. This definition is problematic because it does not consider functional vision. This in fact creates a bias against elderly persons, and may account for the fact that they are among the "hidden blind" — undercounted and frequently outside of the service network, at least in Canada (Goodman, 1985).

Another problem in formally registering elderly people as blind, and thereby eligible for various services, is that ironically, some ophthalmologists are reluctant to inform elderly patients that they are legally blind. From client anecdotal evidence, this seems to be a common occurrence [more so than one would assume] and perhaps, as some have suggested, it may be that ophthalmologists feel that somehow they have failed if they cannot correct the patient's vision. It has been noted that the younger blind population is more likely to take advantage of related services. This may be a result of motivation, greater mobility, or increased referrals by physicians. There could be a physician bias in that they may feel that the elderly person would not benefit from the services provided to younger people.

Many elderly individuals experience the onset of their visual impairment much later in life, and have not developed the adaptations or accommodations used by younger individuals. This leaves the older person suffering more loss of function in ADL [activities of daily living] due to the visual impairment than might exist for someone with a similar acuity level born with or experiencing earlier onset of the impairment (Tuttle, 1984; Vaughan, 1993).

B. A Social Worker's Observation

The lack of physician reporting was illustrated to me while at work in rehabilitation with the CNIB. The daughter of a 78- year-old gentleman living in a small rural town had contacted the CNIB as she was very concerned about her father's reduced vision and his personal safety. Not only was she worried about him crossing streets and being hit by a car, but she was even more anxious about the fact that he was still driving. I learned that although he had recently been seen by an ophthalmologist, he had no idea that he had less than 10 percent vision and should have relinquished his driver's licence.

As stated earlier, the definition used for legal blindness is inadequate. It measures only field of vision and visual acuity, and ignores other important factors such as balance, sensitivity to light, fluctuations in vision, and/or depth perception (Leslie & Meyers, 1996). This clinical but delimiting definition serves as a general standard, but does not take into account the impact on close range activities of daily living for the elderly.

An analysis done in the U.S. by Kirchner and Lowman (1979) highlighted the discrepancy in the subjective, functional measurement of vision as opposed to the objective, clinical definition based on distance acuity. They found that when using the functional definition,

68 percent of all blind people in the U.S. were elderly, whereas a study based on the clinical definition reported an elderly blind population of only 46 percent (pp. 69–73). The subjective or functional view of vision loss is far more important to social workers, since the focus of intervention is upon assessing the impact of vision loss upon ADL and social functioning. This is particularly true as interventions are geared to developing coping mechanisms in these functional areas.

C. Impact on the Individual

In order to function safely in their own homes, elders with vision loss require support, as they are vulnerable to acquiring other disabilities as a result of falls or injuries. These injuries may result in visually impaired elders being prematurely institutionalized. According to a U.S. House of Representatives report (1985), 85 percent of all injuries to people aged 65 and older are caused by falls, and 25 percent of these are due to visual problems. In the same report, the American Foundation for the Blind estimated that 15 percent of the blind population are in long-term care facilities, as opposed to 1 percent of the general population.

The impact of blindness or vision loss is rarely felt in isolation from the other losses associated with growing older. For instance, when there is less ability to rely upon sight, the loss of hearing becomes more apparent. In the same way, balance and steadiness may be affected as a result of vision loss. Further, some may feel that their safety is threatened while moving around, particularly out of doors, which could lead to a feeling of insecurity (Freedman & Inkster, 1976).

Many older people may also minimize their own vision problems because of the social stigma attached to blindness and the social isolation, which is the typical response to sensory loss. During their lives, many may have perceived the blind to be helpless, docile, and dependent on society. These perceptions may reinforce their own perceptions of devaluation. Some elderly clients actually refer to the image of the blind man with the tin cup selling pencils. In reviewing cases of adults that became blind later in life, F.T. Dover of the New York Jewish Guild for the Blind (1959) found that overall, they experienced feelings of worthlessness, frustration, and anger, generally associated with depression. He noted typical responses to be crying, self-pity, loss of appetite, and inability to sleep. Further, common defences against this undesirable situation included denial and projection (Goodman, 1985). For example, during case visits, some newly blinded elders refused CNIB services such as taped library books, stating that they were waiting to see another ophthalmologist, or for stronger glasses that would enable them to have restored vision. Another form of denial is the "faking sighted syndrome." A number of elderly clients declined the opportunity to carry a white cane because they found it more comfortable to pass as a sighted person. Similarly, others did not want to receive any materials that had CNIB labels on the envelopes for fear that neighbours might learn of their visual impairment. In this regard, this tendency to deny, along with increased vulnerability, anxiety, and lowered self-esteem can intensify the impact of vision loss and reduce efforts to adapt/accommodate to it.

Finally, blind elders often struggle with vision loss, which can seriously affect their quality of life in terms of their sense of enjoyment as a result of loss of pleasure in seeing loved ones, natural beauty, and cherished objects. These perceived losses of personal enjoyment and pleasure can in turn affect their self-esteem, dignity, and body image (Goodman, 1985). Thus, vision loss can have a significant impact on the individual in the physical, social, and emotional realms.

D. Impact on Interpersonal and Family Relationships

Vision loss results in decreased ability to perform ADL, which acts to intensify the overall sense of loss experienced by many elderly. Difficulties in cooking, housekeeping, reading, entertaining, recreational activities, and mobility may lead to emotional and physical withdrawal, which leaves family members and friends feeling excluded and unappreciated. An elderly person experiencing these decreased abilities may feel a lack of self-competence leading to anger and frustration. Unfortunately, these feelings are often expressed by blaming others. Friends and family may find the elder to be irritable or rigid, "blowing up" when objects are moved from familiar locations, or when items are inadvertently misplaced.

Based upon these emotional reactions, as well as past attitudes and beliefs about the blind, the elderly person, family, and friends may come to view the vision loss as tragic. The elderly person may become morose and withdrawn, while family and friends may become overly sensitive. They may change their use of language, avoiding words referring to vision (i.e., see, look, view, etc.), resulting in stilted and uncomfortable conversations. They may cease to talk about activities that the elderly person used to enjoy, or quit inviting them to movies, shopping trips, etc., believing these would be uncomfortable or unenjoyable experiences for the individual. When this oversensitivity is compounded by the elderly person's own confused emotions and inability to express his or her own needs clearly, it can contribute to others making assumptions about the elderly person and becoming patronizing in relationships with them.

As well, sometimes friends, family members, and other support groups can be overly helpful or patronizing to the blind individual in an effort to be protective. There is a tendency to treat elderly persons as though their mental capacities are deteriorating. When combined with vision loss, this problem is compounded. For example, a spouse may become overly protective of the visually impaired partner to the point where they do not want the individual to pour hot liquids, cut bread, or go to the bank independently.

Loss of vision may also result in decreased mobility and independence. Of significant impact to many in this regard is the loss of the ability to drive. This can bring about changes in family roles as the elderly person moves from a transportation provider to a person who requires transportation. Issues of timing, availability, and transportation workload sharing may lead to stress and conflict for family and caregivers, while the elderly person may experience a sense of being a burden on others. A conflict may arise when children or other family members lose confidence in the elderly person's ability to drive before the person is able or willing to acknowledge the difficulty. This can result in direct, hostile confrontations or indirect behaviours like refusing to let grandchildren ride with a grandparent, resulting in hurt feelings and/or mistrust. Similarly, spouses, other family members, and close friends may find the visually impaired elderly person to be jealous or clingy due to the insecurity that can develop in social situations. This is true particularly in social situations that are complicated by the inability to gain reassurance from significant others through eye contact and other visual cues normally used by confidants/intimates in these situations. These issues and feelings can be further exacerbated by the elders' lack of confidence in their ability or their actual competence to maintain their personal appearance.

Overall, the anger, self-doubt, and frustration experienced by these elderly persons, along with the changes in abilities and social competence, not only impact their self-esteem and confidence, but also impact their functioning in close relationships. As stated, family and friends can become overly sensitive and helpful, or even patronizing or controlling.

E. A Social Worker's Observation

"M" lived with her husband in a resort town. She had always led an extremely busy life, working professionally, raising children, maintaining an active social life, and participating as a volunteer in the community. At age 74, she began to notice that her vision was deteriorating. The diagnosis of macular degeneration came as a huge blow to her. In the past, she had been meticulous about her appearance and took a great deal of pride in wearing fashionable clothes, wearing makeup, and having her hair done. As her vision slowly decreased, she became extremely depressed and withdrawn. Her husband encouraged her to continue her bridge games using large print cards, and to play golf using bright yellow golf balls and his assistance for distance. "M" found that her confidence level dropped to the point where she did not want to entertain at home in case she spilt something, and did not want to socialize with friends because she felt too self-conscious. She cried often, and stated that she felt badly because she had a tendency to take out her frustrations on her husband. A simple event like pouring orange juice into a glass could erupt into an explosive situation when she missed the glass. She also felt unattractive and worthless, feeling as if she was no longer able to take care of her husband.

F. Implications for Practice

In 1990, 79 percent of the CNIB's new clients were over 60 years of age. Between 1980 and 1990, the number of elderly persons turning to the CNIB for rehabilitation services increased by 141 percent, with more than 100,000 elderly clients expected in the year 2000. Social workers working with the elderly need to dispel myths [see Chapter 2], and increase public awareness of the problems encountered by the elderly blind overall. Providing an education program for in-service training of human service professionals and public service announcements could increase awareness and recognition of the unique needs of these individuals. There is also a need to have materials made available in large print, Braille, and on tape, and to publicize the ability to access taped books from local libraries. Some low-vision services are being integrated into the community through mobile low-vision vans, which provide optical aides to elderly persons located in more remote areas.

Social workers involved with long-term care facilities or residential facilities can take a leadership role in assuring sensitivity to the needs of this population by promoting awareness, and developing specialized programs and procedures to address these needs. Interventions may include reminding staff to announce themselves orally when entering a room or encountering a blind resident, the initiation of support groups to overcome isolation and promote exchange of information, ensuring that notices of coming events are announced orally, and that a balance between visual and auditory entertainment is maintained. Similarly, practitioners conducting home visits to the elderly should take an active role in carefully examining the residential environment, ensuring that elderly persons can adjust lighting in their living space to accommodate their particular vision needs, through to the strategic location of brightly coloured or raised decals to aid in spatial orientation. In short, they need to be sensitive to this population's quality of life and their ADL.

When working with elderly persons with vision loss, the social work practitioner must bring to bear all the knowledge and skills to understand the individual and his or her adaptation/accommodation to this loss. Each individual will respond differently depending upon the situation, and particularly past experiences, family support, and previous coping strengths/weaknesses. Practitioners should consider the following suggestions:

- A safe approach when dealing with blind elderly persons is to ask how they can best be assisted.
- When guiding a blind person, it is best to let them take your arm and walk just slightly ahead so that they can feel the motion of your body.
- When approaching stairs, tell the person if they are going up or down, and describe the environment when appropriate.
- It is very helpful to identify yourself by name as your voice may not be recognizable.
- Use the same vocabulary that you would with sighted people.
- Do not make assumptions about their disability, as every person is unique and will manage their blindness differently.
- It is sometimes the small things that mean the most to the blind elderly. Placing a tactile marker on their stove so that they can continue to cook independently or providing them with a dark felt pen so that they can read a grocery list are often greatly appreciated.
- Magnifiers are often used to assist individuals in reading a label or picking up a stitch while knitting.
- Whereas some elderly may use computers and other technical devices, in many cases the individual may not feel

that it is worth the trouble to learn about new technology. Nonetheless, social workers should familiarize themselves with both simple and sophisticated aids and adaptive techniques.

- Even when family members are close by, loneliness is often prevalent. Listening to their stories and concerns can be more beneficial than focusing strictly on rehabilitation.
- Be prepared to educate family and friends in order to raise their awareness of and sensitivity to the elder's specific needs in order to avoid misunderstandings and unnecessary conflict.

G. A Social Worker's Observation

A few different case examples illustrate these points in a real world setting:

(i) In my travels across Canada visiting newly registered clients of the CNIB, I was always pleased to be able to provide services and products that would assist elders in their homes and their hobbies. One of the generally favoured services was the library talking book service. I was quite unprepared, therefore, when I arrived at an elderly woman's home where I proceeded to bring out the bright blue tape recorder and audio tapes. I knew that this woman was experiencing great sadness over her vision loss, and her daughter thought that talking books would be a great asset for her. When I arrived at the home, the daughter was seated at the table beside her mother. It became evident that her mother did not want anyone to know that the CNIB had been to see her as she was reluctant to reveal to anyone that her vision was failing.

I assured her that this information would remain confidential, and proceeded to explain the services available to her. When I brought out the recorder and pressed the play button, she burst into tears. Her daughter comforted her, and explained that perhaps it was "too soon" to talk about CNIB services. I quickly returned the recorder to my brief case and agreed that perhaps a chat would be enough for this visit. Thus, the focus of intervention quickly became one of building rapport and trust in order to allow her to slowly become comfortable with discussing her vision loss and ultimately accepting it and developing coping strategies to live with it.

(ii) A 69-year-old woman resided with her 70-year-old husband in a rural home about 3 miles from town. Their ophthalmologist had registered her as blind after rapid deterioration of her vision over the past 12 months. In the discussion that followed, they described a pleasant, simple lifestyle revolving around gardening and walks in the woods. They saw no need for any services or assistance. When I asked how she was managing with cooking and making

tea, she responded that her husband would not let her make tea as it was too dangerous. He was afraid that she might burn herself while pouring boiling water into the pot. I described how one could place the teapot in the sink so that if any water missed the pot, it would run into the sink. However, it seemed that the desire was not there to learn even simple tasks.

In this case situation, it became clear that she was accommodating to her vision loss by relying upon her husband to perform responsibilities that had previously been hers. I established a close and friendly relationship with this couple over time, but they continued to refuse any rehabilitative services. They openly talked about anxiety should anything happen to her husband, but felt that for now his change in role and even his overprotectiveness only served to bring them closer together. A key issue for intervention focused upon respecting their right to self-determination, ensuring that it was an informed decision, and holding my own values and concerns in check.

(iii) Finally, I recall a wonderful character who had been blind for about eight years and was in his seventies. His daughter and son-in-law lived upstairs and invited him often for meals. He enjoyed his privacy, and used to laugh when he would have a domestic mishap. I recall the day he called me laughing heartily as he had eaten instant potatoes with milk for breakfast instead of cornflakes. He took up blind golfing and cross-country skiing, and never missed a social dance. His wife had passed away, and he became, as he referred to himself, "a grumpy old man." He became a strong advocate for the rights and services for the elderly blind and provided a great deal of enjoyment to those who knew him.

His situation provided another view of adaptation and accommodation to vision loss. Despite his strong sense of advocacy for the elderly blind and his involvement in consumer groups, he used very few rehabilitation services himself. He certainly accessed recreational programs, but preferred to develop his own adaptations for orientation, mobility, and ADL.

In sum, as can be seen from the above case situations, the range of coping styles with vision loss is quite varied. It is also clear that specific rehabilitation or training for ADL may be helpful, but may not be the paramount area of need. As in most effective practice, the key issue is understanding the meaning of the sensory loss in the context of the person-in-environment. However, in order to achieve this understanding, the practitioner must have knowledge about the nature of sensory losses and their various impacts.

References

Agnew, J. (1986). Tinnitus: An overview. *Volta Review, 88*, 215–221.

Alberti, P.W. (1987). Tinnitus in occupational hearing loss: Sociological aspects. *The Journal of Otolaryngology,* 16, 34–35.

Bienenfeld, D. & Stein, L.M. (1992). Hearing impairment and its impact on elderly patients with cognitive, behavioral, or psychiatric disorders: A literature review. *Journal of Geriatric Psychiatry,* 25, 145–156.

Birren, J.E. & Schaie, K.W. (1985). *Handbook of the psychology of aging,* 2nd ed. New York: Van Nostrand Reinhold Company.

Brinson, W.S. (1983). *Speechreading in practice.* In W.J. Watts (ed.), *Rehabilitation and acquired deafness,* pp. 205–218. London: Croom Helm.

Butler, R.N. & Lewis, M.L. (1977). *Aging and mental health.* St. Louis: C.V. Mosby.

Calvert, D.R. & Silverman, R.S. (1978). *Conversation and development of speech.* In H. Davis & S.R. Silverman (eds.), *Hearing and deafness,* pp. 388–399. New York: Holt, Rinehart, & Winston.

Carlsson, S.G., Erlandsson, S.I., & Hallberg, L.R. (1992). Coping strategies used by middle-aged males with noise-induced hearing loss, with and without tinnitus. *Psychology and Health,* 7, 273–288.

Christensen, J.M., Hutchinson, J.M., Nerbonne, M.A., & Schow, R.L. (1978). *Communication disorders of the aged: A guide for health professionals.* Baltimore: University Park Press.

Cox, B.P. & McFarland, W. (1985). *Aging and hearing loss: Some commonly asked questions.* Washington: Gallaudet College/National Information Center on Deafness.

David, M. & Trehub, S.E. (1989). Perspective on deafened adults. *American Annals of the Deaf,* 133, 200–204.

Delk, M.T. & Schein, J.D. (1974). *The deaf population of the United States.* Silver Spring: National Association of the Deaf.

DiPietro, L. & Wax, T. (1984). *Managing hearing loss in later life.* National Information Center on Deafness, Gallaudet College.

Doty, R.L. (1997). Studies of human olfaction from the University of Pennsylvania Smell and Taste Center. *Chem Senses,* 22, 565–586.

Dover, Francis T. (1959). Readjusting to the Onset of Blindness. *Social Casework,* 40, 334–338.

Freedman, S.S. & Inkster, D.E. (1976). *The impact of blindness in the aging process.* New York: Center for Independent Living, New York Infirmary.

Gant, N.D. & Kampfe, C.M. (1997). The social and psychological challenges faced by persons with Meniere's Disease. *Journal of Applied Rehabilitation Counseling,* 28(4), 40–49.

Gillyatt, P. (1997). Loss of smell: When the nose doesn't know. *Harvard Health Letter,* 22(2), 6.

Goodman, H. (1985). *Serving the elderly blind: A generic approach.* New York: Haworth.

Granick, S., Kleban, M.H., & Weiss, A.D. (1976). Relationships between hearing loss and cognition in normally hearing aged persons. *Journal of Gerontology*, 31, 434–440.

Hallberg, L.R. & Erlandsson, S.I. (1993). Tinnitus characteristics in tinnitus complainers and noncomplainers. *British Journal of Audiology*, 27, 19–27.

Hausman, C. & Rezen, S.V. (1985). *Coping with hearing loss: A guide for adults and their families.* New York: Dembner Books.

Hazen, S. E., Hoot-Martin, J.L., & Larsen, P.D. (1997). Assessment and management of sensory loss in elderly patients. *Association of Operating Room Nurses Journal*, 65(2), 432–436.

Hull, R.H. (1977). *Hearing impairment among the elderly.* Lincoln: Cliffs Notes.

Kampfe, C.M. (1990). Communicating with persons who are deaf: Some practical suggestions for rehabilitation specialists. *Journal of Rehabilitation*, 56, 41–45.

Kampfe, C.M. (1994). Vocational rehabilitation and the older population. *The Southwest Journal on Aging*, 9, 65–69.

Kampfe, C.M. & Smith, S.M. (1997). Interpersonal relationship implications of hearing loss in persons who are older. *The Journal of Rehabilitation*, 63(2), 15.

Kampfe, C.M. & Smith, S.M. (1998). Intrapersonal aspects of hearing loss in persons who are older. *The Journal of Rehabilitation*, 64(2), 24.

Kirchner, C. & Lowman, C. (1979). Statistical briefs: Elderly blind and visually impaired person: Projected numbers in the year 2000. *Journal of Visual Impairment and Blindness*, 73, 69–73.

Leslie, D.R. & Meyers, L.L. (1996). In D.F. Harrison, B.A. Thyer, & J.S. Wodarski (eds.), *Cultural diversity and social work practice*, 2nd ed., pp. 201–231. Springfield: Charles C. Thomas.

Luey, H.S. (1980). Between worlds: The problems of deafened adults. *Social Work in Health Care*, 5, 253–265.

National Center for Health Statistics. (1990). *Current estimates from the National Health Interview Survey, 1987.* Washington: Current Vital Health Statistics Series 10, No. 176.

Orlans, H. (1987). Sociable and solitary responses to adult hearing loss. In J.G. Kyle (ed.), *Adjustment to acquired hearing loss: Analysis, change and learning: Proceedings of a conference held in University of Bristol*, pp. 95–112. Bristol: Center for Deaf Studies, University of Bristol.

Oyer, E.J. & Oyer, H.J. (1985). Adult hearing loss and the family. In H. Orland (ed.), *Adjustment to adult hearing loss*, pp.139–154. San Diego: College-Hill Press.

Rakel, R. (1994). *Conn's current therapy.* Philadelphia: W.V. Saunders.

Ramsdell, D.A. (1978). The psychology of the hard-of-hearing and deafened adult. In H. Davis & S.R. Silverman (eds.), *Hearing and deafness*, 4th ed., pp. 499–510. New York: Holt, Rinehart & Winston.

Robinson, B.E. (1999, June). *National consultation on the crisis in vision loss: Conference proceedings.* Prepared by Canadian National Institute for the Blind, pp. 9–12.

Rutherford, M. (1999). Turbo charge your taste: When flavor falls flat, the problem may lie not in the food but in a waning ability to taste and smell. *Time*, 153(22), 84.

Schiffman, S.S. (1997). Taste and smell losses in normal aging and disease. *The Journal of the American Medical Association*, 278(16), 13–57.

Smith, S.M. (1986). Rehabilitation, aging and employment: Perspectives for the rehabilitation counselor and employer—An action paper. Rehabilitation and Aging (Mary Switzer Monograph No. 11). Washington: National Rehabilitation Association.

Thomas, A. (1984). *Acquired hearing loss: Psychological and psychosocial implications.* London: Academic Press.

Tuttle, D.W. (1984). *Self-esteem and adjusting with blindness: The process of responding to life's demands.* Springfield: Charles C. Thomas.

United States Census Bureau. (1994–1995). *Table 6, Americans with Disabilities: 1994–95.*

U.S. Department of Health and Human Services. (1991). *Aging America: Trends and projections*, 1991 ed., no. FCoA 91-28001. Washington: U.S. Department of Health and Human Services.

U.S. House of Representatives (1985, April). *Blindness and the elderly.* Select Committee on Aging, pp. 5–6.

Vaughan, C.E. (1993). *The struggle of blind people for self-determination: The dependency rehabilitation conflict, empowerment in the blindness community.* Springfield: Charles C. Thomas.

Williams, P.S. (1984). *Hearing loss: Information for professionals in the aging network.* National Information Center on Deafness, Gallaudet College.

Wright, B. (1983). *Physical disability: A psychosocial approach*, 2nd ed. New York: Harper & Row.

Internet Resources

Canadian National Institute for the Blind: Living with Vision Loss
A resource guide for caregivers of the blind.
http://www.cnib.ca/livingwithvisionloss/index.htm

Capital Health—Seniors Health
     http://www.capitalhealth.ca/Health+Services/Health+Topics/
     Demographic+Groups/Seniors+Health/default.htm
Extendicare Consumer Information
     http://www.extendicare.com/consumer/article37.htm

Additional Readings

Doty, R.L. (1997). Studies of human olfaction from the University of
     Pennsylvania Smell and Taste Centre. *Chem Senses,* 22, 565–586.
Kampfe, C.M. & Smith, S.M. (1998). Intrapersonal aspects of hearing loss in
     persons who are older. *The Journal of Rehabilitation,* 64(2), 24.
Kolker, D. (2002). Coping with and adapting to age-related vision loss.
     Canadian Social Work Journal, 4(1), 67–84.
Luey, H. (1994). Sensory loss: A neglected issue in social work. *Journal of
     Gerontological Social Work,* 21(3/4), 213–223.
Nation Advisory Council of Aging. (1990). *Living with sensory loss,* cat. no.
     H71-2/1-8-1990E. Ottawa: Minister of Supply & Services Canada.

CHAPTER 10

ABUSE AND NEGLECT OF THE ELDERLY PERSON

JACQUELINE F.L. BOBYK-KRUMINS

AND MICHAEL J. HOLOSKO

The phenomenon of elderly abuse has only recently surfaced as an area of concern for social workers and clinicians alike. This chapter offers an overview of this troublesome issue, which has cast a shadow on the lives of some of our older citizens in North America. In particular, the nature of abuse, characteristics of the abused and the abuser, etiology, and implications for practice are discussed.

I.   Introduction

This chapter synthesizes existing literature in order to provide an understanding of the growing problem related to the recognition and treatment of elderly abuse in North America. It has two objectives: (1) to identify the nature of abuse, and (2) to present the implications for social work practitioners by offering a model for intervention.

A.   *The Nature of Elderly Abuse*

Prior to defining elderly abuse, it is imperative to first understand its prevalence. Pillemer and Finkelhor (1988) are among the pioneers who systematically studied elderly abuse in North America. Their landmark study in the greater Boston area in 1985–86, designed to determine the level of physical and verbal abuse and neglect experienced in the elderly population, found that 3.2 percent of their sample ($N = 2020$)

had been maltreated. A subsequent and comparably designed study in Canada with 2,000 seniors reported a similar abuse rate of 4.0 percent (Podnieks, 1989).

Recently, a landmark study conducted by the National Center on Elder Abuse in Washington, D.C., released some startling and much needed current information on the prevalence of elderly abuse and neglect. The National Elder Abuse Incidence Study (NEAIS) is the first attempt to establish a national baseline for research purposes, and its results confirm what researchers have been trying to impart for years. In short, elderly abuse in America is largely hidden and underreported. Specifically, their findings indicated that "approximately 450,000 elderly persons in domestic settings were abused and/or neglected during 1996" (National Center for Elder Abuse at the American Public Human Services Association in Collaboration with Westat Inc., 1998, p. 1). Of these cases, a mere 70,942 (16 percent) were reported to state Adult Protective Services (APS). Further, community workers (e.g., volunteers, home care aides, etc.) uncovered the balance of cases (378,982). This study also revealed that: (i) females were abused more frequently than males, and (ii) those 80 years and older were abused at least twice as often as their younger counterparts aged 65+ (National Center for Elder Abuse at the American Public Human Services Association in Collaboration with Westat Inc., 1998).

1. Defining Elderly Abuse

Defining elderly abuse has been a challenge for both researchers and clinicians for a number of years. For instance, Wolf (1988) stressed "from the very beginning of the scientific investigation into the nature and causes of elderly abuse, definitions have been a major issue" (p. 758). A major roadblock to establishing a universal definition has been that investigators have approached elderly abuse from different perspectives—that of the victim, the caregiver, the physician, the nurse, the agency, the social worker, the social policy—and as a result, there has been a lack of clarity and consensus across these domains (Decalmer & Glendenning, 1997).

For the purpose of this chapter, *domestic elderly abuse* is defined as "any of several forms of maltreatment of an older person by someone who has a special relationship with the elder" (e.g., spouse, a sibling, a child, a friend, or a caregiver in the older person's home or in the home of a caregiver) (National Center on Elder Abuse, 1999, p. 1). *Institutional abuse* takes into consideration the above definition with the exception of the locale of abusive events (e.g., nursing homes, daycare centres, group homes, etc.). *Self-neglect* refers to those cases where elderly either deliberately or unknowingly fail to provide for their own basic needs.

Within each type of abuse, researchers have identified several characteristics and degrees of harm. As Figure 10.1 illustrates, currently there are five general areas of investigation (Aitken & Griffin, 1996; Eastman, 1994; McDonald et al., 1991; Mulley, Penn, & Burns, 1998; Ontario Association of Professional Social Workers (OAPSW), 1992; Podnieks, 1989; Quinn & Tomita, 1997; Reis & Nahmaish, 1995; Wolf & Pillemer, 1986; Wolf & Pillemer, 1989).

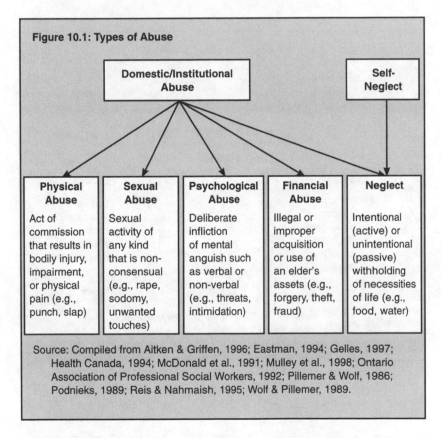

Figure 10.1: Types of Abuse

Physical Abuse	Sexual Abuse	Psychological Abuse	Financial Abuse	Neglect
Act of commission that results in bodily injury, impairment, or physical pain (e.g., punch, slap)	Sexual activity of any kind that is non-consensual (e.g., rape, sodomy, unwanted touches)	Deliberate infliction of mental anguish such as verbal or non-verbal (e.g., threats, intimidation)	Illegal or improper acquisition or use of an elder's assets (e.g., forgery, theft, fraud)	Intentional (active) or unintentional (passive) withholding of necessities of life (e.g., food, water)

Source: Compiled from Aitken & Griffen, 1996; Eastman, 1994; Gelles, 1997; Health Canada, 1994; McDonald et al., 1991; Mulley et al., 1998; Ontario Association of Professional Social Workers, 1992; Pillemer & Wolf, 1986; Podnieks, 1989; Reis & Nahmaish, 1995; Wolf & Pillemer, 1989.

2. Detecting Abuse

Signs of abuse are not always visible. Whereas a black eye, for instance, is likely to generate specific questions, a practitioner who comes into contact with an unresponsive elderly person may consider a number of other factors before abuse is even suspected. In light of the persistent ageist attitudes present in North American society, agitation and unexplained fears, for example, may even be interpreted as part of the aging process or as a sign of dementia.

As with other forms of abuse (child and spousal) and with mandatory reporting laws, service professionals are obliged to respond in those cases where there is tangible evidence (Duffy & Momirov, 1997). However, emotional and financial abuse, for example, are more covert, less obvious types of abuse that can exist for long periods of time before

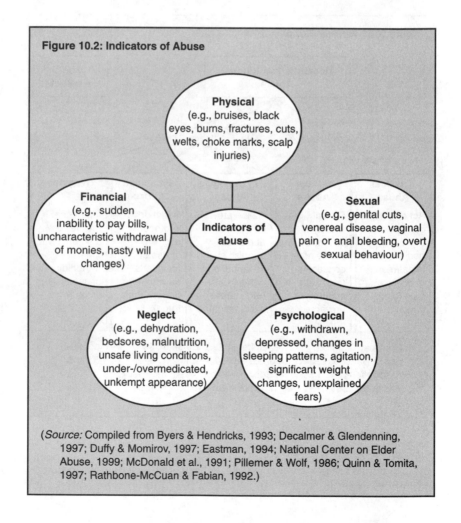

Figure 10.2: Indicators of Abuse

Physical
(e.g., bruises, black eyes, burns, fractures, cuts, welts, choke marks, scalp injuries)

Financial
(e.g., sudden inability to pay bills, uncharacteristic withdrawal of monies, hasty will changes)

Indicators of abuse

Sexual
(e.g., genital cuts, venereal disease, vaginal pain or anal bleeding, overt sexual behaviour)

Neglect
(e.g., dehydration, bedsores, malnutrition, unsafe living conditions, under-/overmedicated, unkempt appearance)

Psychological
(e.g., withdrawn, depressed, changes in sleeping patterns, agitation, significant weight changes, unexplained fears)

(*Source:* Compiled from Byers & Hendricks, 1993; Decalmer & Glendenning, 1997; Duffy & Momirov, 1997; Eastman, 1994; National Center on Elder Abuse, 1999; McDonald et al., 1991; Pillemer & Wolf, 1986; Quinn & Tomita, 1997; Rathbone-McCuan & Fabian, 1992.)

being ascertained. In fact, a significant amount of abuse perpetrated against the elderly requires the professional to look beyond initial presenting problems. Recognizing the indicators of abuse, therefore, is critical.

3. Characteristics of Victims and Abusers

There is always a delimiting tendency when trying to generalize or classify groups of people into discrete categories. Albeit, there is evidence of certain abuse trends; some see the nature of the relationship between the victim and the abuser as "the most telling" in terms of risk for abuse. For the most part, it appears that characteristics of both the abused and the abuser vary with each type of abuse, and it is important to recognize the inherent risk associated with rendering premature assumptions.

Research on the characteristics of victims and perpetrators has been collected for at least twenty years and certain patterns have begun to emerge (Aitken & Griffin, 1996; Beaulieu & Tremblay, 1994; Eastman, 1994; Johnson, 1991; McDonald et al., 1991; Ontario Association of Professional Social Workers, 1992; Podnieks, 1989; Shell, 1982; Wolf et al., 1986; Wolf et al., 1989). (See Table 10.1 for a compilation of studies and their significant findings).

Overall, abuse is more often meted out to the "old-old" (Bristowe & Collins, 1989; Eastman, 1994; McDonald et al., 1991; National Center on Elder Abuse, 1999; National Center for Elder Abuse at the American Public Human Services Association in Collaboration with Westat Inc., 1998; Shell, 1982; Wolf & Pillemer, 1989) and research to date indicates that 68–75 percent of physical, psychological, and financial incidents involve female victims (Lau & Kosberg, 1979; National Center on Elder Abuse, 1999; National Center for Elder Abuse at the American Public Human Services Association in Collaboration with Westat Inc., 1998; Ontario Association of Professional Social Workers, 1992; Penhale, 1992; Podnieks, 1989; Shell, 1982). Pillemer and Finkelhor (1988), however, have cautioned the latter claim, noting that gender is not always a predetermining factor and cite their findings of 52 percent male victims and 48 percent female victims to support their position. Further, Pillemer and Finkelhor (1988) suggested that if the ratio of elderly men to women in the general population were factored into the equation, males rather than females would be found to be at a higher risk in general (McDonald et al., 1991).

Evidence to support a familial relationship between the abuser and abused also exists. For example, Pillemer and Finkelhor (1988)

**Table 10.1: Selected Findings from Research on Elderly Abuse: Victim/
Perpetrator Statistics**

	Research Technique	Victim Statistics	Perpetrator Statistics
Lau & Kosberg (1979)	12 month review of client case records (N = 404)	- 77% female - 54% widowed - 75% at least one physical or mental impairment	- 82% of abusers related to abused
Block & Sinnott (1979)	Mailed questionnaires and analysis of agency records (N = 443)	- 81% female - 76% lived with relatives - 96% physically or mentally impaired	- 53% between 40–60 years of age - 56% female - 80% related to abused and under stress
Wolf et al. (1982)	Mailed questionnaires to human service agencies	- 70+ female - mental/physical disability - lived with and/or dependent on abuser	- male relative under 60 years of age - history of mental illness, alcohol/drug abuse
Gioglio & Blakemore (1983)	Questionnaires administered to elderly (N = 342)	- 70% female - 56% 75 or more years of age - 87% in poor health - 35% living with abuser - 70% of financially abused not living with abuser	- 72% males between ages of 16–69 - 61% part of immediate family
Giordano & Giordano (1984)	Review of cases reported to Adult Services in six Florida counties between January 1976 and January 1982 (N = 650)	**Physical/ psychological:** - 66–83 years of age - white, female, low income **Neglect:** - 72–89 years of age - white, female, low income, lives with buser **Financial:** - 72–89 years of age - white, widower with low income	**Physical/ Psychological:** - primarily white, married, low income **Neglect:** - primarily white male or female **Financial:** - primarily white male or female

con't

Table 10.1: (continued)

	Research Technique	Victim Statistics	Perpetrator Statistics
Podnieks (1989)	Telephone survey(*N* = 2,000)	- more female victims - isolation, limited activity - few supports - health issues	- middle aged/elderly - mental illness - drug/alcohol dependency - financial dependence - more often spouse or a child
Wolf & Pillemer (1989)	*Three Model Project* Assessment of cases of abuse and neglect seen in the Model Projects (*N* = 328)	**Physical/ Psychological:** - independent - poor emotional health - social network intact **Financial:** - single - money problems - loss of support systems **Neglect:** - difficulty with ADLs - decline in mental health - little or no social contact	**Physical/ Psychological:** - lived with victim - history of mental illness - dependency apparent **Financial:** - lives away from victim - alcohol abuse - financially dependent - no other supports **Neglect:** - older females - no history of mental illness/ independent - victim is source of stress
Pillemer & Bachman-Prehn (1991)	Questionnaires administered to nurses and nursing home aides (*N* = 577)	- 36% physically abused in preceding year (restraint highest at 6%) - 81% psychologically abused in preceding year (yelling highest at 70%)	- 10% of nurses/ aides questioned admitted to one or more physically abusive acts - 40% admitted to one or more psychologically abusive acts

con't

Table 10.1: (continued)

	Research Technique	Victim Statistics	Perpetrator Statistics
Administration on Aging: NEAIS (1998)	Data collected from Adult Protective Service agencies and community workers in 20 counties of 15 American states	- 48.7% 80+ years - highest rates among elderly with $9,999 or less annual income - disproportionate number of abused women - 47.9% unable to care for self - 59.5% of abused; somewhat confused	- 52.5% males - 52.4% of neglect perpetrated by women - 60.1% of physical and emotional abuse by males - 65.8% of abusers under 60 years of age - 47.3% adult children - 19.3% spouses - 4% unrelated caregivers - 44.7% self-neglect seen in 80+ females - 44.7% self-neglect in females
Statistics Canada (2000)	Survey of elderly homeowners ($N = 4,324$)	- 1% physical, sexual, or financial abuse - 7% emotional abuse - 9% males reported emotional or financial abuse - 9% of financially abused in rural areas	- spouse most likely implicated in emotional or financial abuse - 43% adult children implicated in physical abuse and 28% spouses - 28% spouses implicated in physical abuse

References for Table 10.1

Kosberg, J. (ed.). (1983). *Abuse and maltreatment of the elderly: Causes and intervention.* Littleton: John Wright, PSG Ltd.

McDonald, P.L., Hornick, J.P., Robertson, G.B., & Wallace, J.E. (1991). *Elder abuse and neglect in Canada.* Toronto: Butterworths Canada, Ltd.

National Center on Elder Abuse at the American Public Human Services Association. (1998). *The National Elder Abuse Incidence Study: Final report September 1998.* Washington: National Center on Elder Abuse at the

American Public Human Services Association.

Podnieks, E. (1989). *National survey on abuse of the elderly in Canada: Preliminary findings.* Toronto: Office of Research and Innovation, Ryerson Polytechnical Institute.

Statistics Canada. (2000). *Family violence in Canada: A statistical profile 2000.* Ottawa: Ministry of Industry for the Canadian Centre for Justice Statistics.

Wolf, R. & Pillemer, K. (1989). *Helping elderly victims: The reality of elder abuse.* New York: Columbia University Press.

reported 65 percent of spouses and 25 percent of adult children as the abuser. Similarly, Shell (1982) found 23.6 percent of offenders to be sons, 21 percent daughters, and 16.4 percent husbands. Furthermore, the NEAIS (1998) reported, "in almost 90 percent of the elder abuse and neglect incidents with a known perpetrator, the perpetrator is a family member, and two-thirds of the perpetrators are adult children or spouses" (p. 1).

Many abusers appear to have characteristics indicative of mental illness, deviant behaviour, cognitive impairments, physical disabilities, and sociopathic tendencies (Busby, 1996; Podnieks, 1990). Lau and Kosberg (1979) described abusers as "non-normal adult child(ren) who (are) mentally ill, retarded or alcoholic" (McDonald et al., 1991, p. 30). Similarly, Wolf, Godkin, and Pillemer (1984) found 31 percent of abusive caregivers suffered from a psychiatric illness and 43 percent from substance abuse. Alcohol in particular is consistently reiterated [in the literature] as a contributing factor to abuse (Busby, 1996; Bristowe & Collins, 1989; Lau & Kosberg, 1979; Shell, 1982). Some abusive caregivers have even attempted to absolve themselves of responsibility for their violent behaviour by suggesting that alcohol was to blame, similar to claims made in other forms of familial abuse (spousal and child).

When examining self-neglecting elderly persons, Rathbone-McCuan and Fabian (1991) cited mental impairment, interpersonal difficulties, and inability to access or lack of information on resources. In fact, isolation (particularly geographical) is a significant factor in all types of abuse. NEAIS (1998) supported these findings reporting depression, confusion, or extreme frailty as contributing factors in self-neglect. For these individuals, expressing needs may be difficult because of a fear of institutionalization or being labelled burdensome to others (Rathbone-McCuan et al., 1991). Drug and/or alcohol abuse have also been found to play a role in self-neglect where managing self-care is even more cumbersome (MacLean, 2000).

While it is true that awareness of the living conditions and resources available to the elderly in institutional settings has increased, there is little documentation in terms of maltreatment of the elderly themselves (Pillemer & Bachman-Prehn, 1991). In one of the few research efforts available, McDonald and Collins (2000) discovered that at least one third (32–37 percent) of nurses and nursing assistants had witnessed one incident of physical or verbal abuse, primarily perpetrated in the hospital (86 percent). With recent restraints imposed on the health care system in Canada, it would be logical to postulate that as noted with caregivers, professionals too are having difficulty coping with an increased responsibility and lack of resources. An American study provided comparable statistics for physical abuse in a nursing home setting (36 percent), but strikingly higher numbers for verbal abuse (81 percent) (Pillemer & Bachman-Prehn, 1991).

4. Causal Factors
A review of empirical and theoretical research indicated that in addition to the characteristics noted above, there are other factors relevant to the understanding of elderly abuse. These are intergenerational violence, dependency, negative attitudes toward the aged, social isolation, and caregiver stress.

(a) Intergenerational Transmission of Violence
Based on social learning theory, the transmission of violence from one generation to the next suggests that as children, abusive caregivers themselves were victims of violence. When the question has been asked, some abusers do report experiencing violence in their childhood. Quinn and Tomita (1997), for example, reported that 25 percent of adult children identified as abusers had been abused themselves in childhood. Gelles and Strauss (1989) estimated 30 percent of confirmed cases to be associated with transgenerational violence. Despite such evidence, many researchers continue to debate the validity of this particularly since very few studies have provided evidence to support this contention (Busby, 1996; Eastman, 1994; Gelles, 1997; McDonald et al., 1991; Quinn & Tomita, 1997; Wolf & Pillemer, 1989). In addition, when examining these data, the inclusion of ad hoc data as a measure of discovery appears highly dependent on the direction of the research being undertaken (Quinn & Tomita, 1997). Further, some researchers have found little or no evidence to support intergenerational violence as a factor in elderly abuse (McDonald & Collins, 2000; Pillemer and Finkelhor, 1988).

Nevertheless, the possibility that survivors of childhood abuse retaliate against their elderly parents is worthy of mention, particularly since tension between parents and children can sometimes last a lifetime (Kosberg, 1983). At minimum, when addressing caregiver needs in intervention, there is real benefit to exploring historical relationships between family members.

(b) Dependence

Early research initiatives have focused on the dependency between the elderly person and the caregiver (Block & Sinnott, 1979; McDonald et al., 1991; Quinn & Tomita, 1997). Specifically, physical and mental impairments seen in some cases suggested that these victims were more vulnerable to abuse based on their dependence with activities for daily living (ADLs). More recent research, however, while noting the dependence of older, frail elderly, has revealed that the abusers themselves are equally or even more reliant on the victim for support with their own ADLs. In short, dependency is a two-way street. For example, Podnieks (1989) found that perpetrators who abused drugs or alcohol and/or were experiencing financial hardship relied heavily on their victim for support. This was particularly evident when the abuser was an adult child (Decalmer & Glendinning, 1997; McDonald et al., 1991; Ross 1991; Wolf & Pillemer, 1989).

(c) Attitudes toward Aging

Ageism and discrimination of the elderly based solely on age is commonplace in North American society [see Chapter 2 of this text]. Isolated by ageist labels such as "frail," "senile," "demented," "ornery," and "wrinkled," many elderly persons struggle to maintain their independent status in a society that associates negative connotations with their very being. Further, the implication of categorizing and marginalizing this segment of the population is noted in the pervasive assumption that the elderly are not competent enough to manage their own care (Duffy & Momirov, 1997; Hampton, 1999) and relinquishing independence necessarily predisposes some elderly to abusive treatment.

A general fear of aging also prevails in North America and strong societal beliefs about independence and self-determination make it "difficult to know how to act in the presence of an elderly individual who is impaired" (Quinn & Tomita, 1997, p. 9). Infantalizing is a common response that is dehumanizing and perpetuates the notion that like children, these adults are not capable of making decisions that protect their interests.

(d) Caregiver Stress
Growing old today in North America is different from what it was 30 years ago. Medical advances have increased the life span and as a result, many of our elderly are living longer and with "deteriorating physical conditions" (Kosberg, 1983, p. 135). *Generational inversion* is becoming a more common phenomenon with adult children now caring for their parents and doing so well into their own middle years.

In situations where the elderly parent requires a high level of care, the potential for stress can be severe. If indeed caregivers are older and dealing with their own failing health, the level of stress is exacerbated. In addition, the struggle for power and control between an elderly person and caregiver poses additional stress. Having to relinquish power is difficult and having to take on unwanted tasks can stir up feelings of resentment. Decision making and problem solving may become increasingly difficult and over time, feelings of love and respect may deteriorate into feelings of hate and/or guilt. Unresolved familial issues may rear and the overall quality of care may be adversely affected.

Although institutional care may be an attractive alternative, for some the cost is prohibitive. Even if cost is not a factor, both the elderly and the caregiver may not consider this a viable option. The former may see this as a means of further restraint and the latter may be more concerned about the financial implications (particularly if he/she is financially dependent on the elderly person).

(e) Social Isolation
Social isolation in old age has been recognized as an issue for some time. In 1984, results from the *Three Model Project* [in the U.S.A.] revealed that one in five had no contact other than with the perpetrator (Wolf et al., 1984). Today, elderly persons are even more likely to live alone and with a greater number of physical impairments, thus intensifying the isolation from others (Kosberg, 1983).

The frail old are at significant risk. Given their decreased mobility, they may fade into the woodwork of their homes, depending on others to bring them what they need to survive. If bedridden, their isolation is complete (Quinn & Tomita, 1997).

For caregivers, the demands of care can also have negative consequences. As an elderly person's condition deteriorates and the level of commitment for care increases, the demands on the caregiver may mean more isolation from their own social contacts (Olshevski et al., 1999). For both the elderly person and the caregiver, these conditions are ripe for elevated frustration and tension. And in some cases, this may lead to abuse.

II.   Social Work Implications

Ending violence against our elderly citizens requires a multi-level commitment that takes into consideration measures for crisis intervention, prevention, education, community awareness, and advocacy. This segment of the chapter begins by highlighting assessment concerns. It follows with an examination of the micro-level aspects of an existing model for intervention and ends with a brief look at strategies for macro-level care.

A. Assessment

Referrals for assessment of the elderly may originate from a number of sources. In the case of physical abuse, for example, an emergency physician may be the professional who first discovers the evidence. In non-emergency situations, a number of sources are implicated. Members of the clergy, family, friends, neighbours, or home care workers may generate a referral, for example, based on their own observations or suspicions.

Social workers who are recipients of such referrals are encouraged to elicit as much information as possible from the initial source prior to making direct contact with the elderly person (Quinn & Tomita, 1997). In some cases these formal and/or informal contacts have had lengthy relationships with the older person and may be more willing to address their suspicions with a professional than with the elderly person themselves. In this way, their relationship is preserved and the risk of alienation is lowered (Hargrave & Hanna, 1997). The benefit for the social worker in this situation is that with prior information, the initial visit can be timely, taking into consideration the identification of the suspected abuser, the need for a safe meeting location, and the demeanour of the potential client.

1. The Elderly
Given the nature of elderly abuse and neglect, it is evident that service providers and practitioners have a number of factors to consider. While it is anticipated that a social worker who engages with an elderly client will explore suspicions of abuse and neglect, violence is never an easy

subject to broach. Sensitivity and respect are paramount and the worker should exercise good measures of tact and diplomacy.

Consider intergenerational violence, for example. Violence may be a fact of life for this client, having been exposed to it for a number of years (Tindale et al., 1994). Denial may present as a significant barrier to recognition of maltreatment. The embarrassment, secrecy, and guilt often associated with abuse (especially when a family member is implicated) compound a client's reluctance to face the reality of the situation.

Further, the worker should be aware of the dynamics in any relationship based on unequal power and control. As witnessed in cases of spousal abuse, some perpetrators exert tremendous power and control to the point where the life of the victim is in jeopardy (Busch & Valentine, 2000; Steinmetz & Straus, 1974; Walker, 1979). Minimizing abuse is common and the client may exert tremendous energy into trying to convince outsiders that "everything is fine." The threat of escalating violence further perpetuates helplessness and the need to always be on guard (Doyle, 1997). Recognizing that safety is of primary concern, the worker must be sensitive to the self-preservation techniques employed by the client when confronting incongruences.

Resistance is common in many cases in the initial stages of contact and among the elderly, this resistance carries with it many years of life experience, coping strategies, and valued independence. As indicated in Chapter 1 of this text, this may be their first formal contact with a social worker, and his/her presence at this stage in life may be a source of confusion and frustration. In fact, any gesture may be viewed as an attempt to undermine autonomy and freedom. To gain the confidence of the elderly client, the practitioner must take deliberate steps to ensure that the rights of the elderly to make choices are protected.

To reduce fear, one goal of the first contact should be to develop a professional, trusting, and friendly relationship (Quinn & Tomita, 1997) and unlike other assessments, those conducted with the elderly may take several visits before enough information is secured to make an evaluation of need. Engaging the assistance of other health care professionals is also highly recommended to address other areas of concern, including medical and mobility issues that could impact an intervention strategy (Blakely et al., 1993; Eastman, 1994; Emlet, et al., 1995; Harelet al., 1990; Johnson, 1991; Mulley et al., 1998; Rathbone-McCuan et al., 1991; Reis & Nahmaish, 1995).

2. The Suspected Abuser

Recognizing that intervention ought to result in as little disruption to the life of the elderly as possible means realizing that in cases where familial members are suspected of abuse, the bond they share is, despite its apparent dysfunctional nature, stronger than any relationship with a professional will ever be. Successful intervention in these cases may hinge upon the practitioner's ability to develop a plan that addresses both the victim and the abuser's issues.

An interview with the suspected abuser should focus on his/her perception of the victim's dependencies as well as their own (i.e., alcohol, drugs, financial). In addition, the abuser's version [or recollection] of events can be compared to the victim's report of details. Further, problem-solving abilities and the degree of isolation experienced by the caregiver (i.e., resource availability, relief, social interaction, etc.) require attention (McDonald et al., 1991; Quinn & Tomita, 1997; Weiner, 1991).

The perceived level of cooperation from the elderly client can also adversely affect the relationship. The caregiver (who may have been thrust into a caretaking role) may be faced with what appears as an uncooperative, ungrateful "patient." The older person, on the other hand, may resent being a "patient" and refuse to comply. The anxiety and fear experienced by the caregiver in light of the situation may result in anger and attempts to "force" the patient to oblige. The elderly person is protesting the lack of self-determination and the caregiver is fearful of the consequences of non-compliance (e.g., death, deteriorating health, incompetence). Opening up the lines of communication is clearly in order under these circumstances. The level of responsibility assumed by the caregiver is haphazard and threatening to the elderly person's independence. Self-neglect may be a consequence (or protest) to the loss of independence. This is also a concern in institutional care facilities (Rathbone-McCuan & Fabian, 1992) where the struggle for self-determination (or choice) is often curbed by the transfer of responsibility to the facility.

In North American society, caregiving roles have often been delegated to women (Hargrave et al., 1997). Given the socialization process and the propensity of women to care for their children, it is sometimes assumed that caring for aging parents is a natural, expected, and/or desired role. Particular family values and beliefs promote gender inequality and devalue the time and energy required to effectively juggle nuclear family responsibilities, the home, and extended family needs. With evidence mounting that women are as likely as men to abuse or neglect the elderly (see Table 10.1), investigating the link between gender inequality and abusive behaviours does not absolve responsibility, but rather opens up an avenue of intervention for the practitioner.

3. The Role of Physicians

Strategies employed to address the issue of elderly abuse require a focus on safety, health, education and prevention, and research generally supports a multi-disciplinary approach (Beaulieu & Tremblay, 1994; Carriere et al., 1991; Emlet et al., 1995; MacLean, 1995; McDonald et al., 1991; Penhale, 1992; Podnieks, 1997; Sadler, 1994; Schoenberg et al., 1999; Tindale et al., 1994) in any intervention plan.

As part of a multi-disciplinary team, physicians are in a favourable position to play a key role in detecting maltreatment. Elderly citizens are known to visit their doctors on a regular basis, thereby providing an opportunity for the physician to explore issues of abuse during a routine checkup (Schoenberg et al., 1999). They are also in a position to recognize changes in behaviour (mental health status) and suspicious physical injuries.

A 1997 study supported a commitment by physicians to address abuse and neglect when suspected. In fact, this study revealed that with education and standard protocols in place, they would refer suspicious circumstances to appropriate agencies (Krueger & Patterson, 1997). A consequence of a relationship between a physician and other professionals, for example, has the potential to be a win-win for the client given the propensity for elderly clients to respect (McDonald & Collins, 2000) and heed the advice of their doctor. As a gatekeeper, the physician may be seen as a catalyst to promoting a healthy, safe environment for older cohorts.

B.   A Model for Intervention

The intervention model highlighted in this section is derived from a Canadian undertaking entitled *Project Care* (Reis & Nahmaish, 1995). It promotes a multi-disciplinary team approach based on empowerment, protection, and prevention of abuse and neglect.

Empowerment, a "process of helping individuals to maximize their confidence, skills and abilities in order to take control of their lives and to make informed decisions that are in their best interests" (Reis & Nahmaish, 1995, p. 10), has gained popularity in the last few decades (Holosko et al., 2001). It is derived from the three areas of powerlessness, power, and oppression (Busch & Valentine, 2000, p. 82). Viewed in the current context, empowerment theory focuses on restoring power and control to the elderly.

Entering into a plan of care based on empowerment where *protection* is needed requires the professional to focus strategic efforts in areas that reflect the preservation of the elderly person's independence as much as possible while providing him or her with a safe living environment. Client-focused prevention strategies recommended by *Project Care* focus on education for both the victim and the abuser: (a) educating elderly about abuse, self-care, and personal rights; and (b) educating caregivers about their abusive behaviours, more appropriate coping strategies, and available community resources (Reis & Nahmaish, 1995). The Model will be discussed here as it relates to both its assessment and intervention efficacy.

1. Assessment Tools of the Model

Any tool used for assessment should be comprehensive and include provisions for an examination of medical history, mental health status, and social interactions (Quinn & Tomita, 1997). *Project Care* recommends the use of three assessment tools: *BASE* (Brief Abuse Screen for the Elderly), *CASE* (Caregiver Abuse Screen), and *IOA* (Indicators of Abuse) (Reis & Nahmaish, 1995) to be used in conjunction with a brief telephone interview, a lengthy face-to-face assessment, and in consultation with interested parties (multi-disciplinary team members).

The *BASE* tool provides the practitioner with a quick, reliable method of screening for the presence of abuse. This one-page questionnaire (composed of five questions) is designed for use by interviewers working with caregivers and elderly clients aged 60 or over. *CASE* is administered to the caregiver, offering a professional a glimpse into the relationship between the elderly person and the caregiver and providing a quick overview of the possibility that abuse exists. Practitioners administer both the *BASE* and *CASE* with clients and caregivers independently. The *IOA* is used by the practitioner subsequent to the *BASE* and *CASE* and focuses on the opinion of the professional based on his or her perception of current events (Reis & Nahmaish, 1995).

2. Intervention Strategies

In keeping with the plan for a multi-disciplinary approach, key stakeholders recommended by Reis et al. (1997) include homemakers, social workers, doctors, rehabilitation therapists, psychogeriatricians, lawyers, police officers, psychiatrists, bank managers, victim/witness personnel, and trained volunteers. To minimize the potential for misunderstandings, Reis et al. (1997) have developed the *AID* (Abuse Intervention Description) that "provides a useful guide to help plan and monitor the progress and success of the intervention techniques to be used in an abuse case" (p. 24). As a generic implement, *AID* helps to maintain focus and can be referred to for clarification of intent.

Each member, as part of a core team, plays a crucial role in working toward ending abusive behaviour. [Table 10.2 outlines proposed teams and accompanying tasks.]

For instance, social workers, as part of the *multi-disciplinary team,* may take on the role of coordinator and procurer of services, monitoring delivery and progress with consideration for the client's needs [i.e., whether or not they are being met]. With direct intervention, the social worker may choose second-order change techniques (e.g., developing a collaborative rather than an adversarial relationship) (Hargrave & Hanna, 1997). Mediation can help both parties cope with stressful situations and reinforce a positive helping relationship. [As a cautionary note, however, when using this technique, the social worker must ensure a thorough understanding of his/her intent to remain neutral and engage in a regular review of the value and effectiveness of such a role on a case-by-case basis.]

Similarly, a bank manager, as part of an *expert intervention team,* could offer financial guidance to prevent or alleviate financial abuse. A lawyer's role as part of the same team may be to review legal documents held by the client or to advise the team or the client of their legal rights. The point is that by involving a myriad of professionals, each benefits from the expertise of another and the clients in question benefit from a holistic approach.

The benefits of using this field-tested intervention plan extend to self-neglect/abuse cases. In particular, the *volunteer buddies team* can be a valuable resource for an elderly person who is alone and isolated. The *community senior abuse committee* can also assist by linking this client to other clients in similar situations.

Likewise, this intervention model can be utilized in institutional settings and, in fact, may be easier to implement given the community connections and multi-disciplinary approach that is characteristic of many of these settings today. Involving the professional community that exists within the facility may provide an avenue for these caregivers to vocalize their concerns.

Table 10.2: Project Care Intervention Teams

Home Care Team	Multidisciplinary Team	Expert Intervention Team	Volunteer Buddies	Empowerment Support Group	Community Senior Abuse Committee
- basic intervention unit - Initial assessment (*BASE, CASE, IOA*) - ecommends *AID* plan	- 3 to 5 home care members review initial assessment - plans and monitors strategies	- volunteer consultants - offer specialized advice and guidance	- matched with victims of abuse - provide non professional support on a regular basis	- works with both victim and abuser - emotional support - practical aid and education	- volunteer community intervention - targets seniors, professionals, and the community at large

(*Source*: Reis, N. & Nahmiash, D. (1995). *A guide to intervention*. North York: Captus Press, Inc.)

From a practical point of view, administering such a comprehensive program can be prohibitive particularly since government cutbacks to social services in the past decade have resulted in the elimination of staff and services. While there are a number of community initiatives underway and new ones being established, few have the resources to commit to such an undertaking. Even so, there is merit to reviewing and captioning portions of this well-deliberated plan.

In addition, the assessment devices of the Model previously presented were designed to assist practitioners in their attempt to screen for the existence of abuse, but are not intended to replace the need for thorough knowledge in the area of elderly abuse and neglect, the aging process, and the life cycle. Further, these tools represent only one component of the assessment process and represent the assessor's professional opinion of present circumstances.

C. Advocacy, Prevention, and Education

Work carried out in the macro-level arena generally focuses on promoting health and well-being in the community. With regard to the elderly population, this implies a proactive approach aimed at ending existing and (anticipated) future violence toward seniors. Lobbying for social policy changes and promoting community-wide education programs geared at awareness and prevention are two methods utilized by social workers to draw attention to issues that impede self-determination and the rights of individuals.

1. Lobbying
With the elderly population growing [see Chapter 1] it is evident that planning is key to health and social welfare. Lobbying for social policy change in the areas of health and social programming with the intent to increase and improve choices and access is important to the preservation of the independence of our growing elderly cohort. With regard to disabled seniors, for example, accessible and affordable housing options and transportation services can reduce dependence on others for self-care, while at the same time improving the chances that community living remains an option for a longer period of time.

In public facilities, given the prevalence rates known about abuse in these establishments (McDonald & Collins, 2000; Pillemer & Bachman-Prehn, 1991), it is crucial that efforts to encourage regulating bodies to re-examine their staffing and hiring procedures be undertaken. Policy makers and planners must be made aware of the current circumstances under which staff operate. For instance, it is not acceptable for elderly residents to be forced to wear diapers because staff do not have time (too many responsibilities) to take residents to the restroom except during prescribed time frames.

In keeping with the empowerment model, seniors themselves must be courted into the advocacy arena as partners. They are the best resources for information on what is needed and the passion with which they can express these needs is key to success. Not only is speaking up for one's rights an empowering experience, the fact that today's elderly "collectively enjoy considerable political power and influence" (Podnieks, 1990, p. 1) also suggests that this cohort possesses the skills to make things happen.

2. Education and Prevention

Perhaps the most significant opportunity for health promotion lies in our ability to educate and be educated. Educating seniors is the first priority and can be initiated before retirement (i.e., retirement planning). Financial planners, real estate personnel, lawyers, and employers, for example, are potential targets for information dissemination activities. Quite simply, a fact sheet can be included in any retirement planning pitch.

Given the current trend toward more community-based services and, in consideration of the preference of the elderly to rely on informal social networks (Health Canada, 1994), it is necessary [for both the elderly and the caregiver's sake] to include caregivers in any educational strategy. It can take on many forms from education on common ailments associated with aging to a list of ongoing resource options in the community and/or through government agencies.

Education of the general public on the reality of abuse in old age and on the aging process itself can help eliminate some of the presumptions and fears associated with getting older. Seniors themselves should be prompted to become a part of endeavours to encourage relationships between generations and to illustrate to recipients the value in appreciating the aging process.

As noted, these are only two areas of opportunity for change. Time permitting, many more could be introduced including an expansion of research, self-help groups, mutual aid groups, and community coalitions, for example. What is of significance, however, is that if elderly abuse and neglect are to be prevented, now is the time to take action.

III.   Concluding Remarks

Opening the door to table this issue has been difficult to say the least. The findings of the NEAIS shatter the beliefs of many—that retirement is a time to relax and reflect on life's accomplishments. Yet, it is crucial to continue with current momentum and further research efforts in the area of elderly abuse and neglect.

As indicated, definitional issues continue to cloud treatment realities. A universal definition is sorely needed to bring clarity and purpose to both assessment and intervention in elderly abuse cases. Apprehension in such cases because of "wishy-washy" wording interferes with preventative efforts and jeopardizes the safety of seniors. Albeit caution is required when investigating suspicions of abuse, being careful should not mean debating what constitutes abusive behaviour.

Working within current constraints, the gatekeeping role becomes crucial. As noted earlier in this chapter, elderly persons may be suspect of intervention motive and resist assistance. As a regular contact, physicians in particular must be provided with education and protocols to follow up when faced with uneasy circumstances. Trust is paramount here as elderly patients trust their physicians, and physicians must be able to trust the system in order to feel comfortable in reporting suspicions.

Gerontological social workers too are in a position of trust. Having taken the time to educate themselves thoroughly on the aging process, they are a unique group of professionals capable of taking on advocacy, coordinating, mediating, assessment, and education roles. Shifting from one role to another and weaving in and out will be commonplace. As part of a multi-disciplinary team, gerontological social workers "bring to the table" their concern for client well-being and appreciation of the role of fellow team members.

It is clear that elderly abuse is not a single-faceted problem. Whereas with children, the state has an obligation to speak for the child and is mandated to protect the child from further harm, in both spousal and elderly abuse cases we are working with adults—individuals who have a responsibility and a right to make choices for themselves. As catalysts for change, it is important to realize that ending violence is a long-term commitment to the promotion of safety and health for all concerned.

References

Aitken, L. & Griffin, G. (1996). *Gender issues in elder abuse.* Thousand Oaks: Sage.

Baron, S. & Welty, A. (1996). Elder abuse. *Journal of Gerontological Social Work,* 25(1–2), 33–57.

Beaulieu, M. & Tremblay, M.J. (1994). *Abuse and neglect of older adults in institutional settings: A discussion paper.* Ottawa: Health Promotion and Programs Branch for Health Canada.

Blakely, B.E., Dolon, R., & May, D.D. (1993). Improving the responses of physicians to elder abuse and neglect: Contributions of a model program. *Journal of Gerontological Social Work,* 19(3/4), 35–49.

Block, M.R. & Sinnott, J.D. (eds.). (1979). *The battered elder syndrome: An exploratory study.* College Park: University of Maryland Center on Aging.

Bristowe, E. & Collins, J.B. (1989). Family mediated abuse of noninstitutionalized frail elderly men and women living in British Columbia. *Journal of Elder Abuse and Neglect,* 1(1), 45–64.

Busby, D.M. (ed.). (1996). *The impact of violence in the family: Treatment approaches for therapists and other professionals.* Toronto: Allyn & Bacon.

Busch, N.B. & Valentine, D. (2000). Empowerment practice: A focus on battered women. *AFFILIA,* 15(1), 82–95.

Byers, B. & Hendricks, J. (eds.). (1993). *Adult protective services: Research and practice.* Springfield: Charles C. Thomas.

Carriere, R., Newton, A., & Sullivan, M. (1991). Elder abuse: The first steps in community prevention. *The Social Worker,* 59(1), 10–12.

Decalmer, P. & Glendenning, F. (eds.). (1997). *The mistreatment of elderly people,* 2nd ed. Thousand Oaks: Sage.

Doyle, C. (1997). Protection studies: Challenging oppression and discrimination. *Social Work Education,* 16(2), 8–19.

Duffy, A. & Momirov, J. (1997). *Family violence: A Canadian introduction.* Toronto: James Lorimer & Company, Publishers.

Eastman, M. (ed.). (1994). *Old age abuse: A new perspective,* 2nd ed. New York: Chapman & Hall.

Emlet, C.A., Crabtree, J.L., Condon, V.A., & Treml, L.A. (1995). *In-home assessment of older adults: An interdisciplinary approach.* Gaithersburg: Aspen Publishers, Inc.

Gelles, R.J. (1997). *Intimate violence in families,* 3rd ed. Thousand Oaks: Sage.

Gelles, R.J. & Strauss, M.A. (1989). *Intimate violence.* New York: Simon & Schuster.

Gioglio, G.R. & Blakemore, P. (1983). Elder abuse in New Jersey: The knowledge and experience of abuse among older New Jerseyans.

Unpublished manuscript, Department of Human Services, Trenton, New Jersey.

Giordano, N.H. & Giordano, J.A. (1984). Elder abuse: A review of the literature. *Social Work* 29(3): 232–236.

Hampton, R.L. (ed.). (1999). *Family violence: Prevention and treatment*, 2nd ed. Thousand Oaks: Sage.

Harel, Z., Erlich, P., & Hubbard, R. (eds.). (1990). *The vulnerable aged: People, services and policies*. New York: Springer.

Hargrave, T.D., & Hanna, S.M. (eds.). (1997). *The aging family: New visions in theory, practice and reality*. New York: Brunner/Mazel.

Health Canada. (1994). Community awareness and response: abuse and neglect of older adults. Ottawa: Ministry of National Health and Welfare. [On-line] Available at: http://www.hc-sc.gc.ca.

Holosko, M.J., Leslie, D.R., & Cassano, D.R. (2001). How service users become empowered in human service organizations: The empowerment model. *International Journal of Health Care Quality Assurance*, 14(3), 41–62.

Johnson, T.F. (1991). *Elder mistreatment: Deciding who is at risk*. New York: Greenwood Press.

Kosberg, J.I. (ed.). (1983). *Abuse and mistreatment of the elderly. Causes and interventions*. Littleton: John Wright, PSG Inc.

Krueger, P. & Patterson, C. (1997). *Detecting and managing elder abuse: Challenges in primary care*. Toronto: Canadian Medical Association.

Lau, E. A. & Kosberg, J.I. (1979). Abuse of the elderly by informal care providers. *Aging*, 10–15.

McDonald, L. & Collins, A. (2000). *Abuse and neglect of older adults: A discussion paper*. Ottawa: Health Promotions and Programs Branch, Health Canada.

McDonald, P., Hornick, J., Robertson, G., & Wallace, J. (1991). *Elder abuse and neglect in Canada*. Toronto: Butterworths.

MacLean, M.J. (ed.). (1995). *Abuse and neglect of older Canadians: Strategies for change*. Toronto: Thompson Educational Publishing.

MacLean, M.J. (2000). *Self-neglect by older adults*. Ottawa: Health Canada for the National Clearinghouse of Family Violence.

Mulley, G., Penn, N., & Burns, E. (eds.). (1998). *Older people at home: Practical issues*. London: BMJ Publishing Group.

National Center for Elder Abuse. (2000). The Basics: What is elder abuse? [On-line] Available at: http://www.gwjapan.com/NCEA/basic/index.html.

National Center for Elder Abuse at the American Public Human Services Association in Collaboration with Westat Inc. (1998). Administration on Aging: The national elder abuse incident study; Final Report, September

1998. [On-line]. Available at: http://www.aoa.dhhs.gov/abuse/report/ default.html.

National Center on Elder Abuse. (1999). The source of information and assistance on elder abuse. The Basics. [On-line]. Available at: http:// www.elderabusecenter.org.

National Center on Elder Abuse. (1999). The source of information and assistance on elder abuse. [On-line]. Available at: http://www. elderabusecenter.org.

Olshevski, J.L., Katz, A.D., & Knight, B.G. (1999). *Stress reduction for caregivers*. Philadelphia: Brunner/Mazel.

Ontario Association of Professional Social Workers. (1992). Elder abuse: A practical handbook for service providers. [Brochure] Toronto: Ontario Association of Social Workers.

Penhale, B. (1992). The abuse of elderly people: Considerations for practice. *British Journal of Social Work*, 23, 95–112.

Pillemer, K. & Bachman-Prehn, R. (1991). Helping and hurting: Predictors of maltreatment of patients in nursing homes. *Research on Aging*, 13(1), 74–95.

Pillemer, K. & Finkelhor, D. (1988). The prevalence of elder abuse: A random sample survey. *The Gerontologist*, 28(1), 51–57.

Pillemer, Karl & Finkelhor, David. (1989). Causes of elder abuse: Caregiver stress versus problem relatives. *American Journal of Orthopsychiatry*, 59(2), 179–187.

Pillemer, K. & Wolf, R. (eds.). (1986). *Elder abuse: Conflict in the family*. Dover: Auburn House.

Podnieks, E. (1989). *National survey on abuse of the elderly in Canada: Preliminary findings*. Toronto: Office of Research and Innovation, Ryerson Polytechnic Institute.

Podnieks, E. (1990). *National survey on abuse of the elderly in Canada: The Ryerson Study*. Toronto: Ryerson Polytechnic Institute.

Podnieks, E. (1997). Introduction. Adults with vulnerability. Addressing abuse and neglect. Paper presented at a workshop presented to service professionals in the Greater Toronto Area, Toronto, Ontario. [On-line]. Available at: http://www.utoronto.ca/aging/awvhome.htm.

Quinn, M. & Tomita, S. (1997). *Elder abuse and neglect. Causes, diagnosis, and intervention strategies*, 2nd ed. New York: Springer.

Rathbone-McCuan, E. & Fabian, D. (eds.). (1992). *Self-neglecting elders: A clinical dilemma*. New York: Auburn House.

Reis, N. & Nahmaish, D. (1995). *When seniors are abused: A guide to intervention*. North York: Captus Press.

Reis, M., Nahmiash, D., Brownridge, N., & Wolfe, R. (1997). Uniting protocol with practice. Paper presented at a workshop presented to service professionals in the Greater Toronto Area, Toronto, Ontario. [On-line]. Available at: http//www.utoronto.ca/aging/aging/awvhome.htm.

Ross, J.W. (1991). Editorial. *Health and Social Work*, 16(4), 227–229.

Sadler, P. (1994). What helps? Elder abuse interventions and research. *Australian Social Work*, 47(4), 27–35.

Schlesinger, B. & Schlesinger, R. (eds.). (1988). *Abuse of the elderly: Issues and annotated bibliography*. Toronto: University of Toronto Press.

Schoenberg, N.E., Campbell, K.A., & Johnson, M.M. (1999). Physicians and Clergy as facilitators of formal services for older adults. *Journal of Aging and Social Policy*, 11(1), 9–26.

Shell, D. J. (1982). *Protection of the elderly: A study of elder abuse: Issues and annotated bibliography*. Toronto: University of Toronto Press.

Statistics Canada. (2000). *Family violence in Canada: A statistical profile: 2000*. Ottawa: Ministry of Industry for the Canadian Centre for Justice Statistics.

Steinmetz, S.K. & Straus, M.A. (eds.). (1974). *Violence in the family*. New York: Harper & Row.

Tindale, J.A., Norris, J.E., Berman, R., & Kuiack, S. (1994). *Intergenerational conflict and the prevention of abuse against older persons*. Ottawa: Health Promotions and Programs Branch, Health Canada.

Walker, L.E. (1979). *The battered woman*. New York: Harper & Row.

Weiner, A. (1991). A community-based educational model for identification and prevention of elder abuse. *Journal of Gerontological Social Work*, 16(3/4), 107–119.

Wolf, R.S. (1988). Elder abuse: Ten years later. *Journal of American Geriatrics Society*, 36(8), 758–762.

Wolf, R.S., Godkin, M.A., & Pillemer, K. (1984). *Elder abuse and neglect: Report from the Three Models Project*. Worcester: University of Massachusetts Medical Center.

Wolf, R.S. & Pillemer, K. (1989). *Helping elderly victims: The reality of elder abuse*. New York: Columbia University Press.

Internet Resources

National Center on Elder Abuse (NCEA).
A national resource for elder rights, law enforcement and legal professionals, public policy leaders, researchers, and the public.
http://www.elderabusecenter.org/

National Clearinghouse on Family Violence (NCFV) Health Canada.
    A national resource centre for all Canadians seeking information about
    violence within the family.
    http://www.hc-sc.gc.ca/hppb/familyviolence

Additional Readings

Johnson, I.M. (1995). Family members' perceptions of and attitudes toward
    elder abuse. *Families in Society: The Journal of Contemporary Human
    Services*, 76(4), 220–229.
Kivnick, H.Q. & Murray, S.V. (2001). Life strengths interview guide:
    Assessing elder clients' strengths. *Journal of Gerontological Social Work*,
    34(4), 7–31.
Matlaw, J.R. & Mayer, J.B. (1986). Elder abuse: Ethical and practical
    dilemmas for social work. *Health and Social Work*, 11(2), 85–94.
Michalski, Joseph H. (1995). *A shelter for abused and neglected older adults:
    Needs assessment and feasibility study*. Toronto: Centre for Studies of
    Aging, University of Toronto.
Pritchard, J. (ed.). (1999). *Elder abuse work: Best practice in Britain and Canada*.
    Philadelphia: Jessica Kingsley Publications.

CHAPTER 11

HIV/AIDS AND THE ELDERLY: IMPLICATIONS FOR SOCIAL WORK PRACTICE

NATALIE ST. JOHN AND

MICHAEL J. HOLOSKO

This chapter presents an overview for social workers practising in this field to become more actively involved in the detection and treatment issues of HIV/AIDS within the elderly population. This issue is discussed from the standpoint of: (1) HIV/AIDS and the elderly; (2) the elderly as caregivers; (3) social work roles in direct practice; and (4) social work roles within indirect practice.

I.   Introduction

HIV/AIDS and the elderly is a rising phenomenon that affects many individuals and society at large. Social workers are in an ideal position to help identify those elderly who may have HIV/AIDS, or who may be at risk to contract this disease. They are further able to help individuals, their spouses/partners, and families cope and adjust to their life situations effectively.

This chapter begins by providing information on HIV/AIDS and the elderly, the prevalence of this disease within this population, and the factors that impact significantly on the likelihood of elderly persons acquiring HIV/AIDS. Social workers in this area must have specific knowledge of this disease, and they need to identify various aspects associated with treating all those involved. There is an opportunity for social workers to be effective in direct practice with the individuals and their families, but there is also the need for social workers to be involved within indirect practice, which will be discussed in the following chapter.

II.　HIV/AIDS and the Elderly

The HIV/AIDS disease is primarily thought of as a disease of the young, and many physicians, along with the rest of us, never even think about an older person with HIV/AIDS. Among men and women over the age of 65, AIDS stands as the 15th leading cause of death (Hillman & Stricker, 1998, p. 483). In the United States, the Center of Disease Control (CDC) stated that 10 percent of all HIV/AIDS cases reported to them occurred in persons 50 years of age or older (Puleo, 1996, p. 2). As the aging population is the fastest-growing age group in North America, this percentage will only increase unless more attention is paid to this issue, and more formal and informal supports are designed specifically for older persons with HIV/AIDS.

The most common forms of transmission in older people are homosexual behaviour (62 percent of all reported cases), intravenous drug use (11 percent), use of tainted blood products (9 percent), and heterosexual behaviour (6 percent) (Hillman & Stricker, 1998, p. 483). According to Puleo (1996), this figure for heterosexual transmission is the highest in any age group. There have also been some reported cases where older people have acquired AIDS by looking after their child who had the disease.

Blood transfusions are the most distinctive transmission source among the elderly compared with other age groups. Blood screening didn't begin until 1985, so those who received transfusions before this time are now likely to be in their later years of life. Many of these people may have received transfusions unknowingly during surgery because hospitals were not obligated to tell the patient; therefore, they may have received infected blood without knowing they were at risk (Linsk, 1994, p. 366). As symptoms usually develop four to seven years after being exposed to HIV, it is expected that the number of cases reported through blood transfusions will decline as blood is screened now, and anyone who received the tainted blood before 1985 should be showing symptoms already.

Two factors impact significantly on the likelihood of elderly persons acquiring HIV/AIDS. These are biological and sociological. In regard to the former, physically there is an increased risk of elderly persons becoming infected as there is a general decrease in the immune system functioning in both men and women as they age. For women, there is a greater likelihood of microscopic or macroscopic tears in the vaginal wall due to dryness that comes with age, which allows easier passage for the HIV virus (Hillman & Stricker, 1998, p. 484). Older adults are also more at risk as they are less likely to wear condoms than younger people because they feel they are not at risk for sexually transmitted disease, and because they no longer fear conception (Hillman & Stricker, 1998, p. 484).

From a sociological perspective, a number of societal myths shroud this issue. For example, it is a common stereotype that the elderly do not have sex, which seems to be widely accepted by both physicians and the rest of society. Hillman and Stricker (1998) stated that a physician may overidentify with the elderly patient as a parent or authority figure who simply could not have sex and therefore could not be at risk for the disease. Another misconception is the notion of "bad things happening to bad people" and the thought of an innocent-looking, kind, older person contracting AIDS is hard for even therapists to conceptualize (p. 486). Although the CDC stated that the use of injection drugs appears to be an increasing risk behaviour for HIV among older persons, it is still the misconception that the elderly do not use non-prescription drugs, they never could have, and that the drug users generally die before reaching old age (Linsk, 1994, p. 365). The next common assumption people tend to make is that elderly people are heterosexual. Because of these widely accepted beliefs, older people are not targeted to receive even the basic HIV/AIDS education. In 1992, a National Health Interview survey was done in the United States, which found 16 percent of those 50 years and older reported having no knowledge of AIDS, and 77 percent thought they had no chance of getting the virus and, as a result, would not get tested (Puleo, 1996, p. 4). Puleo (1996) stated that public education programs that have been implemented for younger persons may not be as successful with the elderly as learning needs and abilities change with age. As cognitive efficiency and visual and auditory acuity may decline, there is a need for one-on-one instruction, frequent summarization, and restatement of what is being taught (p. 5).

The media has relied on fear-inducing messages, which has had little effect on behaviour, and instead has brought unnecessary fear and anxiety to the public (Anderson & Wilkie, 1992, p. 106). Anderson and Wilkie (1992) stated that by the media focusing on "risk groups" instead of "risky practices," those people who are not gay or intravenous drug users may not see themselves as vulnerable to the HIV infection (p. 107). Also, the identification of "innocent victims" with the implied contrast of "the guilty" who have brought it on themselves has created difficulties to those infected to achieve any rational public understanding of the nature of the transmission of the virus (Anderson & Wilkie, 1992, p. 107). As indicated in Chapter 2 of this text (Holosko and Holosko), social workers need to not only help to tell the stories of their clients to society, but also debunk the myths that serve as barriers to their treatment.

The greatest opportunity for risk assessment is in health care settings, but even here neglecting to take a sexual history of elderly patients is the norm. HIV/AIDS risk assessments are rarely done, and minimal HIV/AIDS education occurs. By neglecting these issues, it deprives the elderly of opportunities to reduce their risk with behaviour modification. In a study of AIDS risk behaviours among late middle-aged and elderly Americans, it was determined by Stall and Catania (1994) that when people over the age of 50 are made aware of their risks, they can and will modify their behaviour accordingly (Puleo, 1996, p. 7). This indicates that social workers, nurses, physicians, etc., need to educate the elderly about possible risk factors so that they can modify their behaviours.

As many AIDS symptoms are the same as other diseases, health care professionals tend to try to rule out all other possibilities first before testing the patient for HIV/AIDS, which doesn't allow for a timely diagnosis. In this regard, they typically ignore the array of symptoms consistent with HIV/AIDS, and look at them idiopathically to test for other diseases. The most common symptom that gets misdiagnosed is HIV-associated dementia being mistaken for Alzheimer's disease. Two important differences that need to be recognized are that AIDS-induced dementia often presents with a rapid onset within six months and often includes cognitive and psychomotor impairment in that same time, whereas in Alzheimer's the disease typically manifests symptoms gradually over at least a year, and the psychomotor impairment usually does not begin until the later stages of the disease (Linsk, 1994, p. 485). By doing a sex and drug history at each contact, a health care provider can then suggest testing if necessary to the patient and/or discuss condom use, making them available to all patients and making sure they know how to use them. If an AIDS test is suggested, it is important that elderly persons know about the confidentiality of the test, which is usually very important to them, and they must be aware of the retesting procedures in six months' time.

III. The Elderly as Caregivers

One area that affects the elderly with this disease is the increased demand for them to care for children with HIV/AIDS, grandchildren who may be infected themselves, or have deceased parents due to AIDS. Brabant (1994) recognized that many elderly parents provide enormous support and care to their children with HIV/AIDS who often turn to their parents as the illness progresses (p. 132). This support and care often takes place while the parent is going through a grief and loss process of learning a child has HIV/AIDS and, in some cases, that they are also homosexual (Brabant, 1994, p. 132). There are some issues that affect elderly caregivers, and the first has to do with the demands and the role of caregiving itself. For example, an elderly caregiver may begin to feel primary caregiver strain in keeping up with the demands of household managerial tasks, chores around the house, and personal care of the patient (Brabant, 1994, p. 133). The next issue is financial strain. According to Brabant (1994), elderly persons often live on fixed incomes, especially if they are retired, and this income is typically only planned for one or two persons. Adding another individual to the budget may compromise the elderly person's economic base (p. 134). If employed, the elderly person may also have problems with employment for being absent to care for a child or grandchild, which may contribute to financial problems and frustration. Although elderly persons are living longer and are generally healthier, there are still some certain aspects of aging that may have an effect on their ability to be a caregiver. Some examples are less stamina, reduction in mobility, diminished visual acuity, as well as any physical deterioration from a disease they may have (Brabant, 1994, p. 134). They may also have to give up leisure and social activities that they value in order to care for their child/grandchild, and they may risk losing their social network due to isolation and the stigma attached to the HIV/AIDS disease itself. The caregiver will have to also deal with the fear of becoming infected with the disease and the consequent anticipated loss of the loved one for whom they care (Brabant, 1994, p. 133). Finally, the caregiver also has to deal with the lack of value that society places on the role of caregiver and has to learn to cope with the realization that he or she will outlive the child (Gutheil & Chichin, 1991, p. 239).

In regard to caregivers, for social workers it is important to have knowledge about aging, caregiver issues, and AIDS-related issues when working with these caregivers. A social worker needs to be able to answer questions about transmission, treatments, lifestyles, AIDS organizations, and any support groups available (Brabant, 1994, p. 143). Brabant (1994) stated that it is important to reaffirm the dignity of the caregiver and empower him or her as much as possible by giving choices even if they are limited (p. 144). It is also recommended that touching be used toward the caregiver during counselling and support as it conveys the message that you are not afraid of "catching" anything (see Chapter 2). It is important, however, to ask permission for this, and never pat the person on the back as this is frequently seen as demeaning (Brabant, 1994, p. 144).

When a grandparent takes on the responsibility of caring for a grandchild after his or her own child has passed away due to AIDS, the grandparent experiences the same financial stresses, social stigma, and physical strains, but also have some issues unique to being a caregiving grandparent. They may feel betrayed, ashamed, or guilty as they feel they have failed as parents, and they wonder if they will do any better with their grandchildren (Nazon & Levine-Perkell, 1996, p. 25). They also tend to face issues such as loneliness and depression caused by their loss, and they have to deal with things such as the teenage rebellion and the generation gap when raising their grandchildren with whom they may not know how to deal effectively (Nazon & Levine-Perkell, 1996, p. 25).

IV. Social Work Roles in Direct Practice

At the onset, it should be noted that there are barriers to intervention that are common with the elderly population about which social workers working with these clients should be aware. The first is that older persons with HIV/AIDS often do not feel entitled to help. This is especially common for older gay men who may feel that "they got what they deserved," and they may feel they need to isolate themselves (Anderson, 1998, p. 448). Anderson (1998) stated that older people may feel bad about using the precious few health care resources that should be going to younger people (p. 448). Here, social workers must emphasize that they are not competing for resources with younger people, and that there are still services available for everyone. Also, the elderly need to know that they are worth helping and that their age does not matter. The final barrier is the social stigma associated with HIV/AIDS in our society, which unfortunately may cause older people not to risk coming forward for any form of assistance (Anderson, 1998, p. 448).

In moving the discussion to the reality of an elderly person being tested for HIV/AIDS, if the HIV test comes back positive, the elderly person typically goes into a crisis state requiring crisis intervention and emotional support. There are usually several stage-specific (à la Kubler-Ross) emotional reactions that accompany a positive diagnosis. Shock is the most common initial reaction to the diagnosis (Health & Welfare Canada, 1990, p. 55). This may result in an inability for the patient to talk to anyone about the HIV diagnosis and to isolate himself or herself from all family and friends. The next common emotion is denial. This is when the individual tries to forget or ignore the new diagnosis. Health and Welfare Canada (1990) stated that this can be positive as it may provide the individual with time to gather energy and deal with the subsequent issues. On the other hand, denial can also be dangerous if it prevents the individual from taking care of treatment needs and adopting safer sex practices (p. 56). Another emotion that typically surfaces is anger. Anger can be directed at the person who is responsible for the HIV infection, the situation that led them to the infection or society in general, when they see themselves isolated, alienated, and discriminated against (Health & Welfare Canada, 1990, p. 56). If they lose their routines and relationships with their friends and families as a consequence, this may contribute to the anger. A social worker can facilitate positive ways to express anger, and help the client to maintain existing relationships that are necessary for support. Anxiety is also usual when the person considers to whom to reveal a positive status and what is going to happen in the progression of the disease, all of which evokes more fear and compounding anxiety. The issue must be discussed with clients and their partners who have been exposed, so that they can get tested. Telling partners or family members can be extremely stressful, especially when the person has been leading a homosexual lifestyle that no one knew about, or having multiple sex partners, and/or extramarital affairs that led to the HIV infection. In this regard guilt is a common emotion experienced by people as they blame themselves for the specific activities known to have given them HIV (p. 57).

The final stage-specific emotion in this domino-effect continuum is depression when an infected individual may experience a lack of interest in life, feel unclear about future goals, withdraw from family and friends and all other social support, and may have suicidal ideation or attempt suicide (Health & Welfare Canada, 1990, p. 59). It is important for professionals to screen for self-destructive behaviours and declining mental status, at which time if anything is exhibited the appropriate support and referral(s) can be given (Linsk, 1994, p. 369). Family counselling can be used to help the elderly individual tell family members about the diagnosis, and to help the family members deal with their fallout reactions. Precise information and education about HIV can help the client and his or her family deal with the anxieties and fear surrounding the infection of others. With regard to the issues of depression and isolation, human service professionals can connect the patient and family to resources such as home care and help them develop a schedule of activities.

A social worker can also assist clients in exploring the meaning of HIV for them, and discuss how it is likely to change their lives (Linsk, 1994, p. 368). For clients, support groups for HIV-positive persons may be helpful and for others, involvement in AIDS advocacy groups can become a means of expression, support, and action (Linsk, 1994, p. 369). Developing an ongoing plan of psychosocial intervention is the key to the successful management of HIV (Linsk, 1994, p. 368). The elderly client may need intensive case management to provide assessment and linkage to an array of community services.

Three common areas of care for elderly with HIV/AIDS who seek help are long-term care, home care, and care by a caregiver, usually the clients' partner/spouse or family. Long-term care is formal care that provides not only treatment for the disease, but also helps with various activities of daily living (ADL). The focus here is on how one lives with the illness rather than on the illness itself (Wyatt, 1996, p. 81). As with most services today, the extent of services available to clients depends on where they live, whether their friends and family are able to help with their care, on their financial resources, and (sometimes) if they are over 65 years old. It should be noted that older gay men who acquired HIV/AIDS through homosexual transmission are usually more distant from their families both geographically and emotionally due to their sexual orientation, so this group is generally left only with the option of long-term care or home care (King, 1993). There are no specific long-term care facilities for older people with AIDS. Instead, they either enter into a traditional long-term care facility where they are usually younger than the other residents, or they go into an AIDS-specific facility where they are a lot older than most of these residents. In both settings, the older person may feel isolated, facing a disease that has such a stigma, or lacking the company of older people (Wyatt, 1996, p. 82). It is recommended that when a rehabilitation assessment is done that patients should be assessed and treated not just from a performance perspective (i.e., whether they can do the task), but also by the time of day those tasks are performed, the environment in which they are performed, and the extent to which these tasks are of value and importance to the lives of the patients (Wyatt, 1996, p. 84). When these specific assessments are completed, then the worker will be able to note the physical and psychosocial skills that may require therapeutic intervention for an adapted routine.

Home care is a much more flexible service that can be started, intensified, or discontinued at any time depending on the needs of the client. When home care is combined with housing services, adult day health programs, personal care services, occupational therapists, skilled nursing care, hospice care, and other services available, it becomes an effective form of care. This tends to diminish the isolation of clients by having them still interacting with people through these adjunct programs, but also being able to have care at home, which is preferred (Wyatt, 1996, p. 87). Although hospice care is available, AIDS patients have been reluctant to accept their services as they prefer to continue aggressive treatment for as long as possible (Wyatt, 1996, p. 91). Another obstacle for palliative care is that it provides care to those who are within a few months of dying, but with AIDS it is not always possible to predict when someone has six months to live.

The third form of care is informal caregivers. A study by Raviers and Siegel (1991) found that those with AIDS used informal family caregivers for two-thirds of their total assistance required for ADL, transportation, administrative functions, and home medical care (Levine-Perkell, 1996, pp. 115–116). It has been found that spouses and significant others are the main sources of this care. In some cases, the clients' partners' own advanced age and possible health problems make this group themselves susceptible to serious physical and mental health problems as a result of caregiving (Levine-Perkell, 1996, p. 116). According to Levine-Perkell (1996), research has demonstrated that family caregivers of the elderly or ill person often suffer loss of self (i.e., deterioration of intimate marital relationship or transformation of the "couple identity"), depression, mental exhaustion, and burden. There is also stress associated with performing the household tasks, personal care of the patient, and increase of financial burden and limited social and leisure activities when you are a caregiver (p. 116). Another decision that adds stress is if the infected person asks the caregiver not to disclose that he or she has HIV/AIDS. This deprives the caregiver of the support the caregiver may be able to potentially receive from interaction with others in the same situation, or from other resources. For some, the inability to disclose this information causes increased frustration, stress, isolation, and even a sense of hopelessness (Levine-Perkell, 1996, p. 117). It also often becomes necessary for caregivers to coordinate their efforts with various stakeholders in the care network, which can become overwhelming when trying to seek the necessary services for the patient's acute and chronic needs. In this regard, social workers can work with caregivers to help coordinate their needs and try to eliminate undue stress. Social workers must become familiar with all helping disciplines in this regard, knowing what the needs of the patients are and where they can be referred to. The social worker must also be aware of the community referral services and the eligibility requirements so that they can give caregivers this information.

One area that is a constant challenge for older people when assessing the issue of care is finances. As better treatment and improved care for HIV/AIDS patients evolves daily, even elderly people are living longer with the disease. However, many older people with HIV/AIDS anticipate early death, and deplete their savings in paying for care. Social workers need to assist clients with their finances and advocate for those who cannot afford these treatments and care (Maclean, 1999, p. 8). Another issue affecting older HIV/AIDS patients is pain management. Some people believe that it is natural for someone with a terminal illness to experience considerable pain. In this case, a social worker can encourage the person to seek medication that will provide them with appropriate pain relief, and explain to patients that they do not have to experience these degrees of pain (Anderson & Wilkie, 1992, p. 162). For example, by teaching the client muscle-relaxation techniques and the use of guided imagery, one may reduce some of the anxiety that may be contributing to the level of pain experienced (Anderson and Wilkie, 1992, p. 162).

One important area in which social workers can help the individual patient, their caregivers, and their family is with issues surrounding death and dying. Outside of assisting with the actual psychosocial adjustment issues, elderly people living with HIV/AIDS may require the services of a lawyer to draw up a will, assign a power of attorney, and assist them with financial matters in the event of their pending death (Anderson & Wilkie, 1992, p. 167). When elderly individuals handle these matters, they have a greater sense of control over the process of dying. Client can ensure that property is passed on the way they wish, that the people they want notified of the death are notified, and that funeral arrangements are made in accordance with their wishes (Anderson & Wilkie, 1992, p. 170).

If death occurs, social workers need to address caregivers, friends, and family of the deceased during bereavement through supportive counselling. King (1993) indicated that mourning involves emotional, physical, and spiritual reactions that lead people to feel abandoned, confused, depressed, and sometimes suicidal. The caregiver may present emotions of relief, as well as guilt for feeling these emotions. It is important as practitioners to work through the grief process. It is also important to realize that the death of the individual does not relieve the family of the stigma or prejudice associated with the disease, and family members still may be reluctant to share the true cause of death with other family members or friends (King, 1993). Another commonly held belief in society is that homosexual relationships are less emotionally and socially valid than heterosexual relationships, and this is even a common belief within the gay community (King, 1993). This tends to make society minimize the loss felt by the homosexual partner, who tends, therefore, to receive less sympathy from others for the loss. Social workers need to validate the loss and help the partner through the grieving process (Gallant & Holosko, 2001).

V.   Social Work Roles within Indirect Practice

The whole area of education needs to be addressed as this is no longer a young person's disease. Education is seen as the most effective weapon against AIDS (Gutheil & Chichin, 1991, p. 240). According to Gutheil and Chichin (1991), older people are the least informed about AIDS transmission of all age groups, which leads to unnecessary fear of acquiring the disease when they are not at risk, or they may be unaware of the real risks of transmitting the disease and may put themselves and others at risk (p. 240). Along with education about transmission, education about the symptoms of AIDS has to be presented to the older population, so they may recognize that these symptoms are not a normal part of aging and, hopefully, they will therefore seek medical attention. Education about the course of the disease is also needed, so both the patient and the caregiver can anticipate and plan for future challenges. It is recommended that elderly people be trained to educate other elderly people about HIV/AIDS as this may have more of an impact on the seriousness of the issue (Maclean, 1999, p. 6). As previously indicated, caregivers need to be educated about the various social services available to them and how to gain access to these resources. Some avenues for providing education are through seniors' centres, hospital outpatient clinics, organizations that address older people, and private doctors' offices. Health care providers also need to be educated on all aspects of AIDS in the elderly so that they can begin to perform risk assessments, recognize the symptoms in a timely fashion, and educate their patients accordingly.

It is important for social workers to advocate for new programs for both those patients with HIV/AIDS and for their caregivers. When a social worker is seeing a client in a health setting, it is important that a risk assessment and sexual history be conducted and, if necessary, for the worker to inform the doctor of any concerns. Social workers also need to advocate to make sure that elderly patients are not receiving poor treatment from the medical profession, and make sure that they are not being abandoned as this sometimes happens when health care professionals find it hard to deal with patients who will have no chance of recovery (Gutheil & Chichin, 1991, p. 242). It is important to advocate for elderly people to be allowed access to community and institutionally based long-term care programs. It is important for social workers to educate administration, staff, residents, and their families when patients with AIDS are integrated into facilities predominantly for the elderly. This requires having sufficient knowledge of aging and AIDS to educate and answer questions. Also, respite care, home care, and residential services are all essential components of an adequate service system for older people with AIDS and their caregivers (Gutheil & Chichin, 1991, p. 242). It is also important not to compete with younger people with AIDS for services, as all populations need to have access to any services offered. Social workers can assist both younger and older persons with AIDS in developing a coalition to advocate for better services for HIV/AIDS patients and their families.

For caregivers, more support groups are necessary especially for isolated caregivers so that they can share their experiences with others. It is also important that caregivers have access to all community information and options they need so that they can care more effectively. More respite care programs are required for caregivers so they will be able to obtain short-term relief from their responsibilities. Caregivers may also need transportation services, financial help, or case-management services to assist them. It is far less expensive for a caregiver to care for a patient at home than it would be to care for that same patient in a long-term care facility, but caregivers receive no such financial compensation for their work. One idea here is that caregivers be given an incentive to care for the clients, one example of this being a tax deduction as a supplement to financial support. Another area in which social workers can be involved is in working out a plan of care with the elderly caregiver as well as one for the infected elderly person.

Obviously, more research is also necessary in the area of older people with AIDS. There is very limited North American data on this subject. More knowledge is needed about the sexual practices of the elderly so myths can be debunked and professionals can come to realize that the elderly could be at risk for HIV/AIDS and all other sexually transmitted diseases. Research is also needed to examine the psychosocial issues of the elderly with AIDS, as they have different needs than younger people with AIDS, which are not being acknowledged. Also, caregiver roles and stress need to be examined and assessed in more detail from the perspective of those who are caregivers for people with AIDS (Gutheil & Chichin, 1991, p. 242). Especially in Canada, obtaining more information about the diffusion of AIDS among different subgroups of elderly across cultures would be useful for social workers in preparing their education and prevention efforts (Crisologo et al., 1996, p. 66).

Finally, in terms of policy implications, there is a need for social work advocacy in social, health, and organizational policies in this area. Some are those related to screening and testing patients, reporting cases, protective control measures (for example, quarantine), professional obligations (such as the duty to warn), and the extent of the client's influence over his or her treatment decisions (Crisologo et al., 1996, p. 65).

VI. Concluding Remarks

HIV/AIDS is increasing in the age group over 50, especially in the areas of drug use and heterosexual transmission. As long as the public and the elderly themselves believe that they are not at risk, and social workers and physicians do not do the appropriate risk assessments, the number of cases will increase. It is important to develop and maintain education specifically targeted at the elderly, and for social workers to become case managers to work out a plan of care for the elderly person, thereby removing that burden from the caregivers. It is also important to advocate for respite programs and other support groups and programs for these caregivers.

References

Anderson, C. & Wilkie, P. (1992). *Reflective helping in HIV and AIDS.* Philadelphia: Open University Press.

Anderson, G. (1998). Providing services to elderly people with HIV. *HIV and social work: A practitioner's guide,* 443–450. New York: Harrington Park Press.

Brabant, S. (1994). An overlooked AIDS-affected population: The elderly parent as caregiver. *Journal of Gerontological Social Work,* 22(1/2), 131–145.

Crisologo, S., Campbell, M., & Forte, J.A. (1996). Social work, AIDS and the elderly: Current knowledge and practice. *Journal of Gerontological Social Work,* 26(1/2), 49–67.

Gallant, W. & Holosko, M. (2001). Using music intervention in grief work with clients experiencing loss and bereavement. *Guidance & Counselling,* 16(4), 115–122.

Gutheil, I. & Chichin, E. (1991). AIDS, older people and social work. *Health and Social Work,* 16, 237–243.

Health and Welfare Canada. (1990). *Preparing for HIV and AIDS.* Ottawa: Canadian Association of Social Workers.

Hillman, J.L. & Stricker, G. (1998). Some issues in the assessment of HIV among older adult patients. *Psychotherapy,* 35(4), 483–489.

King, M. (1993). *AIDS, HIV and mental health.* New York: Cambridge University Press.

Levine-Perkell, J. (1996). Caregiving issues. *HIV/AIDS and the Older Adult,* pp. 115–128. New York: Taylor & Francis.

Linsk, N.L. (1994). HIV and the elderly. *Families in society: The Journal of Contemporary Human Services,* 75, 362–371.

Maclean, M. (1999). *HIV/AIDS and older people.* Ottawa: AgeWise Inc.

Nazon, M. & Levine-Perkell, J. (1996). AIDS and aging. *Journal of Gerontological Social Work,* 25, 21–31.

Puleo, J.H. (1996). Scope of the challenge. *HIV/AIDS and the older adult,* pp. 1–8. New York: Taylor & Francis.

Wyatt, A. (1996). Long-term care. *HIV/AIDS and the older adult,* pp. 81–94. New York: Taylor & Francis.

Internet Resources

amFAR AIDS Research
>An article on AIDS in seniors.
>http://www.amfar.org/cgi-bin/iowa/news/record.html?record=105

Geriatrics and Aging Canada.
  Search for HIV.
  http://geriatricsandaging.ca
Health Canada: HIV and AIDS among Older Canadians
  http://www.hc-sc.gc.ca/pphb-dgspsp/publicat/epiu-aepi/hiv-vih/older_
  e.html
The Immunodeficiency Clinic
  A Toronto clinic that provides services to persons with AIDS and HIV.
  http://www.tthhivclinic.com

Additional Readings

Brown, B. (2003). *Strengthening the Canadian strategy on HIV/AIDS*. Ottawa:
  Standing Committee on Health.
Kaufman, T. (1995). *HIV and AIDS and older people*. London: Ace Books.
Liberman, R. (2000). HIV in older Americans: An epidemiologic perspective.
  Journal of Midwifery and Women's Health, 45(2), 176–182.
Rowe, W. & Ryan, B. (1998). *Social work and HIV: The Canadian experience*.
  Toronto: Oxford University Press.

CHAPTER 12

SOCIAL WORK PRACTICE WITH RURAL ELDERLY

PATRICIA MACKENZIE

Elderly in rural areas have been described as disadvantaged, both in terms of community and individual resources. Elderly people prefer to continue meeting their needs in old age as they have throughout their lives by relying on informal exchanges with family, friends, and other members of their life-long social networks. By presenting the results of a qualitative study on elderly women residing in rural Saskatchewan, the author presents a series of implications for social work practice and the challenges currently confronting rural practitioners. It appears that rural practice will require creativity, understanding of community, and respecting and empowering elderly rural people to become involved in the development of effective systems of support.

I.   Introduction

Threats to the sustainability of rural communities is becoming an increasing concern in many parts of the world, but are particularly evident in Canada, the United States, and Australia (Cheers, 1990; Coward & Krout, 1998; Joseph & Martin Matthews, 1994; Kinsella, 2001). As local economies struggle to survive in a changing global marketplace, many rural elders live in communities that experience de-population and job loss with the resultant threat to economic and social sustainability (Bull, 1993; Coward et al., 1993; Keating, 1992; Martin Matthews, 1988).

Only limited research has examined the experiences of rural Canadian seniors. The work that has been done highlights issues that are similar to those in the American studies (Joseph & Martin Matthews, 1994). While many elderly Canadians live in an urban or suburban environment, significant portions of the total population over 65 years of age live in rural communities (Stone & Fletcher, 1986). In particular, a number of small towns, villages, and outlying areas of Canada have high proportions of elderly residents in the general population (Joseph & Cloutier, 1991). Canadian census data indicate that settlements of 1,000 to 4,999 residents had 12.9 percent of their population aged 65 and over compared to 9.7 percent for the country as a whole. At the same time, these communities had a high proportion of persons aged 80 and over—2.9 percent compared to the national figure of 1.9 percent (Statistics Canada, 1996).

"Aging in place" is now the dominant process in virtually every geographical area in Canada, although it interacts with migration in different ways in various parts of the country (Health Canada, 1998). There are significant differences across Canada in both the distribution and rates of growth of the elderly population. In some areas of the country the older residents of small towns and villages have successfully "aged in place." These communities have grown older due to the out-migration of younger populations from rural communities to larger centres. The aging of communities in other areas is often the result of the in-migration of retired people. The greatest rates of community aging can be found in areas of the country where aging in place has been augmented by in-migration. Migration effects include the out-migration of the young from some communities as well as the in-migration of the elderly to areas that are popular as retirement communities. Migration from rural to urban areas has been a significant element of change in the distribution of population in Canada for the last 150 years (Marshall & McPherson, 1994). This movement has been highly age-selective. The implication is that less mobile older people tend to accumulate and increase the rate of population aging in those areas where out-migration is strong, while those areas receiving significant in-migrant flows will tend to maintain younger populations.

Communities that provide the social setting for individual aging have been reported to have difficulty in developing or retaining adequate resources to meet the needs of older people (Cape, 1987; McCullough & Kivett, 1998). These rural communities have both a high congregation as well as a high relative concentration of elderly citizens. Congregation considers numbers of elderly people without reference to the remainder of the population. By contrast, relative concentration refers to the number of elderly people as a proportion of the total population in a community (Joseph & Martin Matthews, 1994).

A. Defining the Elusive Concept of a Rural Community

One factor that makes it difficult to evaluate the pluses and minuses of village life for older people is the lack of specificity in present definitions of rurality and debates over the nature of what is a "community." Rural is often seen as a residual concept (i.e., whatever is small is non-urban). Such descriptions have been criticized as simplistic (Glasgow et al., 1993; Krout, 1994). Rural towns and villages can differ in ways that have little to do with their population size. In order to understand the complexity of aging in a rural community, it is important to acknowledge the heterogeneity of the environments in which rural North Americans find themselves growing old.

While some authors assert that it is impossible to identify precise factors that distinguish rural from urban, others have proposed models to follow. Joseph and Martin Matthews (1994) proposed three discriminating factors to assist in this elusive definition: population size, urban proximity, and migration experience. Population size and urban proximity are easily understood, but the concept of migration experience requires further elaboration. Essentially, communities that have aged primarily through out-migration of the young or "aging in place" are believed to be substantively different from those that have become populated by an in-migration of seniors late in life. Recent studies that examine aging in rural areas tend to describe the concept of community in terms of urban proximity, migration experience, population size, and other factors that may make each community "rural."

Classifying where people live as either urban or rural results in a false dichotomy that blurs the variations that may exist within either setting. Wenger (1995) theorized that the rural elderly might live in very diverse environmental contexts even within a very small geographical area. Significant differences in experiences reported by the rural elderly have been found to exist. These appear most notably in the areas of access to various commercial or health resources and in the use of formal and informal support (Coward et al., 1993; Coward & Lee, 1985; Krout, 1994). There has also been some suggestion that the rural elderly as a group do not fare well economically. Significant socio-economic variations within the rural populations exist. Those who are old and poor have been described as experiencing a "double jeopardy" (Coward & Krout, 1998; Krout, 1994).

Ambiguity and vagueness similarly characterize the very concept of community. Attempts to delineate the exact meaning of the word have resulted in a multiplicity of definitions. Community has sometimes been understood as a group of people who share a defined geographical space, such as a neighbourhood. Community can also refer to group of people who share common traits that identify them as a unique group in society, or can refer to the emotional and sentimental characteristics of belonging to a social group. Stoneall (1983) noted that:

> in terms of locality, the rural community can be variously determined to be a small hamlet, a village or small city, an open country neighborhood, or even an entire county; but the social community, while locality connected, is of the mind; the ideational or symbolic sense of community, of belonging not only to a place but in its institutions and with its people. (p. 53)

Despite the questioning of the concept of community through the 1970s and 1980s, the idea of community is again noticeable in the social work literature. The recent approach sees community as inserted into a structural framework constituted by national political and economic structures. This approach implies that community is not independent of what is happening in the rest of society. Many recent theories of community promote the so-called "convergence perspective" and suggest that rural and urban communities are becoming homogeneous on many dimensions (Ollenburger et al., 1989; Willits et al., 1982).

Some people tend to view rural living as idyllic, peaceful, and tranquil. This does not necessarily mean that rural living is better for older people than urban living. However, for many seniors, continuing to live in a community they have come to know and love as "home" is important. A key concern for rural elders is to have the choice to stay rather than having to relocate to a place where familiar people, places, and routine would not exist. As has been pointed out by Coward and Krout (1998), rural communities in the 1990s are no longer "backwoods places" with poor housing, inadequate sanitation, and high levels of poverty. However, living in a rural community in many areas of the country does present challenges to older residents. Many rural villages are barely hanging on to basic amenities such as shops, post offices, and access to medical care.

The primary importance of staying healthy and having ready access to health care resources has been reported extensively in the literature on rural aging. Several authors have noted that providing service, both formal and informal, requires sensitivity to the challenges unique to rural health service delivery (Keating, 1992; Krout, 1998; Martin

Matthews, 1988; Pugh, 2003). Researchers in Canada, the United States, and Australia have reported on factors that inhibit access to service in a rural area (Bull, 1993; Cheers, 1990; Hodge, 1993). These may include physical barriers such as bad weather, geographic isolation, or poor roads. Other factors that have been reported in the literature as frequent barriers to rural service delivery include the declining economy of many rural areas, the lack of available trained service providers, and inadequate supports for family caregivers (Bull, 1993). Transportation has also been reported in many studies as a critical factor to rural service delivery (Schmidt, 2000). In many areas of the country, the limited availability of public transportation means rural elderly people are limited in their ability to access the range of services that are more available in urban communities.

These combined factors may mean that in many rural communities in North America, the rural elderly often find themselves literally beyond the reach of some services. The availability of formal services, health professionals, and other practitioners is obviously less in rural areas of the province than in urban centres. If any rural resident experiences a severe illness or injury that requires significant intervention on the part of the health care system, that intervention must usually be provided in a community some distance from the rural resident's home. Due to the recent consolidation of some health and support resources by many provincial (and state) governments, it is usually no longer possible for the life-long residents of small communities to remain living in the village that has been their home for so long. If an older person requires ongoing medical attention or residential care, relocation to the nearest [hopefully] larger centre with the associated richer resources and service capabilities is usually required. This new location may be a little as little as a few miles away from the previous village. However, without independent access to transportation for her or her age peer network, the new location might as well be one hundred miles away.

B. An Example of Growing Older in Rural Saskatchewan

A strong system of informal support exists for older residents of rural communities. In an in-depth qualitative study conducted by the author in rural Saskatchewan (MacKenzie, 1999), almost all of the respondents were able to describe their involvement with a varied, responsive, and resourceful social network. The members of this informal support system certainly included family, but friends and neighbours, as well as professional caregivers (non-peer/family supports), were declared by the respondents to be invaluable members of their support network. Of particular interest was that all respondents had at least one member of their large kin network living in close proximity, and thereby available for support and assistance. More often than not, most respondents had several other kin members close by and reported feeling well supported and involved in a large and caring family. This family support network was supplemented by [a] connection to a large network of friends and neighbours. Some forms of social support can be provided by almost anyone, including professionals, community agency workers, and perhaps strangers. However, most social support derives from those with whom one has an enduring relationship, primarily family and friends.

The findings from this study suggested that the older residents of these small Prairie villages were well integrated into their respective communities. Women expressed a certain pride and satisfaction in acknowledging that they were "well known" by people in the village and that they "knew most everyone." This led them to state that they felt "visible" in their communities and were comfortable with the familiarity this social integration into community brought to them. For the most part, the older women interviewed for this study considered their particular rural community to be a "good place" to live. This feeling of affinity for place and a positive perspective on a rural lifestyle has been noted in other studies on rural aging (Cape, 1987; Joseph, 1992). The majority of the women in the author's study reported feeling very safe in their respective communities. This sense of personal safety was a major theme that emerged from the data. Women in the study reported feeling particularly comfortable with the visibility, familiarity, and relative proximity to others that accompanies living in a small community. A repeated sentiment was "everyone knows everyone here and we look out for each other." The implication is that if a "malicious stranger" came to town or "mischief/tragedy/accidents" occurred, people would notice and would intervene to protect and support vulnerable members of the community. However, the women also noted that without a vibrant and sustainable rural community, fewer and fewer people would be available to provide this sense of safety and comfort.

This sense of security also contains a number of additional dimensions, all of which were key to the personal well-being of these older women. Unlike other studies, the women in Saskatchewan expressed tremendous satisfaction with their sense of financial security. None of the women considered herself to be "currently poor." All respondents had a mix of both private investment income and Canadian government pensions. With these resources, the women stated they were able to manage to meet their personal expenses without difficulty. As one woman put it "I've been through worse than this on less than pension pay." One benefit to personal financial security for these women was the ability to act a benefactor to family members and charitable enterprises. This ability to give money was something women reported as helping them to "feel good about themselves." In fact, when directly asked in the in-depth interviews to describe how they felt they made a contribution to others, almost all responded by relating incidents of how they made financial bequests. Sadly, none were able to relate to the concept that they were also contributors to social relationships such as "adviser, volunteer, friend, neighbour, supporter, etc." A few offered the opinion that they might be important to their family as "mother/ grandmother/great-grandmother," but most were fairly self-effacing and minimized the social value of such involvement.

In essence, the women in this Saskatchewan study echoed the findings of other studies on older rural women and social support (Kivett & McCullough, 1998; Shenk, 1987). Many of the women perceived of their village as a "community of communion." Several had been born and raised nearby or had relocated to the area as very young women. For them, the local village and surrounding area was "home" and "home" is where they want to stay. However, the intent of these women to "stay put" and "manage on my own" way was dependent on a number of factors. These conditions included having good health, having a positive attitude, and having adequate resources such as proximate social supports.

C. Roles for Rural Gerontological Social Work

1. Animating, Coordinating, and Supporting Social Networks
There is minimal data that report exactly who a rural senior would choose as the most suitable resource to meet any unmet need. Older people have rarely been consulted about what they think of existing resources, how to improve current programs, or how to meet new needs. It is in this information vacuum that social work practise with elderly people in rural areas occurs.

The body of literature on social support and social networks has grown in recent years. Having readily available social support systems is essential to the well-being of elderly people. Previous research has examined the relationships between social support systems and a number of health factors (Ezell & Gibson, 1989; Keating & Fast, 1997; Phillips et al., 2000). These studies found that social support is important for promoting health and well-being and buffering stress. They suggested that social systems of support, if defined broadly as structured human attachments among kin, neighbours, friends, and members of voluntary associations, may represent one of the largest form of health care. An individual's social network may be best understood as a set of personal contacts through which s/he can receive emotional support, maintain social identity, obtain material aid or services, and access new social contacts. Supporting factors that make for an effective and healthy caregiver/care receiver relationship include feelings of closeness, mutual respect, security, and comfort in the interaction. With regard to the frail elderly, social support systems have been found to be effective mechanisms for providing tangible goods, information, and instrumental help with activities of daily living.

A fairly large body of work exists on the social support provided by friends to aged people and on the effect of such support on well-being (Fischer, 1993; Greenberg et al., 1999). Many rural seniors who have "aged in place" have had life-long relationships with age-peer friends. These social relationships developed over time and there is both continuity and stability to them. The women in the Saskatchewan study reported that these relationships developed through the performance of roles such as spouse, parent, worker, friend, and neighbour. The people who made up their social networks may have changed over time. Factors such as shifts in role responsibilities, finances, residential mobility, and the personal properties of the members of the "support" convoy (age, gender, health status) all interact in these evolving life-scripted networks. All of these factors jointly determine both a person's requirements for social support at any given time and the adequacy of the support convoy to respond to such demands. The relative position of the older person to other members in the convoy may have shifted more to the passive rather than active, but these social networks based on life-long associations certainly exist in rural communities. The associations with the greatest value are those that have a high degree of continuity, familiarity, and stability. The "currencies" used by older people to maintain their social exchanges in these non-kin social relationships appear to be the provision of practical aid, companionship, and a sense of shared history. The "currency" exchanges in kin relationships appear to be related to sharing of both tangible resources (money and other goods and services) and a sense of belonging or kinship.

Current literature on kinship networks and social support tends to both encourage and question the notion that the social environments of both urban and rural seniors contain untapped resources that can be harnessed to meet social needs and relieve social distress. Rural spouses and adult children are likely to have other kin members available to assist them with caregiving duties (Keating, 1992). However, these primary caregivers have been found to face personal costs similar to those of urban caregivers such as high levels of stress, a decrease in social network size, lack of respite services, and feelings of guilt and loss (Martin Matthews, 1988). Cape (1987) suggested "rurality, added to incapacity, may lead to premature institutionalization for older people" (p. 51). Given the greater life expectancy of women, it is reasonable to expect that rural widowed, divorced, or single women are particularly vulnerable. The problems of aging are further complicated for women by the fact that they often outlive their helping network of family, friends, and neighbours. An older person's ability to remain in the community is threatened when there is an absence or erosion of such social supports.

Greenberg et al. (1999) found that the number of emotionally close local friends reported by elderly women to be present in their social network convoys were positively related to well-being. This sentiment was also found in the Saskatchewan study. Age-peer friends played a major role in the happiness and life satisfaction of rural older women. The respondents in this study reported that it was much easier for them to both give and receive support from the individuals with whom they had a long-term relationship. Specifically, respondents named other older women as the people they viewed as those they preferred to rely upon for instrumental and emotional support. This reliance on support from age peers has been noted in other studies of relationships in old age (Phillips et al., 2000; Shenk, 1987). Same age peers, particularly those from similar cultural backgrounds or local environments, may have a shared perspective and therefore understand each other better. Interestingly, their feeling of immediate well-being was found to be influenced more favourably by time spent with friends rather than by time spent with family. However, these women also admitted that family contacts provided more stable sources of practical and physical support than friends can, and that these benefits add to their overall well-being.

Gerontologists have often characterized progression from the middle to the later years of life as a series of losses of roles and choices. However, one needs to question the view that older people suffer "role loss" as years go by. Elderly persons usually have few "required" contacts with the general community. Instead, they associate on a daily basis primarily with people they know and who know them. Typically, then, they continue to function in their usual roles within the family and in their network of friends—they are just older, as are many of the other people involved in these social exchanges.

The Saskatchewan study suggested that the roles older women occupied in rural communities did not appear to the young or to the outsider to be of "great status." On a few occasions, the older women also seemed to share this perception. Other women in the study stated that they "were as involved as they had ever been" in various social roles. It seemed that most of the respondents were well integrated into the community and occupied the same roles as a family member and friend that they had occupied for many years. Friendship was one such enduring role and was seen by the respondents as an important factor that contributed to their overall well-being and gave them a sense of personal worth and value. During the course of the data-gathering process, it was observed that rural older women appeared to rely on individuals in their life-long friendship circles for affirmation of their self-worth as well as conviviality. A spirit of true "sisterhood" seemed to exist between the women in this study and other age peers who had experienced similar life events and processes over the years.

2. Working with Families

The available literature on family networks and family supports of the rural elderly suggests that most aid is provided in a family-based environment (Kivett, 1990). Non-familial informal support also exists for large numbers of elderly people. Such support can confer social, emotional, and functional benefits to elderly women. Non-familial informal supports are most commonly friends and neighbours, but also include clergy and social acquaintances. As well, formal service providers such as home health aides, social workers, and local merchants may participate in the informal network of an elder by providing social support or concrete assistance that is not integral to their formal or customary roles.

It has been reported that a strong sense of familial obligation, personal regard, and trust exists between elders and their families (Black, 1985; Kivett, 1988; McCullough, 1998). However, this may not be the case for everyone. Reports of domestic violence and severe conflict between seniors and their adult children are not uncommon. Support and counselling programs for elders experiencing these stresses in rural areas are rare. In fact, such resources are not readily available to anyone in many rural communities. The mental health systems appear ill prepared to deal with the intergenerational issues that accompany an aging population. As well, caregiver support, respite care, and adult day care programs may be readily available in urban centres in North America, but few such programs exist in rural communities.

As noted by Keating (1992), the provision of aid by family members, although appealing, involves cost to both caregivers and recipients. Typically, women are on both sides of the caregiving equation. As older women age, responsibility for meeting their escalating need for assistance is likely to fall to another woman—usually daughters who are aging themselves [see Chapter 19]. Many authors have criticized as unrealistic and ungrounded the belief that informal social support systems contain untapped resources that individuals can activate at the "drop of a hat" (Beggs et al., 1996; Ehrlich, 1985; Keating & Fast, 1997). Questions are beginning to emerge in the literature concerning the way interdependency, equity, and obligation enter into the "give and take" of supportive networks. The relationships among persons in any given social support system are both dynamic and complex. Social workers have much to offer in terms of providing counselling and educational programs to elders and their families.

3. Revisiting Community Social Work, Developing and Coordinating Community Programs
While professional care continues to be the exception rather than the norm when it comes to the provision of day-to-day support and basic caregiving for rural elders, there is a need to provide access to health and social programs for rural elders. The likelihood of a rural older person requesting access to formal care is mediated by many factors. These include "intrinsic" factors such as the views people hold on the acceptability of asking "whom" for "what kind" of assistance, delivered in "what way." Other factors are more "extrinsic" and include household structure, socio-economic circumstances, and the nature and availability of a "user-friendly" formal social support system in rural areas. Other studies have reported that the rural elderly use more informal helpers, and fewer paid helpers provide assistance with fewer instrumental activities of daily living (Coward et al., 1990; McLaughlin & Jensen, 1993). These studies have suggested that while this may reflect the preferences of rural elders, it may also reflect the relatively limited availability of formal services. Other research has demonstrated that service providers have often found that rural elderly may resist formal

services because they want to avoid getting caught up in bureaucracy and perhaps lose some control over their life (Cockerham, 1997).

The women in Saskatchewan said that they would prefer to get help from their informal networks and would like to be able "pick and choose" the formal services they require. These women [like many other people] seemed to prefer care-receiving situations that had elements of reciprocity, which allowed them to preserve their independence and honoured their resilience. In this way, the women were responding to my questions in ways that were similar to other research (Kivett, 1985; Sherr & Blumhardt, 2002). For example, the women in my study who obtained assistance from friends and neighbours seemed to have a clearer sense of "what amount" and "what kind" of assistance from friends and neighbours is/was acceptable. They were generally more comfortable if there had been some ongoing reciprocal relationship where they had previously been of assistance to the other party.

The women in this study also acknowledged that circumstances might arise that would make support from the informal networks of family and friends no longer accessible or suitable for their needs. All agreed that having locally available help from the formal sector would be desirable, but stressed that this involvement would be a "last resort." This reluctance to become involved with the formal care system has also been reported elsewhere in the literature (Keating & Fast, 1997). The principle of frontierism, independent living, and "rugged individualism" has been described as one of the central tenets of rural ideology. Shenk (1987) completed an interesting study and found that older rural women placed certain conditions on participating in formal programs. She found that older rural women would participate if the program would:

a)   meet their needs without involving them in elaborate social service systems,
b)   not associate them with welfare programmes, and
c)   not pose a threat to their control over their own environments. (p. 3)

Krout (1988) noted that rural elders placed a high value on independence, but often happen to live in environments that make it difficult to maintain that independence. Many of the older women in the Saskatchewan study certainly exhibited features of rugged individualism. Most were very reluctant to see themselves as recipients of help and appeared reluctant to become involved with formal home support programs unless it was "absolutely necessary." As has been noted elsewhere (Cockerham, 1997; Phillips et al., 2000), the single most important determinant of the quality of an elderly person's life is health. Health matters affect all other areas of life, including social roles and relationships.

The women in Saskatchewan certainly understood that their ability to live independently in a rural community was dependent on "keeping well." It should come as no surprise, then, that these older rural women considered themselves to be "very lucky to have their health." Stoller (1984) suggested that:

> older persons may expect a decline in health as they age, but when the deterioration does not take place at the rate or to the extent they had anticipated, they may begin to assess their health above the rating they would assign to their peers. (p. 262)

It is also understandable that these women may indeed "underreport" any health concerns. For these women, there seemed to be the attitude that admitting to poor health may lead others to assume their health needs were significant enough to warrant an intervention. As these interventions might curtail their activities or lead to relocation to a care facility, the women typically claimed that "I keep my aches and pains to myself." All respondents agreed that "having your health" was essential to living successfully and independently in their respective village. The fact that they had survived into late old age in a relatively healthy condition when others have not encourages them to feel that they can be positive about their health.

The data certainly suggested that, by and large, these older women would rather see themselves as "able" rather than "disabled," "well" rather than "ill," and "participant in" rather than "recipient of" supportive interactions in social networks. In other words, the social consequences of reporting poor health or physical problems for older women often seemed to mean to them that they would lose some measure of independence and therefore lose personal control over their day-to-day lifestyles and decisions. Regular family contact from both proximal and distant kin was reported as important. However, it appeared that on occasion, families were much more enthusiastic to provide assistance than the older women were about receiving such help! And during the course of some interviews, respondents admitted to performing certain tasks in their own homes that they believed were sure to be viewed with alarm by family members! These tasks were usually associated with activities that might put the older woman at some physical risk. Such perceived "risk-taking" activities included getting in and out of the bathtub without help, climbing up and down basement stairs, or standing on chairs to wash windows, change lightbulbs, or get things down from high cupboards. These generally fiercely independent women stressed that they were not about to waste their days "standing around waiting" for someone to lend a hand with these tasks and would rarely "put someone out" by asking for help.

It appears from these stories that these older women were exercising their right to live with a certain measure of risk. Many implied that discussions around these issues had occurred between themselves and their families and the women more or less decided that the less the caregiving family knew about their "risk-taking behaviour," the better it would be for the whole family. While grateful for the concern the adult children expressed over their well-being, many women claimed that their families "worried too much"! The most successful family relationships seemed to be those in which extended family members were prepared to live with a certain degree of discomfort over whether "mother" was "all right." In fact, it seemed that many families had learned "not to interfere too much" with the older women's "ways" and choose to err on the side of valour rather caution when intervening or offering to do some particular task. However, this "opportunity" for them to live "at risk" seemed dependent on the relative physical vigour of the respondent. Several of the women were really quite fit and they were the ones who claimed that they still "did whatever they damn well pleased"!

As noted by Keating and Fast (1997), increasing emphasis is placed on keeping seniors in the community. The goal of government has become helping seniors to remain at home and involved with their informal networks. Keating and Fast (1997) pointed out that:

> Over the last twenty years ... health and social services for elderly people have stressed the importance of moving from institutionally-based provision to community based care. This shift (is) explained in both humanitarian and economic terms: elderly people are thought to prefer being cared for in their own homes and care in the community is ... thought to be less expensive than in hospitals, nursing homes and chronic care facilities. As governments have been increasingly driven by deficit reduction and cost-cutting objectives, community care has been embraced with mounting urgency ... it is presented as

an uncontroversial, sensible way of responding to elderly people's
needs while also averting demographic and fiscal crisis." (p. 3)

It is a concern that decreased spending on social programs by
government creates situations that marginalize older persons. This
age of economic restructuring and devolution of previously available
"safety net programs" create anxiety and suffering for those elderly
who are without accumulated assets and non-work-related incomes.

4. Research on Rural Aging

There is still much that we do not know about other older women's
lives, attitudes, and experiences. For example, little is known about
the experiences of older First Nations women, older women who more
recently immigrated to Canada, older lesbians, or other older women
who chose to live their lives in non-traditional ways. Conducting
studies that involve a more diverse pool of informants would help to
fill in the gaps of the existing knowledge base. Social workers are well
equipped to become engaged in such research.

Studies about older women would also benefit from incorporating
multiple data gathering procedures and using triangulations of method.
There would be great value in providing a more active role for the
informants at every point in the research design, perhaps using focus
groups and participatory action research methods.

Although families, friends, community groups, and agencies
provide an array of supports to the rural elderly, additional data
on the composition and nature of such support systems is required
(Krout, 1994). Minimal research has been conducted on differences in
community size and informal support systems. In addition, the use of
friends for assistance among the elderly has been studied very little.
Other studies have found that while the rural elderly seem aware
of formal services, their use of these services may be quite minimal
(Ehrlich, 1985; McCullough & Kivett, 1998). Distance from formal
services is a major concern for the rural elderly, particularly when
coupled with terrain, weather, and the lack of public transportation
systems. Krout (1988) discovered that the rural elderly are less
knowledgeable about available social services and are often resistant to
accepting what help that does exist. Very few people feel comfortable
being the "passive recipient" of care and attention. For example, in
the Saskatchewan sample, most respondents expressed a reluctance to
accept offers of rides to places *unless* they could "pay something." This
usually meant that they insisted on offering cash to the "volunteer."

This action/reaction of an offer of a lift versus an insistence on the part of the older woman to contribute financially is just one example of how resource exchange was seen to take place between people in these rural communities.

Most were fearful of "being a burden" to their family. Several described the impact on their self-worth when they came to the realization that they were no longer able to do a particular task on their own. Most stated that it was only after they had exhausted all other creative solutions to the problem that they accepted the position of acting as a recipient of help. Few admitted feeling comfortable with the position. Given the above, we certainly have our research work "cut out for us" as a profession.

5. Family Counselling and Grief Work

The women in my study keenly felt the repetitive loss of "old-time friends." The losses of old friends to death or relocation out of the community (usually to obtain care not available in the under-resourced rural settings) meant that their peer network was shrinking each year. The diminishing size of a network of long-time friends and associates has implications for the continued well-being of those who remain behind. Several respondents reported that this component of their social networks had become less able to provide the quantity and quality of social contacts that had previously been enjoyed. A diminishing of resources in any social support system has a deleterious effect on the ability to continue to manage to live on their own in a rural aging community.

Finally, while expressing a preference for continuing to live in a small community, many of the respondents expressed concerns about the continued viability of rural Saskatchewan in general. In order to discuss the social policy implications that arose from this study [many of which can be generalized to other rural communities], three questions will be addressed in the remainder of this chapter:

1. Can rural communities survive?
2. What is the role of older people in rural communities? and
3. What do rural communities need in order to provide adequate supports to an increasingly aging population?

The implications for these questions hopefully will shape a more evidenced-based approach to rural gerontological practice.

(a) Can Rural Communities Survive?

As has been noted, community is a complex term that can have several meanings. As a geographic term, community refers to particular locales or settlements. Community can also refer to localized social and political systems, or to the social network of a particular locality. Community may also be used to refer to a certain quality of human relationships such as feelings of identity, mutuality, and affinity that may not depend on physical proximity but often do. Traditional concepts of community are based on life-long residence in one locale, tight and well-defined geographic or ethnic boundaries, frequent face-to-face interactions, and an ordered set of common experiences, allegiances, and roles (Beggs et al., 1996; Schmidt, 2000).

Despite rural de-population, it can be expected that many Canadians of all ages will continue to reside in rural regions. However, there have been significant changes to rural settlements over the past century. Older people are very cognizant of the changes that have occurred over their lifetimes. A strong affinity "for place" was an essential ingredient for the personal and social well-being of these rural women. Meaningful connections to people and place are the essence of what rural communities have to offer. These women hold valuable historical information in their memories, little of which is being recorded by others. As the "knowledge bearers" of the historical roots of the province, it would be a wonderful idea to involve rural school children in oral history projects. In this way, younger people can learn of this particular view of the history of Saskatchewan and other rural communities in North America. The relationships that might emerge from these intergenerational contacts could have mutual benefit to senior and child alike.

(b) What Is the Role of Older People in Rural Communities?

Several studies have been done which seek to discover the opinions of older persons on what services are most important to them. These studies have identified the following key concerns:

- *Housing:* Many studies identify the preference for seniors to remain in their own home and community for as long as their health needs are safely met.
- *Independence:* Seniors treasure their independence, including privacy, just as much as the rest of the population. Even limited reliance on family members for care can evoke

feelings of indebtedness that conflict with the senior's ideal self-image of being independent and self-reliant.

- *Choice:* The ability to make choices is also important. Within the context of care and the elderly, choice implies that informal caregivers "are seen to do their caring work by choice and that elderly people are seen to choose to rely on them" (McCullough & Kivett, 1998). According to these same authors, the possibility of choice is greatest where financial resources are sufficient to purchase services on the market, a spouse is present and in reasonably good health, and the care needs of the elderly person are minimal.

- *Socialization and caregiving and receiving:* Socialization and support networks are essential to the emotional well-being of all, and the elderly are no exception. The support relationships among seniors tend to be mutually beneficial and based on equal partnerships. Aging must be thought of in terms of the crucial roles that elders play in their kinship and community groups.

- *Planned dependency:* Due to diverse losses, the elderly tend to make decisions about which activities they will prioritize for energy investment. According to this study, what is important is to generate social supports and other aids that acknowledge loss in capacity but also permit individuation and selective optimization.

One must ask whether policy-makers and service planners are really paying attention to what the data indicate. Elderly people in rural communities are rarely consulted or allowed to assume responsibility for charting their own futures and/or creating services that reflect their needs and desires. Like many other places in North America, Saskatchewan has a predominant pattern of designing service systems in a "top-down" managerial style. Many expensive service delivery systems have been organized around a medical model of care and intervention. A model of service delivery that addresses social as well as physical needs and is based on a consultative approach has largely been ignored to date.

The paternalistic and "expert"-led policy and program development approach needs to be changed. One specific recommendation from my study was to create opportunities to have seniors involved in the process of developing social and health policy, particularly in areas where the decisions made can directly affect their lives. This would involve getting together a number of seniors and others and having them co-construct a system of community care that would make sense to current and prospective consumers. Many community-based services have successfully used the "well" senior as a volunteer to deliver Meals-on-Wheels, act as peer counsellors, and the like. We also need to make places for seniors in the planning and decision-making boardrooms as well.

(c) What Do Rural Communities Need in Order to Provide Adequate Support to an Increasingly Aging Population?
Similar to other places, rural Saskatchewan faces formidable barriers to the provision of services to elderly people who live outside the core urban areas. The reasons for this are similar to those that have been reported elsewhere (Krout, 1994). These include low population density, lack of economies of scale, lack of financial or human capital, an urban bias in government funding, and a view that there is a culture of self-reliance in rural communities that leads individuals to eschew formal services for informal supports. The remainder of this chapter will discuss recommendations for improving services for the aging residents of rural Saskatchewan. This section will address modifications or reinforcement of the current service systems as well as proposing some services that do not currently exist in rural regions of the province.

Seniors have been described as heavy users of health services (Bull, 1993; Keating, 1992). However, the women in my study appeared to make only infrequent trips to physicians. Few had experienced recent hospitalizations and most had only limited involvement with home health care. When asked about any health care concerns, the women identified four related issues as troublesome.

The first related to difficulties *accessing* physicians, particularly specialists. It was relatively easy for these rural women to get medical attention if they could wait until the physician arrived at the local health centre on his/her weekly visit, or if they could travel to the doctor's office. However, getting to see a specialist, having an eye examination, or seeing a dentist or a surgeon, means travelling to the city.

The second issue raised was *access to preventive* or "maintenance" health care services. Many of the women had various health concerns that they believed "weren't serious enough to bother the doctor about." Several stated that they did want information or support about health maintenance strategies. Several women had questions about breast self-examination, control of blood pressure, diet, exercise, and other issues related to self-care. When I asked about access to the local health nurse, most reported that the rural nurses were too busy looking after "the really sick" and were not available to them. One community had a nurse who ran a weekly "wellness clinic" in the senior activity centre. Indeed the women who used that service found it extremely helpful.

The third [and most pressing concern] was related to the recent consolidation or *closure of small hospitals and long-term care services* in rural regions. This concern has been raised elsewhere in the literature and is presented again here to highlight the importance of this issue to older rural residents.

The fourth and final concern was the *relative absence of community-based programs* that went beyond the usual array of homemaking help and home care nursing. There was no adult day programming, little respite care, and only marginal mental health service available in rural Saskatchewan. These gaps in service are being acutely felt in many rural communities and it can be expected that this situation will remain problematic. Significant evidence exists that rural settlements will continue to have escalating numbers of aging residents while at the same time losing younger populations. The net result of this is increasing numbers of persons who need care and decreasing numbers of people to provide it. However, the rural community may be so small and have very few persons in need at any one time. Full-scale "age-specific" programs are usually not viable. However, the needs of elders and their caregivers may be similar to those of other populations. For example, visiting nurses and support groups are both services that are used by many age groups. If these services already exist, they can be adapted to fit the needs of both the rural elder/caregiver and other members of the rural community.

II. *Some Recommendations*

Several recommendations that specifically identify services or resources that would benefit rural seniors include:

1. *Provide financial and/or other incentives for physicians, particularly specialist and allied health professionals (e.g., physiotherapy, occupational therapy, dentists/denturists, optometrists, podiatrists, and mental health practitioners), to provide enhanced services to residents.* While it is unlikely that personnel will relocate to rural communities, mobile clinics could be arranged that would bring the specialist personnel to rural regions on a regular basis.

2. *Introduce health technology to rural regions.* An interesting
    and exciting idea that is becoming increasingly popular
    in both the United States and Australia is the notion of
    telemedicine. Much of the technological infrastructure exists
    already. For instance, both Saskatchewan universities use
    the Saskatchewan Telecommunications Network to deliver a
    variety of university credit courses to students in rural and
    remote areas. Since the province is well served by satellite
    television transmission and there is a medical school in
    Saskatoon, rural general practitioners could be taught and
    supported to deliver services to rural residents. In this way,
    procedures could be done that would otherwise require
    rural residents to travel to the large urban centres where
    most specialist practitioners usually congregate.
3. *Create opportunities for nurse health practitioners, rather than
    doctors, to provide significant preventive and maintenance
    health services.* For example, the School of Nursing at the
    University of Saskatchewan could be encouraged to begin to
    offer nursing education to residents of rural communities,
    thereby training personnel on "their home ground" with the
    hope that they would remain in their rural community to
    practise. It would only take a relatively minimal expenditure
    of funds to make a nurse practitioner service available. The
    physical setting for the delivery of such care could be in the
    local health clinic for communities that have such facilities.
    Other communities could use the senior centre or the local
    parish church, a vastly under-used building in many rural
    communities.
4. *Provide funding for locally available adult day care programs.*
    This would be particularly beneficial to the residents
    of rural communities who are socially isolated or those
    who are providing family care to the physically frail or
    cognitively impaired older person. Once again, adult day
    care programs could operate from the local church or
    church hall or one of the abandoned school buildings that
    are increasingly obvious in many rural communities. In
    addition to professional and paraprofessional personnel, the
    programs could be expanded to provide a role for volunteer
    counsellors, some of whom may be "young seniors" who
    could be trained in a peer-counselling model.

5. *Reconsider the closure and consolidation of nursing home beds in rural communities like Saskatchewan.* Examine the possibility of having a few beds remain open for short-term use, such as "swing beds" or for overnight care, to support caregivers who can manage an older person during the day but need respite at night.

    If it is really not feasible to have even a few beds available in rural communities, consider developing adult foster care homes (both family and non-family based). Creating such a service in small villages would allow rural residents to receive the care they need within their home communities. Funding adult foster care would also provide a source of employment and income to care providers.

6. *Develop a cost-shared or publicly funded transportation service to enable rural residents to travel to nearby or distant communities for both medical appointments and social opportunities.* Mobility is clearly a key to quality of life for the rural elderly, but many of them are dependent upon others for transportation. The women in this study raised lack of access to public transportation as a major concern. Without transportation services, their experience of independent living in rural communities appeared to be "isolation living." None of the communities even operated something as simple as a taxi service and it was therefore not possible for women to even hire a ride when required. This issue has been reported in other rural regions (Kinsella, 2001; Schmidt, 2000). Transportation is not important in and of itself but because of the services to which it provides access. The problems with adequate transportation essentially mean that rural residents are in position of dependence on those with private transport and reliant upon having the courage and determination to ask for lifts from family, friends, or acquaintances. A partially subsidized or private transportation service with reliable and predictable hours of operation would be a boon to the independence of rural seniors.

7. *Enhance caregiver support groups.* In rural communities this could involve churches, senior centres, and/or local health care personnel. Rural families who experience emotional distress often find it difficult to find the time and energy to attend groups in person. However, many rural families,

such as the ones in Saskatchewan, are using computers for both business (cyber-farming) and pleasure. Developing Internet "chat rooms" or funding a 1-800 telephone line may facilitate access to such support. Volunteer peer or non-peer counsellors could also manage both of these resources in part.

8. *Expand the range of housing options in rural communities.* While many small Canadian communities have a seniors' lodge (small self-contained apartments that share a common recreational space), they do not meet the coming needs for alternate accommodation. At present, the elderly residents of most rural communities can either live in their own houses, live with children, or occupy one of the few apartments in "the lodge." Many urban centres have developed a range of sheltered accommodation for older people such as free-hold or "life-lease" condominiums, "Abbeyfield-style" housing, "granny houses" erected on the property of adult children, home sharing, etc. Little of this has been done in rural Canada. Given the increasing numbers of rural residents who intend to age in place, it appears that the time is ripe for the development of new housing options in rural settings.

III. Conclusion

The voices of the women in this study challenge policymakers to make a commitment to create (or recreate) and implement innovative patterns of community life that reflect the new realities of rural living and that serve the diverse interests of the rural community. Given the aging of the population, there is a need to more fully explore the rich variety of experiences of older women before it is too late and these women have departed from our lives. Outcomes from this study provide valuable new information and the opportunity to understand more fully the choices, constraints, and context under which the older female residents of rural Saskatchewan communities conduct their lives. Most importantly, the study findings allow the soon-to-be disappearing voices of our elders to be heard. Their voices reminded me to treasure both the historical successes and the present opportunities of this rural province. Their challenge to all of us is to work to retain the commitment they have had to others, to community, and to the land. The women in this study believed that accepting this commitment will enable people to continue to experience their community as a vibrant, healthy, and compassionate place in which to live well and age successfully. Hopefully, social workers working with the rural elderly may benefit from these experiences.

References

Beggs, J., Haines, V., & Hurlbert, J. (1996). Revisiting the rural-urban contrast: Personal networks in non-metropolitan and metropolitan settings. *Rural Sociology*, 61(2), 306–325.

Black. M. (1985). Health and social support of older adults in the community. *Canadian Journal on Aging*, 4(4), 213–226.

Bull, C.N. (1993). *Aging in rural America*. Newbury Park: Sage.

Cape, E. (1987). Aging women in rural settings. In W. Marshall (ed.), *Aging in Canada: Social perspectives*, 2nd ed. Toronto: Fitzhenry & Whiteside.

Cheers, B. (1990). Rural disadvantage. *Australian Social Work*, 43(1).

Cockerham, W.C. (1997). *This aging society*, 2nd ed. Englewood Cliffs: Prentice-Hall.

Coward, R.T. (1987). Poverty and aging in rural America. *Human Services in the Rural Environment*, 10, 41–47.

Coward, R.T. & Cutler, S.J. (1989). Informal and formal health care systems for the rural elderly. *Health Services Research*, 23, 785–806.

Coward, R.T., Cutler, S.J., & Mullens, L. (1990). Residential differences in the comparisons of helping networks of impaired elders. *Family Relations*, 39, 44–50.

Coward, R.T., Horne, C., & Dwyer, J.W. (1992). Demographic perspectives on gender and family caregiving. In J.W. Dwyer & R.T. Coward (eds.), *Gender, families and elder care*. Newbury Park: Sage.

Coward, R.T. & Krout, J. (1998). *Aging in rural settings: Life circumstances and distinctive features*. New York: Springer.

Coward, R.T. & Lee, G.R. (eds.). (1985). *The elderly in rural society: Every forth elder*. New York: Springer.

Coward, R.T., Lee, G.R., Dwyer, J., & Seccombe, K. (1993). *Old and alone in rural America*. American Association of Retired Persons. Washington: Public Policy Institute.

Cullen, T., Dunn, P., & Lawrence, G. (1990). *Rural health and welfare in Australia*. Centre for Rural Health Research. Charles Stuart University-Riverina.

Ehrlich, P. (1985). Informal support networks meet health needs of rural elderly. *Journal of Gerontological Social Work*, 9, 85–97.

Fischer, L.R. (1993). The oldest-old in rural Minnesota. In C. Neil Bull (ed.), *Aging in rural America.* Newbury Park: Sage.

Glasgow, N., Holden, K., McLaughlin, D., & Rowles, G. (1993). The rural elderly and Poverty. *Rural Sociological Society Reports.* Boulder: Westside.

Greenberg, S., Motenko A., Roesch, C., & Embelton, N. (1999). Friendship across the life cycle: A support group for older women. *Journal of Gerontological Social Work,* 32(4), 7–23.

Health Canada. (1998). *Fact book on aging in Canada.* Ottawa: Minister of Supply and Services.

Joseph, A.E. (1992). On the importance of place in studies of rural aging. *Journal of Rural Studies,* 8(1), 111–119.

Joseph, A. & Cloutier, D.S. (1991). Elderly migration and its implications for service provision in rural communities: An Ontario perspective. *Journal of Rural Studies,* 7(4), 433–444.

Joseph, A. & Martin Matthews, A. (1994). Growing old in aging communities. In V. Marshall & B. McPherson (eds.), *Aging: Canadian perspectives.* Peterborough: Broadview Press.

Keating, Norah C. (1992). *Aging in rural Canada.* Toronto: Butterworths.

Keating, N.C. & Fast, J.E. (1997). Bridging policy and research in eldercare. *Canadian Journal on Aging,* 16(supplement), 22–41.

Kinsella, K. (2001). Urban and rural dimensions of global populations aging: An overview. *The Journal of Rural Health,* 17(4), 314–322.

Kivett, V. (1990). Older rural women. *Journal of Rural Community Psychology,* 11, 83–102.

Korte, C. (1990). The elderly in rural environments. *Journal of Rural Studies,* 4, 103–114.

Krout, J. (ed.). (1994). *Providing community based services to the rural elderly.* Thousand Oaks: Sage.

Krout, J.A. (1983). *The rural elderly: An annotated bibliography of social science research.* Westport: Greenwood Press.

Krout, J.A. (1986). *The aged in rural America.* Westport: Greenwood Press.

MacKenzie, P.A. (1999). Ageing in place in ageing communities: Elderly women's accounts of growing older in rural Saskatchewan. Unpublished Ph.D. dissertation, University of Edinburgh, Edinburgh, Scotland.

Marshall, V.D. & McPherson, B. (eds.). (1994). *Aging: Canadian perspectives.* Peterborough: Broadview Press.

Martin Matthews, A. (1988). Aging in rural Canada. In E. Rathbone-McCuan & B. Havers (eds.), *North American elders: United States and Canadian perspectives.* Westport: Greenwood Press.

McCulloch, J. & Kivett, V. (1998). Older rural women: Aging in historical and current contexts. In R.T. Coward & J. Krout (eds.), *Aging in rural settings: Life circumstances and distinctive features.* New York: Springer.

McLaughlin D.K. & Jensen, L. (1993). Poverty among older Americans: The plight on non-metropolitan elders. *Journal of Gerontology: Social Sciences,* 48, S44–S54.

Ollenburger, J., Grana, S., & Moore, H. (1989). Labor force participation of rural farm, rural non-farm, and urban women: A panel update. *Rural Sociology,* 54, 533–550.

Phillips, J., Bernard, M., Phillipson, C., & Ogg, J. (2000). Social support in later life: A study of three areas. *British Journal of Social Work,* 30(6), 837–853.

Pugh, R. (2003). Considering the countryside: Is there a case for rural social work? *British Journal of Social Work,* 33(1), 67–85.

Rowles, G.D. (1984). Aging in rural environments. In I. Altman, J. Wohlwill, & M.P. Lawton (eds.), *Human behaviour and the environment: The elderly and the physical environment.* New York: Plenum Press.

Rowles, G.D. (1990). Place attachment among the small town elderly. *Journal of Rural Community Psychology,* 11, 103–120.

Rowles G.D. & Johansson, H.K. (1993). Persistent elderly poverty in rural Appalachia. *Journal of Applied Gerontology,* 12, 349–367.

Schmidt, G.G. (2000). Remote, northern communities: implications for social work practice. *International Social Work,* 43(3), 337–349, July 2000.

Shenk, D. (1991). Older rural women as recipients and providers of social support. *Journal of Aging Studies,* 5(4), 347–358.

Shenk D. & McTavish, D. (1988). Aging women in Minnesota: Rural, non-rural differences in life history text. *Journal of Rural Studies,* 4, 133–140.

Sherr, M.E. & Blumhardt, F.C. (2002). Rural elderly women: Application of human behaviour theory and issues for social work education. *Journal of Human Behaviour in the Rural Environment,* 6(4), 47–64.

Statistics Canada. (1996). *Population projections for Canada, provinces and territories,* cat. no. 84-537. Ottawa: Minister of Supply and Services Canada.

Stoneall, L. (1983). *Country life, city life: Five theories of community.* New York: Praeger.

Wenger, G.C. (1995). A comparison of urban with rural support networks: Liverpool and North Wales. *Ageing and Society,* 15, 59–81.

Willits, F., Bealer, R., & Crider, D. (1982). Persistence of rural/urban differences. In D. Dillman & D. Hobbs (eds.), *Rural society in the U.S.: Issues for the 1980's.* Boulder: Westview Press.

Windley, P. & Scheidt, R. (1980). The well-being of older persons in small rural towns. *Educational Gerontology,* 11, 353–373.

Internet Resources

American Administration on Aging
    Information regarding the needs of the elderly in rural areas.
    http://www.aoa.gov/prof/notes/notes_rural_aging.asp
Rural Aging: Global Action on Aging
    Presents information on the aging in rural communities around the
    world.
    http://www.globalaging.org/rural_aging

Additional Readings

Ginsberg, L. (ed). (1998). *Social work in rural communities*, 3rd ed. New York: C.S.W.E.

Scales, T.L. & Streeter, C. (eds.). (2003). *Rural social work: Building and sustaining community assets*. New York: Wadsworth.

Zapf, M.K. (1985). *Rural social work and its application to the Canadian north as a practice setting*. Toronto: University of Toronto Press.

CHAPTER 13

RETIREMENT: PREPARATION, PLANNING, AND PARTICIPATION

LAURA TAYLOR AND

MICHAEL J. HOLOSKO

This chapter examines the role of social workers in the area of retirement counselling. This will be an expanding area for social work practice as the baby boomer generation reshapes our knowledge and perceptions of retirement. This chapter offers a review of phases and types of retirement, and provides a framework for anti-oppressive generalist practice. It suggests areas for development of assessment and intervention knowledge, and skills for gerontological practitioners.

This chapter explores retirement processes as they impact upon the retiree, his/her family, and the expected or anticipated quality of life. Based on demographic projections in North America and elsewhere [see Chapter 1], it is inevitable that retirement will be a "growth industry" well into the middle of the twenty-first century.

Skill sets for working in the retirement area will be reviewed, and some of the value dilemmas presented by retirement will be considered. We will also present assessment and intervention perspectives in keeping with an anti-oppressive, generalist social work practice model [the current iteration in the development of the generalist practice model]. Readers will note that practice, policy, and practice effectiveness evaluation issues are intertwined in retirement counselling.

I.   Retirement and Social Aging

Retirement is defined as the time when regular full- or part-time paid employment ceases, private and public pensions related to the conditions of employment are collected, and a major lifespan transition to life after employment begins (Matcha, 1997). There is no law mandating retirement at age 65 in Canada; however, retirement is often forced upon workers at age 65 by current employment policies. Two mandatory retirement challenges by university professors in Ontario (1990) and Alberta (1992) went to the Supreme Court of Canada. It ruled that while mandatory retirement violates *The Canadian Charter of Rights and Freedoms (1982)*, such violations were considered a "reasonable limit on an individual's rights" (Ont.) and that "discrimination on the basis of age was reasonable and justifiable" (OCUFA, 2003, p. 1). The U.S.A. eliminated mandatory retirement in the *Age Discrimination Employment Act of 1967* and subsequent amendments in 1978 and 1986 (Clark & Quinn, 2002). Nevertheless, in North America, old age pensions and old age security often set 65 as the benchmark age of eligibility. This provides a socially constructed definition of aging that may be about to be deconstructed by the current baby boomer generation.

Retirement begins long before the proverbial "golden handshake" and the required watch or lapel pin is received. It embodies a set of processes beginning from the time one enters the workforce and is given (or not) the first benefits package The concept of retirement itself is relatively new. The 20th century saw the boom of industrialization along with improved health conditions. With the development of influential unions, more and more people began to live long enough to retire and receive employee pensions and benefits. In turn, these benefits have become an increasingly important part of employment contracts (Achenbaum, 1978). In the early part of the 20th century, only 7 percent of adulthood time was spent in retirement. At the beginning of the 21st century, about 25 percent of adulthood time will be spent in retirement (Price, 2000). Furthermore, the profile of retirees and retirement has changed significantly. In the past 50 years, more women have entered the workforce and will retire from full- and part-time employment, and more men and women plan for early or delayed retirement.

Early retirement is relatively recent outcome of corporate downsizing of the 1980s (Clark & Quinn, 2002). It is usually based upon a formula of age plus years of service, enabling retirees to leave the workforce prior to age 65. Early retirement has been popularized in the media, whereby the virtues of retirement planning allow retirees to bask in the so-called "Freedom 55" lifestyle. It appears that the baby boomer generation may reverse, or at least decrease, the trend of early retirement as they have introduced the concept of delayed retirement. Statistics indicate that 80 percent of American baby boomers who make up 28 percent of the population in the U.S.A. and 38 percent of Canadian baby boomers plan to ignore both early retirement incentives and expected retirement age frames and want to work past age 65. Their reasons for delaying retirement generally include financial need, quality of life issues, and, enjoyment of work (Chappell, 2001; Clark & Quinn, 2002; Korczyk, 2001).

II.   Social Work Practice in the Retirement Process

Social work skills and knowledge will be called upon in three major areas of retirement: (1) employee-assistance programs, (2) pre-retirement planning programs, and (3) retirement adjustment and lifespan planning.

A. Employee-Assistance Programs

Policy initiatives focused on eliminating discrimination on the basis of age provide opportunities for older persons to remain in the workforce past age 65. As the workforce broadens the types of retirement packages available, more older workers may be involved in phased-in retirement whereby the employee gradually reduces the time spent at work by working half or fewer days per week, leading to full retirement. Another option is part-time retirement where an employee continues to work regularly but on a part-time basis for as long as is feasible. Employee-assistance services may see an increase in the need for services focused on older worker issues such as caregiver stress, reduced income, adjustment to phased-in or part-time retirement, and time-management issues in the lifespan of the older worker. The literature reveals that "older workers' issues have not been a primary focus of gerontological social work practice effort, social work literature, or social work associations" (Dooley, 2001, p. 158). Dooley cautions that "the issues and conditions of older workers are of critical importance to social workers concerned with the quality of life of the older population" given that there are 8.6 million older workers and 2.5 million retirees (60 and older) in the U.S.A. (National Academy on an Aging Society, NAAS, 2000, cited in Dooley, 2001, p. 158).

Two issues that are relatively new for retirement counselling here are the impact of retirement on identity for older women and the "unretirement" of the disabled worker. One usually thinks of women's retirement issues in terms of interrupted work patterns. However, a greater number of women [than in the past] are likely to have continuous work histories and professional careers. Price (2000) found that the loss of a "professional role" for women was a significant factor in their transition to retirement. Four components to be considered in this regard include: "1) initial transition [to "non-professional status"]; 2) loss of social contacts; 3) loss of employment challenges, and 4) confronting social stereotypes" (p. 86). Price also noted that professional women struggle with social perceptions that once retired, they are no longer competent in their work and/or social milieu.

The second issue of "unretirement" previously noted involves disabled workers who because of improvements in medical treatment are able to move from retirement back into the workforce. This has already been seen in the case of some workers with HIV/AIDS and/or physically or mentally disabled persons. Such individuals pose unique challenges to counsellors in the areas of re-entry to the workforce, accommodations necessary to do the job, employee benefits, career development, and workplace stressors.

B. Pre-retirement Planning Programs

Pre-retirement planning (PRP) is considered a significant risk-reduction factor for many employees. According to Tice and Perkins (1996) "pre-retirement planning is probably the single most formidable means of prevention against post-retirement hardship known to many older adults" (p. 156). They suggest that pre-retirement planning "can help insure economic, social, and psychological well-being in late life" (p. 156). There is considerable agreement in the field that such planning is critical to a successful adjustment to and the experience of retirement.

Pre-retirement planning programs were first developed in 1948 by Hunter at the University of Michigan (Dennis, 2002). Initially aimed at people who were already retired, Hunter developed an educative model that included both psychosocial issues and financial issues, the cornerstones of all retirement planning (Dennis, 2002). However, as recessions and downsizing hit the North American workforce, financial planning and retirement benefits issues began to dominate retirement-planning workshops. There is now a growing awareness for the need to re-emphasize psychosocial education and planning for the retirement years. Indeed, the need to consider retirement planning linked to the aging process is important. There is increased recognition for what is termed a balanced social portfolio reflecting diversified social involvement and activities, composed of group and individual activities and high- and low-mobility activities. Thus, when retirees' social networks change through death of friends and/or spouses, they can turn to individual activities until their social networks begin to expand again, and as health factors limit activity levels, the retiree has in place a repertoire of low-mobility activities (Cohen, 2002).

The relevance and importance of the social planning aspect of retirement is further emphasized when one reflects upon the implications of current demographic patterns of increased life expectancy. In the past two decades, the number of seniors between 75 and 84 years of age has almost doubled and one in ten seniors are 85 years of age or older (Statistics Canada, 1999, cited in Wells & Taylor, 2001). When linking increased life expectancy patterns with early retirement, it is now possible for a retiree to take early retirement at age 50, live to be 100+, and spend 50 or more years as a retired person. This retiree could actually spend more time retired than he or she spent in the workforce! A retirement lasting 50 or more years has forced many financial planners to consider life planning as part of their role. The National Endowment for Financial Education (NEFE, 2001) defined life planning as "a process of: 1) helping people focus on the true values and motivations in their lives; and, 2) determining the goals and objectives they have as they see their lives develop" (Dennis, 2002, p. 57). It also involves "3) using these values, motivations, goals and objectives to guide the planning process and provide a framework for making choices and decisions in life that have financial and non-financial implications and consequences"(p. 57).

Pre-retirement planning workshops are currently offered in many North American work settings. Social workers should advocate for inclusion in such workshops. In addition, social workers could play a valuable leadership role in the educative process for retirement planning as part of career education in universities and/or colleges. We need to embrace the idea that retirement planning should begin the first day one enters the workforce. For retirees who have not had the opportunity to attend pre-retirement seminars, there is an overwhelming amount of information readily available on the Internet. For instance, Dennis (2002) found 962 books and some 287,000 to 1.2

million listings for retirement planning and on-line courses, newsletters, and e-mail counsellors.

C. Retirement Lifespan Counselling

Assessment and Intervention

As with any social work intervention, the need for a good assessment of retiree strengths and needs is essential. The *Life Domains Assessment* helps a retiree focus upon current and longer term needs, strengths, and resources related to: (a) living arrangements, (b) social supports, (c) relationships, (d) leisure and recreation, (e) health and mental health , and (f) finances. It is recommended that legal issues and spirituality) be added to a comprehensive *Life Domain Review* (Hyde, 1992; Tice & Perkins, 1996). In addition to individual, group, and family counselling skills, knowledge of and the ability to provide linkages to community resources is an essential skill for workers in the retirement counselling field.

It is often helpful in the onset of retirement counselling to establish the type of retirement that the retiree has or is experiencing. The literature indicates eight retirement scenarios as follows: (1) *early retirement,* which is usually established by a formula of age and years of service where it is possible to retire somewhere past age 40 but before age 65; (2) *mandatory retirement* or the age set by the employer, usually at age 65, which coincides with the beginning of the Old Age Pension or Social Security; (3) *delayed or late retirement* taken after age 65 and now becoming a trend with a shortage of skilled personnel in many areas of employment and a withdrawal of early retirement packages; (4) *voluntary retirement* where a person has decided to leave the workforce and use the income of previous employment; (5) *involuntary retirement* where a worker must leave the workforce earlier than anticipated often due to poor health or inability to find another position after layoffs; (6) *partial retirement* in which a person works part-time or does consulting work or establishes a small business; (7) *phased-in retirement* where the employer actually facilitates a transition from full-time work to full-time retirement and can include job-sharing, reduced work hours, a leave of absence to try out retirement, transfers to a job with less stress or fewer hours, and/or having the worker serve as a consultant or temporary worker (Wiatrowski, 2001); and, finally, (8) *spoiled retirement* where the illness or death or a partner results in giving up a lifetime of retirement plans (Dorfman, 2002).

Retirement itself is a process of eight recognized phases, although not all people will experience all stages or experience the stages in the order outlined. Atchley's phases of retirement (1976), widely acknowledged in the literature, include: (1) *pre-retirement—the remote phase:* the worker is fairly new to the workforce; (2) *pre-retirement—the near phase:* the plans for leaving employment and retirement are made in affective, cognitive, and behavioural ways and financial issues are assessed; (3) *the retirement event:* at which the employee is officially declared retired, which is usually marked with a celebration; (4) *retirement—honeymoon phase:* the joy of not having to work regularly is appreciated, a routine is developed, and the degree of satisfaction depends on the extent of post-workforce; (5) *the disenchantment phase:* where the losses of routine, work colleagues, and income become more evident, the joy of "free" time fades, and a meaning for the retirement years is sought; (6) *the retirement—reorientation to life as a retiree phase:* this may include developing a second career or volunteer sector involvement; (7) *the stability phase:* where patterns for life in retirement have been established; and (8) *the termination phase:* in this phase the patterns of a retirement lifestyle may change as the person becomes reliant on formal care and long-term care facilities to maintain a quality of life (Atchley, 1976, p. 68, cited in Matcha, 1997, p. 120).

Each sequential stage presents unique issues for the retirees, their families, and their immediate social networks. For instance, retirees who appear for counselling frequently present with feelings of isolation, loneliness, health issues, boredom, feelings of worthlessness, and depression. They also may have family adjustment issues or may seek advice around financial issues or concerns related to changes in lifestyle and/or living arrangements. As well, some retirees are bitter about having to leave work when they still consider themselves productive individuals with much to offer. In such cases, this positive energy and drive needs to be re-channelled, a significant challenge for the retiree and the counsellor.

Since retirement signifies a role loss, it may help the retirees, unresolved in their retirement status, to focus on roles in order to set a plan for using the retirement years in a way that provides satisfaction and fulfilment. Here, the authors offer the following questions, called the PEERS Inventory, as a starting point, particularly for students new to the field, to facilitate further exploration of retirement with a retiree. The PEER Inventory used the following five questions: (1) What was your Pre-retirement role/lifestyle? (2) What brings you meaning and Enjoyment now? (3) Would you consider Exploring how you might use your skills and expertise in a volunteer or entreprenerial capacity? (4) What new *Roles* or activities would you like to explore? and (5) What is causing you *Stress* or dissatisfaction in your new life and/or what symptoms reflect this dissatisfaction?

While individual counselling helps clients develop a focus for retirement and their lifestyle, a major goal of any effective counselling involves linking with resources. The strengths perspective (Glicken, 2004; Saleebey, 1992; Tice & Perkins, 1996) offers a model that has proven effective in retirement counselling. It focuses on: (1) empowerment or discovering power within the person; (2) dialogue and collaboration or determining the needs and then working as agent, motivator, facilitator; (3) membership or encouraging connections with the community, be it as a volunteer, a consultant, a part-time worker, a participant, or a mentor; (4) synergy or the retiree forming relationships with purpose and reciprocity; and (5) regeneration or the new lifestyle developing (Tice & Perkins, 1996).

D. Issues in Retirement across the Lifespan

Regardless of the type or phase of retirement, there is considerable agreement on the issues that have the greatest impact on one's quality of retired life. The two major and pervasive issues are financial security as retirement income may be one-half to one-third less than working income, and health status, which involves continued mobility, independence, and freedom from pain and physical limitations (Tice & Perkins, 1996).

Retirement truly affects all family members. For instance, a stay-at-home partner with set routines may find these altered by the presence of the new retiree, particularly if the new retiree has not planned for retirement. Interestingly, according to the literature, retirement does not lead to a major realignment of household roles (Dorfman, 2002). When both partners work, one partner may retire considerably earlier than the other. The full implementation of retirement plans, such as moving to a warmer climate, simpler housing arrangements, or travelling, must wait for the first retiree; life goes "on hold," waiting to commence. The illness of a partner, particularly in the early stages of retirement, dramatically shifts the initial retirement plans from a concept of freedom and shared activities to the stresses and constraints of caregiver. A caregiver role for parents, relatives, or a dependent adult child may also restrict retirement activities. [See Chapter 19 in this text.]

Within the family, adult children may welcome their parents' retirement, expecting retired parents to be more available for child care and to provide affective and instrumental support. While some retired grandparents find the increased role in their grandchildren's lives rewarding, others may feel that their children are expecting too much. Conversely, adult children may feel that their retired parent(s) are becoming too dependent on them, or are becoming overly involved with their grandchildren.

Common retirement plans often include relocating: (1) to be near children and grand children, (2) to benefit from a warmer climate, or (3) to become reacquainted or be nearer siblings and relatives. In pre-retirement planning, retirees need to carefully evaluate the pros and cons of leaving a known community and their long established social networks. Selling the family home and downsizing or moving into a retirement community may be a part of the retirement plan. Pre-retirement planning helps retirees think through the impacts of these major and sometimes traumatic decisions. As many retirees have found, reversing major relocation decisions is often not a viable option for a variety of reasons (Dorfman, 2002).

III. From Micro to Macro Social Work Practice

At the micro level of practice, role loss, status loss, and drastic changes in life circumstances are all significant issues in retirement. A gerontological social worker should also be prepared to conduct periodic risk assessments for suicide and/or depression. "Depression and depressive behaviour are the most common mental health complaints of older people" (Tice & Perkins, 1996, p. 49). Furthermore, the suicide rate for seniors is higher than that of the general population; older men are at particular risk with a suicide rate that increases with age and is three times that of the general population (McIntosh, 1992, cited in Tice & Perkins, 1996). Thus, it is recommended that all new social workers in this field attend suicide-prevention workshops as part of their preparation for this work. In addition, the ability to conduct assessments around issues such as addictions, including alcohol, drug, and gambling [with casinos erupting all over North America], are relevant for retirement counselling. Social workers in all forms of retirement counselling must also be prepared to be involved in assessments that may result in involuntary retirement, involuntary admission to a hospital or care facility, or removal of driving licences or licences to practise a profession. Social workers working with retirees should also be vigilant in their appraisal of the risk for elder abuse. Retirement can make a senior largely invisible. The potential for undetected elder abuse and self-neglect [see Chapter 10] also needs to be addressed in working with retirees.

At the mezzo level of practice, social workers will find it important to have an extensive network of community sources and resources to facilitate the training, educative interests, and community involvement interests of retirees. Retirees are sought after to provide training in Third World countries, and many health and human service programs rely on volunteers for a variety if reasons [see Chapter 1]. Helping retirees access information, resources, and contacts is an important part of effective involvement of retirees in their community and in the global society in which we now live. In this regard, the Internet offers a wealth of information for both the social worker and for the retiree.

At the macro level of practice, social workers need to follow the tenets of anti-oppressive social work practice and identify, document, and advocate for changes in policies and programs that create barriers for retired persons. The "global village" in which we now live suggests that not only must we concern ourselves with anti-oppressive social work practices for retirees in our own countries, but we must also work for policy changes to prevent discrimination for all retirees worldwide.

At all levels of practice, we need more research to augment social work knowledge, skills, and interventions in retirement lifespan planning. There are many practice research questions to be explored with the baby boomer generation looming. We do not know, for example, what the implications of delayed retirement will be. Will social workers be called upon to develop competency or risk assessments to screen older workers in the workforce? What is it like to be retired for 40 or 50 years? For persons with limited pensions, what services are most needed? These questions need to be explored to enhance our knowledge and skills for work in retirement counselling.

Retirees have developed resiliency, expertise, and life experience, and can be a particularly intimidating group for new social work practitioners. This expertise and experience can be mobilized to formulate creative problem-solving solutions and offer social workers challenging but rich and varied counselling experiences. Spiezia's (2002) article entitled "The Greying Population: A wasted human capital or just a social liability?" stresses the importance of ensuring that our seniors are not "wasted" but rather are empowered to recognize themselves and be recognized as a most highly valued resource.

In this reframing, the following represents a partial list of opportunities available for retirees:

a) opening a new business or becoming a consultant to businesses;

b) taking a course—Elder Hostel programs for seniors offer courses all over the world; many universities have seniors' courses or allow seniors to enrol in courses at free or reduced tuition;

c) becoming a volunteer—many non-profit agencies cannot afford to pay "experts" and many seniors have extensive business, human sector, or experience in trades that would be invaluable to agencies;

d) becoming a consultant to an agency as a volunteer;

e) becoming either a peer mentor or an intergenerational mentor or a foster grandparent;

f) joining a seniors' centre and learning a new activity;

g) finding a way to use the skills acquired over a lifetime in overseas volunteer work; and,

h) becoming more active in a faith community—many retirees are drawn to spirituality, life review, and to reflections on life and end-of-life issues (Koenig, 2003).

IV. Concluding Remark

Retirement processes are made up of new endings and new beginnings. Development of alternative types of retirement will offer increasingly varied opportunities for retirees. This may also trigger many psychosocial issues for older persons and require a wide range of anti-oppressive social work assessment and intervention skills. The baby boomers will have considerable power in their abilities to challenge discrimination on the basis of age or retirement status at both a personal or an institutional level. Their collective will shall inevitably influence policies, programs, resources, and services for retirees.

Social work practitioners using a strengths-based perspective and anti-oppressive social work practice techniques, in addition to providing individual, group, and family counselling, need to serve as information sources and linking agents to community resources. As retirement extends into longer periods of adult life, the need for long-range retirement planning both financially and socially is essential. Schools of social work and social service agencies need to develop educational programs to foster the development of skills necessary to work in the area of retirement planning and to foster life-long retirement planning as a part of career preparation. Effective social work practice in the area of "retirement social work" draws on a wide range of social work assessment and intervention techniques, skills, and knowledge. It also offers the challenge of ensuring that older persons are valued and value themselves in their retirement years.

References

Achenbaum, A. (1978). *Old age in the new land*. Baltimore: Johns-Hopkins University Press.

Atchely, R.C. (1976). *The sociology of retirement*. Cambridge: Schenkman.

Chappell, R. (2001). *Social welfare in Canadian society*. Scarborough: Nelson.

Clark, R.L. & Quinn, J.F. (2002). Patterns of work and retirement for a new century. *Generations, 26*(2), 17–24.

Cohen, G.D. (2002). Retirement: Advising older adults who are contemplating this change. *Geriatrics, 57*(8), 37–38.

Dennis, H. (2002). The retirement planning specialty. *Generations, 26*(2), 55–60.

Dooley, A. (2001). Older workers' issues and social work practice. *Journal of Gerontological Social Work, 36*(3/4), 157–164.

Dorfman, L.T. (2002). Retirement and family relationships: An opportunity in later life. *Generations, 26*(2), 74–79.

Glicken, M.D. (2004). *Using the strengths perspective in social work practice*. Toronto: Pearson Education Inc.

Hyde, P. (1992). *Case management training handbook*. Columbus: Ohio Department of Mental Health.

Koenig, H.G. (2003). *Purpose and power in retirement: New opportunities for meaning and significance*. Radnor: Templeton Press.

Korczyk, S.M. (2001). Baby boomers head for retirement. *Journal of Financial Planning, 14*(3), 116–123.

Matcha, D.A. (1997). *The sociology of aging: A social problems perspective*. Toronto: Allyn & Bacon.

OCUFA. (2003). Mandatory retirement discussion paper, pp. 1–3. [On-line] Available at: http://www.ocufa.on.ca/retire.asp.

Price, C. (2000). Women and retirement: Relinquishing professional identity. *Journal of Aging Studies*, 14(1), 81–101.

Saleebey, D. (1992). *The strengths perspective in social work practice*. White Plains: Longman.

Spiezia, V. (2002). The greying population: A wasted human capital or just a social liability. *International Labour Review*, 141(½), 71–113.

Tice, C.J. & Perkins, K. (1996). *Mental health issues & aging: Building on the strengths of older persons*. Toronto: Brooks/Cole.

Wells, L. & Taylor, L.E. (2001). Gerontological social work: A Canadian perspective. *Journal of Gerontological Social Work*, 50(3/4), 33–50.

Wiatrowski, W.J. (2001). Changing retirement age: Ups and downs. *Monthly Labour Review*, 124(4), 312.

Internet Resources

American Association of Retired Persons
　　A non-profit membership organization dedicated to addressing the needs and interests of persons 50 and older.
　　http://www.aarp.org

Boomers International, World Wide Community for the Baby Boomer Generation
　　Canadian Association for the Fifty Plus.
　　http://www.fifty-plus.net

Canadian Association of Pre-retirement Planners (CAPP) Ontario
　　An association dedicated to a holistic approach: financial and lifestyle to pre- and post-retirement planning.
　　http://www.retirementplanners.net/

Elder Hostel
　　An educational and travel organization for seniors.
　　http://www.elderhostel.org

Guide to Retirement Living Online
　　A guide for seniors and their families in the mid-Atlantic.
　　http://www.retirement-living.com/

Additional Readings

Bronfman, E. (2002). *The third act: Re-inventing yourself after retirement*. New York: Putnam.

Glicken, M.D. (2003). *Using the strengths perspective in social work practice.* Toronto: Pearson Education.

Koenig, H.G. (2003). *Purpose and power in retirement: New opportunities for meaning and significance.* Radnor: Templeton Press.

Savishinsky, J.S. (2000). *Breaking the watch: Meanings of retirement in America.* Ithaca: Cornell University Press.

CHAPTER 14

FACILITATING A GOODNESS-OF-FIT BETWEEN OLDER VOLUNTEERS AND THEIR COMMUNITIES

JUDITH A. WHEELER

At the turn of this century, paralleling trends set by North American governments and an aging society are promoting volunteerism among older adults in unprecedented ways. This is mainly due to the devolution of social programs by government and its shift from professional intervention to that of the non-profit sector in the community to meet social needs. As well, today's older adults are healthier, more economically independent, better educated, and younger at retirement than seniors of past generations. Adults (65-plus) tend to devote more voluntary time to their community on average than any other demographic group. The potential for social work intervention to facilitate a goodness-of-fit between older volunteers and their communities is optimal.

I.   Introduction

Volunteerism gained unprecedented worldwide recognition in the year 2001 as the United Nations declared the International Year of Volunteers (IYV). In Canada, this recognition emerged through IYV as a way to spotlight the significant voluntary contributions Canadians have made to society. Additionally, IYV served as the tool "to expand our thinking of what we can accomplish through voluntary action, and how we can more effectively involve Canadians" (IYV, Projects, 1999, p. 1). This focus is timely since it coincides with the devolution of our social service industry by government throughout the 1990s. Gordon and Neal (1997) contend that the government, in its attempts to reduce costs, markedly shifted social responsibilities to the community and its non-profit sector. In 1998 seniors devoted the greatest sum of formal volunteer contributions employing the smallest number of volunteers. Reportedly 23 percent of individuals aged 65+ contributed 202 hours on average per annum compared to 33 percent of those aged 15–24, who provided an average of 125 hours (Statistics Canada, 1998).

Volunteerism, which is typically defined as freely offering one's time, energy, and skills, is the foundation of both formal and informal volunteerism (Figure 14.1). Although the prevalence of *informal* voluntary action contributions has been less examined, it is an area of growing interest and recognition (Chappell, 1999). Given the current societal trends by all levels of governments and an aging population, it is conceivable that the potential for growth in the seniors' volunteer sector is phenomenal. Yet this phenomenon requires professional intervention if it is to succeed as planned. Social workers are in an ideal best position to facilitate older volunteers achieving a goodness-of-fit within their communities. That is, the malleability of the social work profession, based on its inherent knowledge, values, and skills, is essential to the linking process that must take place.

This chapter provides an overview of the role volunteerism plays in the lives of adults aged 50 years and over, and explores how social work intervention can facilitate the process effectively. It begins by examining the current trends faced by an aging society paralleled with that of all levels of government. It further explores the broader definition of volunteerism to include not only formal but informal volunteerism as a substantial area of contribution. Thus, for ease of clarity, both formal and informal voluntary contributions are defined and examples are given to help guide future social work intervention. Next, the motivational factors related to formal voluntary action by older volunteers are outlined, followed by a summary of the benefits gleaned by all those involved in the volunteer experience. The chapter continues by listing the assumptions inferred by this overview concerning the role of volunteerism by older adults, social work intervention, and government support. Suggestions for social work intervention are offered. The chapter concludes with a list of Internet resources focused on voluntary action by older adults at national and local levels.

II.   Current Trends

North Americans are retiring earlier and spending nearly equal time in both their work and post-work years (MacMillan, 2000). Additionally, it appears that the growing numbers of healthier, economically independent, and better educated older adults, along with an ever-increasing reduction in social programs in society, account for the greatest increase in voluntary service (Gordon & Neal, 1997; Kent, 1989). For instance, in the 1960s, older volunteers commonly lacked education and were "viewed as an intrusion into the well organized functioning of an agency" (Lambert et al., 1964, p. 50). Conversely, in the 1980s, services provided by elder volunteers were considered widespread and significant (Jones, 1986; Kent 1989). This trend is expected to accelerate (Jones, 1986; Manser, 1987) since more than 70 million North American "baby boomers will be entering their seniors years by the year 2010" (Dychtwald, 1986). As funding for social programs declines and the demand for public services increases, the necessity for senior volunteers escalates. Thus, society is being forced to find a goodness-of-fit between its seniors and its communities.

Romero (1986) suggested that the increasing numbers of retired individuals have prompted community planners and agency administrators to explore ways of using the time, talents, and energy of older adults in voluntary efforts. At the turn of this century, government is indeed trying to change the mindset of its society by highly encouraging all Canadians to provide some act of volunteerism, whether formal or informal. This is especially evident in regard to older volunteers. For instance, as one way to promote voluntary action among this sector, Volunteer Canada, in partnership with Manulife Financial, the Canadian Centre for Philanthropy, and Health Canada, are highly promoting their new "emotionally charged inward thinking piece" entitled: *Volunteering ... A Booming Trend*. It ends with "Volunteering is a booming business." This booklet is designed to change the mindset of society by encouraging older adults to "put a lifetime of skills and experience to good use" (MacMillan, 2000, p. 4). Moreover, an increasing number of websites exist that promote voluntary action among older adults and stand ready to assist, in various ways, all those who access them.

Although voluntary action is highly recognized and promoted today, problems exist with it. For instance, due to funding cutbacks by the provincial government in Ontario, six volunteer centres have been forced to close, while remaining centres try to survive by scrambling for other revenue sources. The executive director of Volunteer Ontario stated that the government "talks of encouraging voluntarism while systematically destroying its infrastructure" (Nyp, 1996, p.1). This complaint appears to be echoed across Canada. For instance, Nyp (1996) continued to explain that the executive director of the Canadian Association of Volunteer Bureaux and Centres agreed as she stated that the governments "don't seem to realize that ... volunteers don't just show up at an agency and find the right job to do. They need to be recruited, screened, matched and trained" (Wheeler, 2000, p. 3). For seniors, further problems exist as well. For example, seniors expressed a common concern that they feared volunteering "because [they] are afraid of being stuck. [They] see it as a life sentence with no one to take their place if they leave" (Wheeler, 2000).

III.   Formal and Informal Volunteerism

Informal voluntary action, which "refers to individuals helping other individuals without a mediating institution," is increasingly being highly recognized and promoted (Chappell, 1999, p. 4) (see Figure 14.1). However, Chappell (1999) points out that no actual research regarding this area of volunteerism has been conducted other than that of the *National Survey of Giving, Volunteering and Participating* (NSGVP). In 2000, NSGVP reported that 16.7 million Canadians assisted others in a variety of tasks like babysitting, assisting with letter writing, visiting the sick, driving, and/or shopping for others (Chappell, 1999). The benefits of such voluntary action are generally reported in the social support literature, especially in reference to caregiving (Chappell, 1999; Motenko, 1989).

Although social support literature concerning caregiving has reported positive effects on caregivers, social workers must be cautioned that the caregiving role can and does lead to tremendous caregiver stress and elder abuse as well (see Godkin et al., 1989; Jary & Jary, 1991). It is conceivable that for a number of caregivers, caregiving is being provided only because no one else is available to provide such services. Thus, care provision could be given out of obligation, which might ultimately turn to resentment. Perhaps these situations would improve if those caregivers were provided with either formal or informal voluntary service by others in their circles of support (see Brody et al., 1989; Chappell, 1998; Deimling, 1991).

Finally, there is a growing trend to involve older volunteers in intergenerational volunteer programs. For instance, members of a seniors' centre taught grade six students at a nearby school to knit in a program called "Knitting Generations Together" and was met with great success (Wheeler, 1998).

As indicated in Figure 14.1, formal volunteerism occurs when one "volunteers through an organization" (Chappell, 1999, p. 6). According to NSGVP (2000), formal volunteering among Canadians aged 15 years and over increased 5 percent between 1987 and 1997. Thus, 7.5 million or 31 percent of Canadians reportedly devoted their time to organizations. To give a flavour of the diverse areas in which older volunteers devote their time, a number of positive testimonials have been provided (see MacMillan, 2000). For example, diverse areas of formal volunteering include: Breast Cancer Support Services, Head Injury Association, Dog Shelters, hospitals, Refugee Programs, School Programs at the Canadian Museum of Nature for Children, and one by a gentleman (76 years old) who volunteers for the Tetra Society which "designs and builds items for people with disabilities that are not available commercially" (MacMillan, 1999, p. 13).

Figure 14.1

Volunteerism: "Prosocial action, involving people devoting substantial amounts of time and energy to helping others, often for extended periods of time and at considerable personal costs" (Snyder, 1993, p. 253).

Informal Volunteerism: "Individuals helping other individuals without going through a mediating institution," e.g., caregiving, shopping for others, driving others, babysitting, helping to write letters, visiting the sick, yard work, and housework (Chappell, 1999, p. 4); intergenerational volunteer programs (Wheeler, 1998); peer leaders in health promotion programs (Wheeler, 1997).

Formal Volunteerism: "Volunteering through an organization is typically studied as volunteering," e.g., through the United Way, Cancer Society, in hospitals.

Voluntary opportunities continue to expand. For instance, Wheeler (1997) found that the level of a participant's involvement in seniors' health promotion programs (HPPs) significantly affected the contribution of the elder individual in future HPPs. Thus, striking differences emerged between programs involving elder peer support and leadership within a community and those in which seniors were passive recipients of health promotion education. Programs promoting peer support and leadership roles appeared to lead to greater community-oriented involvement that fostered expansion of their existing HPPs (Penning & Wasyliw, 1992). As a result, promoting goal setting leading to possible elder volunteerism is suggested as one future component of HPPs. Moreover, it is worth noting that social workers contributed as multidisciplinary team members in some of these HPPs. The possibilities remain endless regarding volunteerism by older adults in either informal or formal voluntary settings. Much depends on the motivation behind such a giving act.

IV.   Motivation to Volunteer

Since motivation is a subconscious construct, it is a difficult concept to either observe or chronicle (Cnaan & Goldberg-Glen, 1991). That is, if individuals are not asked what motivates them to volunteer, such information remains unknown (Gillespie & King, 1985). Snyder (1993) categorized motivation as being personal or social, while Clary and Orenstein (1991) identified it as being altruistic (other-centred) or egoistic (self-concerned). When values underpin altruistic motivations for volunteering, individuals score relatively high on empathy, nurturance, and social responsibility (Snyder & Omoto, 1992). Conversely, when personal needs are the motivating factors for volunteering (e.g., esteem enhancement due to low self-esteem or low social supports), these egoistic motivations result in volunteers feeling better about themselves (Synder & Omoto, 1992).

Regardless of motivational rationale, one must maintain a "feeling of being in control, of having a say over what happens in one's life, [as it] has far-reaching consequences for physical and mental health" (Goleman, 1986, p. C1). Older adults from all socio-economic levels maintained an element of control in their lives by expressing their desire for interpersonal, meaningful, volunteer assignments over mechanical or physical tasks (Kuehne & Sears, 1993; Lambert et al., 1964; Newman et al., 1985). Thus, an egoistic motivation (i.e., need for control) may be fulfilled. Volunteers who contributed the most altruistically to society may, ironically, be volunteering for egoistic reasons (Snyder, 1993). Yet egoistic motivations were reported as the primary reason for volunteering at the Red Cross (Gillespie & King, 1985), while self-interest was indicated as the primary motive for volunteering with AIDS victims (Snyder, 1993).

Recently, to determine the motivation for volunteerism among older adults in a formal setting, the *National Survey of Giving, Volunteering, and Participating* provided respondents with a "list of possible reasons" for volunteering (NSGVP On-line, 2000, p. 2). The findings are provided in Figure 14.2 below.

Figure 14.2: What Motivates Older Volunteers?

	45–54 years	55–64 years	65+ years
Belief in a cause	97(%)	98(%)	97(%)
To use skills/experience	76	75	71
Personally affected	70	70	66
To explore own strengths	50	46	37
To fulfil religious obligations	32	40	49
Friends volunteer	20	25	31
To improve job skills	12	9	3

Source: Volunteer Canada, Health Canada, and Manulife Financial. (2000). *Volunteering ... A Booming Trend,* p. 6.

V.   Benefits of Volunteering

Voluntary action among older adults has been found to be mutually beneficial for elder volunteers and those they served. In a meta-analysis of 37 independent studies (1965 to 1996) regarding elderly volunteerism, Wheeler, Gorey, and Greenblatt (1998) found that 70 percent of older volunteers and 85 percent of those they served reported beneficial outcomes. Seniors providing formal volunteer services (in conjunction with care provision by helping professionals "scored higher on quality of life measures than the average non-volunteer did") (p. 75). For example, elderly volunteers indicated they experienced greater life satisfaction, had a "stronger will to live, and reported less somatic, anxious, and depressive symptoms than non-volunteers" (Hunter & Linn, 1980–1981, p. 211). This was found to be especially true for older volunteers who were disadvantaged by personal and social resources (Fengler, 1984). Moreover, Wheeler et al. (1998) reported that nine of the

37 studies inferred that 85 percent of the recipients of their volunteer service (e.g., peer counselling of nursing home residents) scored better on dependent measures (e.g., diminished depression) than did persons in comparison conditions (p. 75).

Moreover, meaningful involvement in voluntary action by older adults is regarded as a key to healthy aging. Being a volunteer allows an older individual to maintain status, structure, and social contact. In turn, meaningful involvement leads to a positive mental outlook and an increased social network (Heller, 1993; Kerschner & Pegues, 1998). That is, volunteer work allows for socialization outside of one's family with people who share similar interests. Particularly for retirees, such social interaction outside the family promotes their health and well-being (Moen, 1995), a significant component of life satisfaction (Choi & Dinse, 1998). As well, the benefits of volunteering across settings, such as peer support in health promotion programs or for AIDS victims, can produce a status-bearing role and contribute to one's feeling of usefulness, self-respect, and socialization (Salmon, 1985). Due to the positive health benefits older adults reap by volunteering, volunteerism is implicitly counted among the individual and social determinants of health that guide the Healthy Communities Model. (For information concerning the Healthy Communities Model, see the World Health Organization Web site at http://www.who.dk).

VI. Assumptions

Five major trends undergird present-day assumptions that are seemingly made by the Canadian government concerning its supportive role in social service provision, volunteerism by older adults, and intervention by professional social service providers. These trends include: (1) the growing numbers of healthier, economically independent, and better educated older adults who are retiring earlier than seniors of past generations; (2) the devolution of social service provision in which the government markedly shifted social responsibilities back to the non-profit sector in communities; (3) the recognition and promotion of volunteerism through IYV among older adults as a way to increasingly involve older volunteers to meet community need as the so-called baby boomers enter their senior years; (4) the decreased funding by the government for recruiting, training, matching, and screening of volunteers by social organizations; and (5) the increased use of the Internet by the government to provide information and direction as a way to recruit volunteers and aid those who wish to work with volunteers in general.

Given the above trends, it appears that the Canadian government assumes that:

- older adults who wish to volunteer will simply use the Internet to link them to their area of interest(s),
- all social workers and volunteer managers possess an awareness of the Internet and will access it for information and direction in working with volunteers or promoting volunteerism, and
- older volunteers of the so-called baby boomer generation will not require training due to being more highly educated than seniors in past generations.

However, it is conceivable that such assumptions lead to the following problems as well:

- the government expects that prospective volunteers and/or agency staff will access the Internet, which may not be the case in most situations,
- the Internet is not accessible to everyone, especially to older adults,
- it is difficult to bring information on the Internet down to a personal level,
- the Internet cannot provide the training, screening, and matching of volunteers within a social organization,
- the government "talks of encouraging voluntarism while systematically destroying its infrastructure" (Nyp, 1996, p.1), and
- the government implicitly wants to replace current social service provision by professionals, wherever possible, with older volunteers.

For instance, Street contended that "the attitude seems to be 'there's no money, let's get a volunteer to do it.... The whole notion of voluntarism is being challenged. Is it only about getting work done? Or is it about providing a service, achieving a sense of meaning through altruistic endeavors, civic duty and moral responsibility?" (Nyp, 1996, p. 3). On the other hand, Wheeler et al. (1998) reported beneficial effects for nearly 80 percent of the elder volunteers who engaged in meaningful voluntary action and 90 percent for those they served. They further suggested that "... gerontological social work practice may be more effective—perhaps as much as 10 to 20 percent more so, as indicated by incident client improvement rates—when older volunteers concomitantly work with such clients" (p. 76).

VII. Implications for Practice

Social work intervention is built on *the two cornerstones of theory and practice*. Yet updated models and theories concerning intervention to facilitate a goodness-of-fit between older volunteers and their communities appears to be lacking since this is a relatively new area for social workers and health professionals alike. In this regard, social workers could become familiar with their employment surroundings and the levels of elder voluntary contribution within them. Prior to developing programs and services involving older volunteers, social workers could develop goals, objectives, and action plans that would specifically meet needs in agencies. Moreover, such plans could emerge from a theoretical basis specific to the action being discussed. Once discussed, it could be beneficial to represent a model by constructing a diagram to explain the model at a glance. It is recognized that any new model and theory must be tested and modifications made as required by actually designing and implementing a program that works within a newly developed model and theory. Information such as this is meant to be shared among social workers in general. Thus, it follows that social workers need to contribute to scholarly literature regarding their contributions to agency needs.

Existing or developing theoretical models and theories are major requirements for designing volunteer programs and services. In general, social workers should consider the needs of both the volunteer and the agency staff when designing programs and services. Due to the heterogeneity of the older population and their need to maintain control in their lives, no one program will likely suit all older volunteers. It is, therefore, imperative to design quality volunteer programs that include older adults in the planning and participation of such programs (see Heller, 1993). Moreover, social workers who work closely with older adults find that "entering into a person's life space ... requires delicacy, knowledge, compassion, careful planning and skill (Germain & Gitterman, 1980, p. 35). Through an ecological approach, programs and services must provide "opportunities for successful supports which includes resources and knowledge required for effective task accomplishment; regulate the rhythm and pace of the work; and manage passivity and dependent-independent issues" (Germain & Gitterman, 1980, p. 102).

Salmon (1985) noted that "volunteers should not be used as unpaid staff members to cover budgetary problems" (p. 220). However, it is conceivable that if older volunteers wish to assist in a specific area, e.g., teaching a child to read, then a written contract between the volunteer and the agency specifying that activity may be in order. Social workers could aid in negotiating those concerns upfront until each party is satisfied. The social worker's objective here is to facilitate linking older volunteers into a goodness-of-fit within their communities. Their goal is to both enrich the lives of all persons concerned, while safeguarding job security for employees.

Social workers, to date, have not conducted sufficient research regarding voluntary action by older adults. Practice research is needed, however, to identify the areas of interest in which seniors desire to be involved in a voluntary capacity. Paralleling this, research must be conducted to investigate the needs of agencies, organizations, and the community at large requires keeping in mind that volunteer efforts are not to impinge on the employment opportunities of younger individuals. That is, volunteers must not replace an employee's position in any agency. The inclusion of open-ended questions in such research could promote a flexible, broader scope of involvement, thereby enhancing greater opportunities to facilitate the desired goodness-of-fit between older adults and their communities. This basic research would also become the foundation for the more rigorous studies required to support social policy changes.

Mellinger and Holt (1982) suggested that it would also be beneficial to understand the behaviour of people who do not volunteer. Stevens (1991) believed that social workers could benefit a greater number of elderly volunteers by researching the educational levels of a large number of newer volunteers in relation to their placements. Similarly, Chappell (1999) provided a comprehensive listing of the gaps in the research literature regarding both formal and informal voluntary action. For instance, Chappell (1999) reiterated Mellinger and Holt's (1992) suggestion that important questions remain as to why some people volunteer and "why some do not; and whether those who do not would do so under different circumstances" (Chappell, 1999, p. 7).

VIII. Policy Development

Policy development is required at both micro and macro levels. At present, Volunteer Canada is developing ways to promote volunteerism among older adults and is open to suggestions based on research and experiences. Accepted contributions and resulting policies are provided on its website, http://www.volunteer.ca. Thus, social workers could be counted among those who wish to contribute to this endeavour by identifying the needs of both agencies and organizations, as well as those of older volunteers. Moreover, it is conceivable that recommendations providing achievable goals could be among the first to be considered. For example, if social workers would conduct research as suggested by Chappell (1999) to determine why some people volunteer and "why some do not; and whether those who do not would do so under different circumstances" (p. 7), they could prove to be a highly valuable profession in the eyes of the government, in the area of research, and possibly program development. Social workers cannot overlook the fact that this area of concern was important nearly two decades ago as well. For instance, Perry (1983) suggested that "policy-makers and program planners should focus on creating more helper/volunteer roles for those persons who are not traditionally attracted to volunteer positions" (p. 116).

Further, increased involvement by older volunteers in the social service sector has also increased concerns among agency staff that their jobs may be in jeopardy. Thus, there is an ever-growing need to develop policy and procedures manuals for volunteers within organizations. Social workers, especially those working as private consultants, are in an ideal position to develop agency policies that could allow for harmonious working relationships between agency staff and volunteer contributors. This type of intervention would require interviewing staff, volunteers, and those being served to guide how such policies could be designed to achieve a more favourable working environment for all concerned.

How one advocates on behalf of older volunteers is determined by one's social work role. Social workers in senior centres could conduct research or various intergenerational programs that could appropriately meet both the needs of the centre's members and those within their communities. For example, "Knitting Generations Together" was an intergenerational program that invited older volunteers to teach grade six students to knit. In a case like this, a social worker could present the idea to members of the centre and, if accepted, could then go to the school to advocate on behalf of the senior volunteers, thereby facilitating the linking process needed for this voluntary action to take place. On the other hand, social workers who conduct practice research and provide recommendations that direct voluntary action by older volunteers, by the nature of this process, are advocating on behalf of older volunteers. However, gerontological social workers in private practice must advocate on behalf of older volunteers on an individual basis. Such individuals may desire to volunteer in service areas that are not yet opened to them in their communities. Thus, social workers in this capacity must advocate on their clients' behalf to the appropriate party that could most efficaciously accommodate and utilize the skills and generous offer being made by their clients.

References

Brody, E.M., Saperstein, A.R., & Lawton, M.P. (1989). A multi-service respite program for caregivers of Alzheimer's patients. *Journal of Gerontological Social Work*, 14(1–2), 41–74.

Butler, R.N. & Schechter, M. (1995). Productive aging. In G. Maddox (ed.-in-chief), *The encyclopedia of aging*, 2nd ed. New York: Springer.

Chappell, N. (1998). *Evaluation report: National respite care project*. Ottawa: Canadian Association of Community Care.

Chappell, N. (1999). Volunteering and healthy aging: What we know. Keynote address at the Canadian Forum on Volunteerism in Montreal. [On-line] Available at: http:www.volunteer/dev/projects/healthy_aging/english_text.html

Choi, N.G. & Dinse, S.L. (1998). Challenges and opportunities of the aging population: Social work education and practice for productive aging. *Educational Gerontology*, 24(2), 159–173.

Clary, E.G. & Orenstein, L. (1991). The amount and effectiveness of help: The relationship of motives and abilities to helping behaviour. *Personality and Social Psychology Bulletin*, 17(1), 58–64.

Cnaan, R.A. & Goldberg-Glen, R.S. (1991). Measuring motivation to volunteer in human services. Special Issue: Methods for research and intervention with organizations. *Journal of Applied Behavioral Science*, 27(3), 269–284.

Damron-Rodriguez, J. & Lubben, J.E. (1997). The 1995 WHCoA: An agenda for social work education and training. *Journal of Gerontological Social Work*, 27(3), 65–77.

Deimling, G.T. (1991). Respite use and caregiver well-being in families caring for stable and declining AD patients. *Journal of Gerontological Social Work*, 18(1–2), 17–134.

Dychtwald, K. (1986). Speculations on the future of ageing, wellness, and self-care. *Impact of Science on Society*, 36.3(143), 245–254.

Fengler, A.P. (1984). Life satisfaction of subpopulations of elderly: The comparative effects of volunteerism, employment, and meal site participation. *Research on Aging*, 6(2), 189–212.

Germain, C.B. & Gitterman, A. (1980). *The life model of social work practice.* New York: Columbia University Press.

Gillespie, D.F. & King, A.E.O. (1985). Demographic understanding of volunteerism. *Journal of Sociology and Social Welfare*, 12(4), 798–816.

Godkin, M.A., Wolf, R.S., & Pillemer, K.A. (1989). A case-comparison analysis of elder abuse and neglect. *International Journal of Aging and Human Development*, 28, 207–225.

Goleman, D. (1986, October 7). Feeling of control viewed as central in mental health. *The New York Times*, pp. CI, CII.

Gordon, J. & Neal, J. (1997). Voluntary non-profit organizations: A new research agenda. *Society/Société* (Newsletter of the Canadian Sociology and Anthropology Association), 21(1), 15–19.

Heller, K. (1993). Preventive activities for older adults: Social structures and personal competencies that maintain useful social roles. (Special section: A paradigm for helping, consultation II, section 6). *Journal of Counselling and Development*, 72(2), 124–130.

Higgin, J. (1992). "Health for all" and health promotion. In B. Wharf (ed.), *Communities and social policy in Canada*, pp. 152–180. Toronto: McClelland & Stewart.

Hunter, K.I. & Linn, M.W. (1980–1981). Psychosocial differences between elderly volunteers and non-volunteers. *International Journal of Aging and Human Development*, 12, 205–213.

IYV Projects. (1999). International Year of Volunteers (2001). Volunteer Canada. [On-line] Available at: http://www.volunteer.ca/dev/projects/ international year of vol/iyvl.html.

Jary, D. & Jary, J. (1991). *The HarperCollins dictionary of sociology*, p. 497. New York: HarperCollins.

Jones, S. (1986). The elders: A new generation. *Aging and Society*, 6, 313–331.

Kent, J. (1989). Volunteers in health organizations. *Voluntary Action*. Ottawa: Ministry of Supply and Services Canada.

Kerschner, H. & Pegues, J.M. (1998). Productive aging: A quality of life agenda. *Journal of the American Dietetic Association*, 98(12), 1445 (8 pages). [On-line serial] Available at: Article A53479831.

Kuehne, V.S. & Sears, H.A. (1993). Beyond the call of duty: Older volunteers committed to children and families. *Journal of Applied Gerontology*, 12, 425–438.

Lambert, C., Gubberman, M., & Morris, M. (1964). Reopening doors to community participation for older people. How realistic? *Social Service Review*, 38(1), 42–50.

MacMillan, D. (1999). Older adults and volunteering: A booming trend. Volunteer Canada. [On-line] Available at: dmacmillan@volunteer.ca.

MacMillan, D. (2000). Volunteering: A booming trend. Volunteer Canada. [On-line]. Available at: dmacmillan@volunteer.ca, or contact Volunteer Canada at 1-800-670-0401.

Manser, G. (1987). *Encyclopedia of social work*, 18th ed., vol. 2. Washington: National Association of Social Workers.

Mellinger, J. & Holt, R. (1982). Characteristics of elderly participants in three types of leisure groups. *Psychological Reports*, 50(2), 447–458.

Moen, P. (1995). A life course approach to post-retirement roles and well-being. In L.A. Bond, S.J. Cutler, & A. Gram (eds.), *Promoting successful and productive aging*, pp. 239–256. Thousand Oaks: Sage.

Motenko, A.K. (1989). The frustrations, gratifications, and well-being of dementia caregivers. *The Gerontologist*, 29, 166–172.

Newman, S., Vasudev, J., & Onawola, R. (1985). Older volunteers' perceptions of impacts of volunteering on their psychological well-being. *Journal of Applied Gerontology*, 4(2), 123–127.

Norris, T. (1997). [no title]. On-line journal: National civic review, 86(1), 3 (8 pages). [On-line serial] Available at: Article A19532653.

NSGVP On-line. (2000, September) National survey of giving, volunteering and participating, (5 pages). [On-line] Available at: http://ccp.ca/nsgvp/n-f6-ca.htm.

Nyp, G. (1996). The real cost of voluntarism. Front & Centre On-line, 3(3), 1–2, 4. [On-line] Available at: http://www.ccp.ca/information/documents/fc84.htm.

Penning, M. & Wasyliw, D. (1992). Homebound learning opportunities: Reaching out to older shut-ins and their caregivers. *Gerontologist*, 32(5), 704–707.

Perry, W. (1983). The willingness of persons 60 or over to volunteer: Implications for the social services. *Journal of Gerontological Social Work*, 5(4), 107–118.

Romero, C.J. (1986). The economics of volunteerism: A review. In Institute of Medicine/National Research Council, *America's aging: Productive roles in an older society*. Washington: National Academic Press.

Rowe, J.W. (1997). The new gerontology. Online journal: Science 278(5337), 367 (2 pages). [O-line serial] Available at: Article A20006378.

Salmon, R. (1985). The use of aged volunteers: individual and organizational considerations. *Journal of Gerontological Social Work,* 8(3–4), 211–223.

Snyder, M. (1993). Basic research and practical problems: The promise of a "functional" personality and social psychology. *Personality and Social Psychology Bulletin,* 19, 251–264.

Snyder, M. & Omoto, A.M. (1992). Volunteerism and society's response to the HIV epidemic. *Current Directions in Psychological Science,* 1, 113–116.

Stachenko, S. (1994). National opportunities for health promotion: The Canadian experience. *Healthy Promotion International,* 9(2), 105–110.

Statistics Canada. (1998). National survey of giving, volunteering and participating (NSGVP), 1997. *The Daily,* 3–7, cat. no. 11-001E. Ottawa: Statistics Canada.

Stevens, Ellen. (1991). Toward satisfaction and retention of senior volunteers. *Journal of Gerontological Social Work,* 16(3–4), 33–41.

Wharf, B. (ed.). (1992). *Communities and social policies in Canada.* Toronto: McClelland & Stewart.

Wheeler, J.A. (1997). Elder's involvement in health promotion programs: A qualitative review. (Unpublished manuscript) Available from: J. Wheeler, 65 Cameron Ave., Essex, ON N8M 2L2.

Wheeler, J.A. (1998). Essex retirees social club: Assessment of programs and services. (Unpublished manuscript) Available from: Essex Retirees Social Club, 32 Russell St., Essex.

Wheeler, J.A. (1999). Improving the quality of life of older adults: A sourcebook for social work practice based on a healthy communities model. Book proposal in progress. Information available from: J. Wheeler, 65 Cameron Ave., Essex, ON N8M 2L2.

Wheeler, J.A. (2000). Seniors' quality of life project. Available from: South Essex Community Centre, 215 Talbot St. E., Leamington, ON N8H 3X5.

Wheeler, J., Gorey, K.M., & Greenblatt, B. (1998). The beneficial effects of volunteering for older people and the people they serve: A meta-analysis. *International Journal of Aging and Human Development,* 47(1), 69–79.

Internet Resources

AARP: The Volunteer Experience
http://www.aarp.org/volunteerguide/
Canadian Volunteer Centres Experts in Volunteerism
Volunteer Opportunities Exchange (VOE)
http://www.voe-reb.org/index.jhtml

e-Volunteerism
  The Electronic Journal of the Volunteer Community.
  http://www.e-volunteerism.com
Volunteer Canada
  A comprehensive resource guide for volunteers and organizations.
  http://www.volunteer.ca/
Volunteer Work Program: Seniors in Service to Seattle
  Clearinghouse in linking seniors to volunteer opportunities and
  identifying seniors who are seeking volunteer opportunities.
  http://www.cityofseattle.net/humanservices/mosc/sis/default.htm

Additional Readings

Haddon, D. (2003). *The 5 principles of ageless living: A woman's guide to lifelong health, beauty, and well-being.* New York/Toronto: ATRIA Books.

Hodgson, H. (1999). *Smart aging: Taking charge of your physical and emotional health.* New York/Toronto: John Wiley & Sons, Inc.

Koenig, H.G. (2002). *Purpose and power in retirement: New opportunities for meaning and significance.* Philadelphia/London: Templeton Foundation Press.

McDonald, J. & McDonald, O. (2003). *Get up and go: Strategies for active living after 50.* Toronto/Oxford: The Dundurn Group.

Midlarsky, E. & Kahana, E. (1994). *Altruism in later life.* Thousand Oaks: Sage.

SECTION II

SELECTED PRACTICE SETTINGS

CHAPTER 15

SOCIAL WORK PRACTICE WITH INSTITUTIONALIZED FRAIL ELDERLY

RON MARTYN AND

LEN FABIANO

The dramatic increase in the number of older people in recent years and on into the first part of the twenty-first century has heightened awareness of the need for increased and improved institutional services for the elderly. The field of social work has and will continue to change to meet the new demands placed on it by the system and by the older frail clients. This chapter focuses on the changes and expectations of social workers in response to the special needs of the frail elderly in both generic and age-specific institutions. The skills required of the social worker for this specialized area are presented along with strategies for future development in the field.

I.   The Clientele

A.   *The Numbers*

In recent years, the dramatic increase in the number and percentage of people over 65 years of age in both Canada and the United States has been a major focal point for demographers and service providers alike. Expectations of an ever-increasing cohort of senior adults have heightened concern for the demands that will follow in the health care sector. The reality is that the percentage shift of elderly persons has already begun. The number over 65 years of age will accelerate to over 22 percent of the total population (as compared to an average of

11 percent in 1986) by the year 2030 (Chappell et al., 2003; Marshall, 1987) and continue to rise at a steady rate beyond this period.

The institutionalized frail elderly account for between 3 percent of the population over 65 years (e.g., United States) and 8 percent of the population over 65 years (Canada, Sweden) (Berg et al., 1988; McPherson, 1983). This major variation in percentage terms reflects a combination of several factors. Where there are insufficient affordable institutional services, the rate of institutionalization is lower. Similarly, where there is an availability of extensive home support services, the rate of institutionalization will be decreased. Conversely, where there are limited home supports, combined with affordable available institutional services, the percentage of institutionalized frail elderly will be increased.

The percentage of seniors living in long-term care facilities is misleading in terms of the likelihood of an older person living in such a facility. While the percentage ranges from 3–8 percent in most regions, the reality is that the majority of people will, at some point in their lives, live in a long-term care setting. The low percentage refers to how many are living there at the moment. Over one's lifetime, however, the chances are much greater that one will live in a care facility than not. This further emphasizes the important role that long-term care services provide to this population.

A further consideration is that the major increase in this age group falls into the category of the "old-old"—those over the age of 85 years. This age group is the fastest-growing segment of the older population and represents the largest portion of the institutionalized frail elderly (Atchley, 2000).

The implications for the future are obvious. Not only will the numbers of older persons increase significantly, but also the number of "old-old" (and consequently the frail institutionalized elderly) will increase even more dramatically. This shift has already resulted in changes to the health care delivery system, and it will force even more dramatic changes over the next 30 years.

B. Profile of Institutional Care Settings

The institutionalized frail elderly are found in both general population or generic health care settings and age-specific facilities. General or generic settings include acute-care hospitals, psychiatric facilities, and special treatment centres. Age-specific settings or long-term care facilities include nursing homes, homes for the aged, and, to some extent, retirement facilities. The roles and functions of social workers in relation to the frail elderly will be examined relative to both types of settings.

C. General Population (Generic) Care Institutions

By their very nature, general population institutions were never specifically geared to a particular age group. Their intent has been to provide care for all regardless of age. However, as a result of the recent surge in the numbers of older adults, such institutions have increasingly recognized that this segment of the population constitutes a disproportionately high number of the total clients being served.

The impact of an increasingly older clientele has presented new challenges for the generic facilities. Not only do the special needs of this clientele present special demands, but there are also increased operational pressures on the system that impact the entire organization. Older clients require longer recovery times for most treatments and as a result the turnaround time from admission to discharge increases significantly (Novak, 1985). Generic settings today are finding that their costs are increasing as more and more clients become long-term in nature—not only is there added cost for the longer treatment program, but there is added pressure for more bed capacity to resolve the shortage of bed space for those awaiting admission. Increasing the bed capacity puts added pressure on an already financially taxed system.

Social workers are employed in most generic settings. They provide services to the broad range of clients within such institutions, but they too feel the impact of encountering an increasing number of older clients. The need for more time to serve these long-term-stay patients adds pressure to the job. Likewise, this segment of the population requires from the professional new skills and knowledge to effectively deal with their complex problems. Some generic facilities have responded accordingly by providing an increased psycho-geriatric perspective in treatment plans, upgrading staff, and hiring gerontological specialists within each discipline area (Becker & Kaufman, 1988).

D. Age-Specific Care Institutions

Up until the early 1970s, few social workers were employed in age-specific care institutions. The focus of care in such settings was quite limited. Further, programming, supports, and resources were at a minimum. The average age of resident populations was typically mid to late 70s, and although the clientele were frail, they were provided few supports. In the late 1980s, a different resident profile has emerged. The average age of the resident population was now late 80s, with a new mandate for care that employs concepts such as quality of life, individualized care, and home-like environments (Novak, 1985).

Generally speaking, there are two distinct groups of long-term care facilities:

- There are those that are responding to the added demands of an increasingly complex clientele through a clear and progressive focus in their philosophy, programming, staff supports, and resources. Such organizations are setting new standards of care through innovation and a client-centred focus on care.
- The other group is comprised of those that are mired in past practices and, without clear direction, are struggling to meet the new demands of residents. While representing the minority of care providers, this group fits the long-held negative stereotypes of such settings. They have been delinquent in keeping up with the knowledge, trends, and expectations within this specialized area. With increasing demands for quality care through government legislation, public accountability, and demanding accreditation expectations, such facilities are struggling to continue functioning, let alone provide quality of life for this unique clientele (Grossman & Weiner, 1988).

Long-term care is very diverse not only in its progressiveness but in its configuration. For example, working in a 600-bed facility creates different demands from working in a 60-bed facility. A facility located in a major urban setting is quite different from one located in a remote rural setting. Likewise, the configuration of the resident population within any one facility can vary dramatically. Most facilities have three distinct groups: those clients who are cognitively well but physically disabled; those who are mentally impaired; and those who are both physically frail and mentally impaired.

Furthermore, one cannot guarantee a homogeneous age group even in what are usually considered age-specific institutions. Some facilities in some regions have individuals as young as 14 mixed with others as old as 105, all under the same roof. Some even have a mixture of seniors and long-time institutionalized mentally handicapped individuals of a variety of age ranges.

When one speaks of becoming involved in age-specific, long-term care institutions, there are many options and levels of quality from which to choose. While many long-term care facilities participate in national accreditation programs, the expectations from state to state or province to province vary, and such participation is generally optional. As a result, there are no guaranteed standards of services and supports within long-term care facilities. Direct care staff in most long-term care facilities consists mostly of nurse's aides, with registered nursing staff generally assuming leadership functions. Recreation staff play an integral part in direct care provision in this setting as well. In the typical age-specific, long-term care setting, every member of the facility from housekeeper to aide, from maintenance person to administrator, is an integral part of the care process and team (Fabiano, 1989). This is especially important when one considers that staff come from a variety of backgrounds and disciplines and many possess minimal training in this specialty. This is an approach that is not generally encouraged in the acute-care or generic setting.

It must be recognized that the majority of residents in today's long-term care settings are identified as suffering from some degree of mental impairment, with physical frailty seen as a secondary issue. Such residents present special demands on care providers (Washburn et al., 2003) and cannot be overlooked on the part of social workers or other health care providers.

Today the majority of age-specific, long-term care facilities employ social workers. This is in marked contrast to the realities of limited social work practices in long-term care prior to the 1990s. Even though the need and desire may be present to have such a specialist on a full-time basis, most generally receive funding to support only a part-time position to their staff complement.

What is evident to this point in the evolution of the social workers' role within long-term care is that the limits and scope of the role within any one facility often depend on the initiative and creativity of the individual social worker involved. The challenge for the field of social work is to anticipate the changes before they happen and incorporate new and innovative strategies in response to the increased demands and changes.

E.   The Clientele

The institutional setting in which the older adult is located determines to some extent the problems presented. In other words, the differences associated with the social, psychological, and physical environment of different institutions may result in varied responses with any one client. Therefore, it is important to consider the frail elderly in relation to the type of settings in which they are found.

The elderly admitted as short-term-stay patients (a few days) in generic settings do not create the same problems as those who become long-stay patients (a period of weeks or months) in an acute-care setting. Further, the older adult seldom exhibits one distinct impairment. Rather, s/he typically demonstrates a variety of disabilities. When placed in a setting that includes younger clients, the differences can cause problems.

The contrasting profiles of younger versus older patients/clients, their reason(s) for being in generic settings, and the impact and prognosis of their diagnoses are contributing factors to difficulties they will inevitably encounter in assessment, treatment, and rehabilitation.

For example, a younger person may be admitted to the hospital with a leg fracture suffered in a football game at school. In the bed next to him is an elderly man who fell at home and broke his hip. While the injuries are of the same general nature, these individuals' needs and responses will be quite diverse. The energy, resilience, and recuperative powers of the young man may result in his fracture having little more impact than restricting him to bed. His cognitive and physical energy level is still intact, resulting in his need to be active and occupy his time to relieve the boredom. As a result, he does those things he likes to do—play his radio (loudly), watch television, do his homework, and visit with his friends (which periodically seem to occur all at the same time!).

Meanwhile, the effect of the fractured hip on his elderly roommate is much more severe. This older patient is not so quick to bounce back to his normal self. The demands now placed on him both physically and emotionally may be taxing his remaining resources to the limit. In fact, the combination of the injury, its restrictiveness, and the effects of the medication given for pain may cause bouts of confusion and disorientation. Any added noise or disturbance in his room presents further stress that he cannot easily deal with at this time, hence the conflict. Both patients become increasingly frustrated and agitated with each other. This places demands on staff to resolve the conflicts and smooth over the differences in this imposed relationship.

Furthermore, the older client can constantly challenge the pace that staff normally maintain. As a person ages, his or her functioning levels decrease. Reflexes, muscle strength, coordination, cognitive processing, etc., are still intact and working, but are not as fast or as resilient as when the person was younger. This does not create a handicap to older persons in their life course, as they simply learn to adapt to the gradual changes as they occur. But when they experience a new disability, that limitation now often taxes those resources to their limit.

Adding further to such problems may be the approach, perception, and focus of the facility and staff toward the long-stay older adult in the general population care centres. In a setting that is focused on treatment and recovery, and that measures its successes by major positive changes in a person's condition, performance, or behaviour, working with the long-stay older patient may be seen as counterproductive to the organization's mission.

The improvements of the older patient experiencing multiple long-standing problems associated with a decrease in physical energy, stamina, and recuperative power are often less dramatic than that to which staff are accustomed. When the prognosis shows little gain, those staff who are trained to "cure" are frustrated in what they perceive as the waste of intense and aggressive efforts.

For facilities and staff who are geared and trained under the medical model of care, the older client can be seen as a source of frustration (Henderson & Vesperi, 1995). Such frustration is manifested both overtly and subtly. Overtly, the facility can point to the backup of treatment and long waiting lists as evidence of the negative impact older people have on the care system and the reason for the institution's inability to cope. In a way, the older clients are often seen as the source of institutional paralysis.

Negative consequences of staff frustration with older clients can be more subtle and consequently more difficult to identify. Seldom will staff openly express their frustration about the older long-term patient. However, it becomes difficult to contain one's frustration over a long period of time. Eventually, staff may not be able to control their feelings and frustrations when performing care with this client. Although it is hoped that the quality of physical care is not jeopardized, the emotional and psychosocial components may be. The older client will often find that the staff spend decreasing amounts of time with him or her.

In some settings this can be understandable. Generally, the majority of generic institutions are not environmentally equipped to handle a long-stay patient. The best example is an acute-care hospital. Many medical floors where such a patient will be found do not have lounges, dining areas, etc. The patient is then restricted to his or her room for extended periods of time because there is really nowhere else to sit.

The general expectation is that the patients will wear hospital gowns rather than being dressed, perpetuating for the older patient "the sick role." Staff on such units do not normally consider how a patient must occupy his or her day. The usual expectation in the generic setting is that patients are too ill to be concerned about fulfilling their time or are well enough to occupy it themselves. The older long-term patient is usually not ill enough that s/he is oblivious to the hours passing, nor well enough to be independent in filling those hours. This boredom and isolation can only complicate the patient's frailty, resulting in withdrawal or behaviour outbursts in order to break the pattern and routine of this setting.

The care of older clients in generic institutions will not only continue in the future but will be accelerated. The implications for such settings are that both the institutional and staff approaches to care for the frail elderly will require significant changes in order to best serve this clientele.

II.   Age-specific Institutions and the Frail Elderly

One of the most common stereotypes of aging is that all "old people" are alike. In actual fact, there are as many differences among the older population as there are between the young and the old (Keith, 1982). This is perhaps easier to appreciate when one thinks in terms of age spans. It is easy to accept that the needs and interests of the 15-year-old are different from that of the 35-year-old. For example, they don't even recognize the names of one another's favourite musical performers, let alone appreciate the music. On the other hand, there can be an expectation that the person who is 70 years of age has a great deal in common with the person who is 90. Just as there is a 20-year span and differences in interests and needs in the younger age comparison, there are similar differences between these older groupings. They don't all like the same old tunes. The difficulty for staff in an institution for older clients is to not only recognize and support these differences, but also be aware that over time the institution must change as the age cohorts change.

One problem that may be perpetuated in an age-specific, long-term care facility is that if all clients are older and disabled to some degree, the range of expectations made by the clientele, the institution, its staff, and the clients themselves can be narrower. The obvious detriment of such settings is that there can be an "age-ghettoization" process.

There are few, if any, younger people within the facility (other than the caregivers themselves), and the older clients are surrounded by a diminished level of expectation—a "what else can I expect at my age" response (Fabiano, 1989). This becomes a self-fulfilling prophecy, of course, because the client does not expect to be able to do more and, it becomes difficult to motivate the client to try harder, to go beyond the current functioning level. While the personal lifestyles of the younger population can pose frustrations and difficulties for the older client in the institutional setting, the older person can also long for some contact with age groups other than the elderly. It is common in age-specific settings to hear an older client comment about visitors "breathing some life into this place" following a visit by a group of young persons or family members.

Upon entry to the age-specific, long-term care facility, the person does become a "resident." The name itself is indicative of the institutional expectation of the person's tenure—this is not for recovery, rehabilitation, and return home—this is for recovery and rehabilitation to the point where the person will be able to function at his or her maximum level in the setting. This perception and expectation is reinforced by the operating norms (most people stay long term, and the staff reinforces the person's settling in and making this home). Residents are encouraged to bring in mementos and some furnishings from home. There are no restrictions on visiting hours, and there are more offerings of seemingly non-therapeutic recreational activities, much like what one would find in the outside community.

The net result of this process has the potential of reinforcing the client's loss of control and choice. Now that the person is in an institutional setting, there generally is little discussion or acceptance of the idea of a return to home. The negative responses (fight or submission) may be heightened upon introduction to this new environment (Fabiano, 1989).

Social workers within the age-specific institutions face many problems that are similar to those experienced in generic settings. Both residents and family members are the key target groups for the social worker's efforts. Residents in the long-term care settings exhibit the same responses of resignation, unrealistic anticipation, and a realistic acceptance combined with the determination to try to deal with the disability as well as possible. However, there may be differences in the intensity of the responses. The focus in long-term care is a different one than what most are accustomed to in an acute-care setting. The question arises: What do you do for the person who has virtually lost all of the major components that have provided him/her with a desired level of quality of life? The client who experiences compounded grieving is one who has gone from one major loss to another without the opportunity to resolve the initial loss. This has a domino effect, where the emotional experience of the first loss only compounds the second, weakening the person's coping skills and support systems (Fabiano, 1989). In these circumstances, there is seldom the opportunity to work with the person toward rebuilding a life. Rather, there is the potential to patch life together with what is remaining—probably one of the greatest challenges for those in the "people professions."

The converse of the resident's acceptance of his or her functioning level provides the social worker with the next challenge. Once the resident has accepted the status of "resident," the problem of resignation and giving up may become more of an issue. The social worker now must work to provide encouragement for the person to continue to try to be involved in the face of recognizing that things may not get a whole lot better.

Again, the client must come to understand that making the choice to do nothing also has consequences. The result of doing nothing will inevitably be further deterioration. As bad as things may seem now, the resident must understand that they can get worse if nothing is done and there is withdrawal from the surrounding people and activities of the facility. The social worker provides both individual and group supports for residents in the long-term care environment. While the bulk of these interactions may take place in the early stages following admission, there will also be the need for ongoing support for different residents at different times (Burnside, 1984).

The function of helping residents understand their own responsibilities in their personal care plan is an important element in the process of motivating residents. It is one in which the social worker plays a key, but not the only, role. The social worker functions as a team member, coordinating approaches and strategies with all members of the care team. Not only does this have implications for the obvious functioning areas in the facility, such as nursing, O.T., physiotherapy, and recreation, but also the not-so-obvious areas such as housekeeping and dietary. The social worker must work with all other team members as equal partners in the care process. The dietary aide can either reinforce or undermine the team's efforts with casual comments or actions in the course of serving a meal. Similarly, the housekeeping aide can have a dramatic impact on the resident's outlook and approach to life. People who work in long-term care generally concede that residents will often disclose more to the housekeeper who comes into their rooms every day than to any other member of the care team. Without encouragement and recognition that they have such valuable insights, the housekeeping staff will often not be aware that they have this exceptional vantage point and will not come forward with their observations. The social worker must not only be open to talking to the housekeepers about what they have seen and heard, but they must also reinforce with them the important role they can serve and encourage them to share this input with others.

Times have changed in long-term care. In the past the main concern centred on physical issues—programming to prevent bedsores and contractures and deal with issues of the bowels and bladder. The field then progressed to centre attention on social issues such as supports and activities. While there has been an increased focus on socio-emotional concerns, further progress is still required.

One hundred percent of the clientele in long-term care is vulnerable to depression, one of the predominant disorders of the frail elderly (Butler & Lewis, 1982). Given the variety and severity of losses experienced within a short period of time, from widowhood, to a change in lifestyle, to relocation, disability, and so on, it is no wonder that these individuals experience what can aptly be termed "compounded grieving" (Fabiano, 1989).

Chemical interventions continue to be the first and primary response to emotional disruption in the lives of seniors within the community and in long-term care. According to Atchley (2000), 15 percent of those over 65 years of age need mental health services to deal with depression or chronic illness in the United States, while only 2–4 percent receive psychological, psychiatric, or community mental health services. Effectively dealing with the emotional side of these lives through psychosocial therapeutic interventions is still too infrequent in long-term care, and the role of the social worker is crucial to help enrich and expand these caring processes and approaches.

III.   Practice Roles and Responsibilities

Social workers face the same moral dilemmas as other health care professionals when confronted by the prospect of working with the elderly in long-term care. For many, the reasons for getting into the field are the same as those that repel them from working with the institutionalized frail elderly. There is generally a desire to help those who are in need; however, the frail elderly can present too much need. Some care providers find it difficult to deal with people with as many impairments and limitations as those living in long-term care. When confronted with clients whose prognoses present only short-term marginal gains before their condition is further eroded or they are eliminated by death, the care provider's need for personal gratification may take precedence over the desire to assist the clients.

Most professionals believe that working with other populations in the health care sector more attractive, glamorous, and exciting because the clients have more potential for improvements that they can use for a long period of time. In a society that highly values designer clothes, exotic foreign cars, and life in the fast lane, and where people are inundated by a media blitz focused on drugs, alcohol, domestic violence, sexually transmitted diseases, and child abuse, the realities of the needs of the frail elderly are often lost. People working in the health care sector, including social workers, are obviously influenced by the culture. It is difficult for health care professionals to be motivated by wrinkles, sagging body parts, incontinence, prostate problems, memory loss, and the constant presence of death.

The frail elderly represent one of the social worker's greatest challenges. The social worker must both help the client respond positively to various impairments and obstacles, while thinking and feeling his or her own way through notions and prejudices about the elderly, growing old, and death.

The philosophy of age-specific institutions is one featuring holistic care, which is consistent with the mandate of the social work profession. The skills the social worker brings to the setting are viewed as not only fitting within the philosophical perspective, but also equal in value to the provision of physical care. The social worker in a non-age-specific institution is usually seen as a member of the larger health care team. Theoretically, the social worker has as much input and importance as any other member of that team—be it the physician, nurse, occupational therapist, or others (Edelson & Lyons, 1985); this often falls short in actual practice. The social worker may find that the hard facts, such as patient temperature, blood pressure, and bowel movements, carry more weight within the medical model of health care than the less measured and calibrated observances of the social sciences. The position the social work department and personnel on the organizational chart should help to shed some light on the status of the program within the facility. If it is located under the medical umbrella, there may be a realistic expectation that there will be a dominant role to be played by the medical staff.

The social worker in long-term care generally has an active role with many functions undertaken with an eclectic approach. Almost any activity can be called for in this setting, including counselling residents family and staff, assessment and placement coordination of prospective residents, case management, policy development, leading support groups, evaluating practice, and educating. The range of responsibilities and duties of the social worker depends very much on the size and attitudes of the facility and the ability and drive of the individual social worker. Such a professional may be expected to cover any or all of the following components:

1) Working with the client:
   • direct counselling
   • group support
   • behavioural assessment and intervention
   • advocacy
   • education
   • resource utilization
2) Working with the family:
   • direct counselling
   • support group
   • education
   • integration into care
3) Working within the organization:
   • assessment and placement
   • employee-assistance program
   • policy development
   • volunteer coordination
   • mediation and conflict resolution
   • research and evaluation
   • coordination with other organizations services
   • staff training
   • community outreach coordination

IV.   Potential for Role Development

The social worker's roles and responsibilities within institutional settings have evolved considerably and will continue to expand in the immediate future. In generic settings, there are opportunities to facilitate the organizations' attempts to come to grips with serving an increasingly elderly dominated clientele. In age-specific settings, the standards or expectations of the social worker's role remain fluid with tremendous latitude for development. The role of the social worker depends primarily on the individual facility; the perception of the need and benefits of such a professional; the philosophy and progressiveness of the facility; the resources and time made available to the individual social worker; and the creativity, initiative, and personal drive of the individual fulfilling the role.

In an ever-changing area of specialization such as long-term care, each facility is compelled to evolve in multiple directions at the same time in order to keep up with the increasing demands and expectations placed upon on it. In the planning of some facilities, the social worker's role is seen as a part of such progression. In other facilities it has been a long-established and integrated role, while yet others see the position being rather tangential in that it is there only because of specific funding. The reality is the changing clientele [changing in terms of needs and numbers] is forcing the requirement for the increased availability of social workers within such settings.

In the near future the older adults that will be served are today part of the "me generation," the postwar baby boomers. This cohort has been a dominant group throughout their lives in our society and one that has been comfortable and successful in shaping policy directions; there is no doubt that they will continue to do so into the future as well. Therefore, there is a great likelihood that services for older adults will increase in magnitude and quality as these baby boomers approach their own old age and expect excellence in service. There is also less hesitation on the part of many in this cohort to seek out professional help in dealing with emotions and relationship issues as compared to those who are presently over 75 (Lasoski & Thelen, 1987). This help will be integrated into the service package expected by those entering institutional care settings in the future.

As has already been identified, areas such as resident advocacy, case management, and community outreach and coordination are recognized as crucial in the health care continuum. These are areas that are ideally suited to the skills of the social worker, and there are opportunities to develop and be involved in such services.

The ever-increasing numbers of mentally impaired residents in long-term care facilities present ongoing challenges and opportunities for social workers. Through the acquisition of specialized skills in response to the needs of these residents, the social worker can serve as a valued member of the care team. By focusing on issues such as the physical environment, social groups and interactions, awareness of behavioural triggers, cultural sensitivity, and the employment of interpersonal approaches suited to this special population, social workers can provide a critical link to the residents' satisfaction with their home.

As indicated in all of the chapters in Section II of this text, success in long-term care is dependent upon an interdisciplinary or multidisciplinary approach to care. While vestiges of the medical model still linger (Henderson & Vesperi, 1995), a more holistic approach to care is becoming the norm.

> Many groups have useful contributions to make to the development of health care for older people, and some practitioners in nursing, social work, occupational therapy, gerontology and other professions have training and experience in health aspects of aging that far exceed the average physician's. (Atchely, 2000)

In such a milieu, the social worker who makes meaningful contributions and values the perspectives of others will play a major role in the lives of residents, families, and employees. Awareness, understanding, and respect of the roles others play in the care setting are required to achieve such success. The social worker must acquire a reasonable knowledge of the other disciplines in order to participate and contribute. Within long-term care, resident assessment and measurement of progress is moving toward the utilization of the Minimum Data Set (MDS), a universal and comparable measurement process used extensively in the U.S. and some parts of Canada. Social workers will need to familiarize themselves with such tools and processes as they emerge in order to continue to add to the therapeutic process.

References to an area provide an indication as to the evolution of the discipline, and for social work in long-term care, the recent text entitled *A Guide for Nursing Home Social Workers* (Beaulieu, 2002) suggested that there has been clear progress (albeit a U.S. perspective). Beaulieu's detailed descriptions of the many functions of the social worker in long-term care point to the emergence of common understandings and expectations, and provides a valuable resource to the field.

Much of the impetus for the increased utilization of social workers in age-specific institutions is likely to come from within such organizations in the future. This can only help to reinforce the need for the expansion of services to include social work. This self-advocacy on the part of social workers should be facilitated by networking among both practising social workers and non-practising social workers who are functioning in related capacities (Karuza et al., 1988). If social workers recognize the pioneering role that they are serving in the age-specific institutions, the need and value of networking will be obvious, and this will become an increasingly important area of involvement for them in the future.

V. Concluding Remarks

Throughout this chapter focus has been on the current and future role of social workers in institutional settings. At times, the roles appear quite established and clear. In other instances they are seen as being marginalized or almost non-existent—social work practices and skills being implemented through the auspices of other disciplines and functions. Both scenarios are visible in the workplace today. The challenge for social workers of the future is to determine where in this scenario they will be able to function most effectively. Some will personally find the established positions to be what they are seeking, and they will benefit most by moving in that direction. Others will be excited by the crusading nature of becoming involved in the less well-defined areas of service and will embark on this more uncertain career path. Either route offers tremendous scope and opportunity for the social workers of the future.

Case Example

Mr. Jones has had a history of relative affluence. He was a bank manager for 42 years until he was forced to retire (with many misgivings) at the age of 65. In retirement he initially had considerable difficulty filling his time and defining his role. He interpreted retirement as "being old." He believed he had little purpose. His pre-retired life was predominantly occupied by his job, and without it he had difficulty defining his personal self-worth and identity.

His relationship with his wife was always strong. In retirement that relationship only intensified. She filled the void, challenging him to become involved, becoming his main companion. For three years she directed him into rewarding activities, with much of their time spent travelling. He was beginning to enjoy his changed status and the freedom it provided him.

At the age of 68 Mr. Jones experienced his first stroke. Although the residual effects of that stroke were minimal, it hit him hard, only further reinforcing his previously held misconceptions of "being old" and his changing role. Again it was his wife who became his main motivational support. It was her encouragement and persistence that drew him away from the abyss of emotional collapse. Two years later he experienced his second stroke. The residual effect this time was much more severe. He lost movement on his right side, as his right arm and leg were completely paralyzed.

He was devastated. His time in hospital was a difficult one. His emotional response was expressed in chronically aggressive behaviour. He resisted physiotherapy, activities, and almost everything he needed in order to effectively cope and achieve his maximum independent state. The result was that there was little progression beyond being able to transfer himself to a wheelchair. Within a short time, he was ready for discharge. The options given to his family were home or admission to a long-term care facility. His wife decided she wanted to take him home.

Within three months she worked with him to the point that he was able to walk with a quad cane. She had him active to a certain degree. Her constant support became the catalyst to move him through his grieving state to a point where he began to see a light ahead in the tunnel. Within a year of his second stroke he still presented angry outbursts, but maintained a more livable state. It was at this time that his wife died suddenly.

His inability to care for himself resulted in immediate placement in a long-term care facility. He was allowed to bring in only minimal personal belongings. To him each item he sold or gave away represented a permanent separation from his past—a further loss of his wife and a part of himself.

He now not only had to deal with the loss of his wife, his companion, and his mentor, but he also had to forfeit the lifestyle to which he was accustomed. As someone who was used to being in control, he would not accept nor participate willingly now when confronted by directives and routines. The only accommodation available was a semi-private room. He was required to share this room with another man in his 90s who was very frail and non-communicative due to a recent stroke.

Mr. Jones's daughters were beside themselves as to what to do. Their mother was the dominant figure within their family and the only one who "controlled" Dad. Dad's aggressive response only made them feel hopeless and frightened. They had never encountered the full extent of his emotional outbursts before. Mom had always buffered his emotions so they never totally saw this side of him.

Staff in the facility found themselves with an increasingly difficult resident. His aggressive outbursts resulted in avoidance behaviour on their part. Staff spent only as much time with him as was necessary. The more Mr. Jones was left alone, the deeper he sank into his depression and grief.

His involvement within any functions of the facility was almost non-existent. From admission, he sat himself in a wheelchair and refused to walk or even to stand on his own. He would not transfer from bed to chair and back without assistance. Whenever he did receive help, he was belligerent and vulgar, making accusations that staff moved him the wrong way or were not quick enough to respond. Some nursing staff suggested that he be administered sedation to make him more manageable. There was concern that Mr. Jones's frustration and aggression might be taken out on other residents if they disturbed him.

The social worker became the intermediary within the facility. Her initial assessment of Mr. Jones consisted of reviewing his past history, lifestyle, family dynamics, and his response to his two strokes. She started working with him in one-to-one counselling. Initially her attempts to establish any rapport were thwarted. As she got closer to any delicate issues, his aggressive response became more intense. During this initial work-up, she met with the daughters to help them understand their father's behaviour and to assist them in learning how to cope with his outbursts and emotions.

With the background information in hand, the social worker began working on establishing a positive relationship with Mr. Jones. During the same period, contact was made with another long-established resident who had indicated an interest in participating as a "resident buddy." The social worker discussed Mr. Jones with the other resident buddy, and he agreed to start visitations with Mr. Jones in the hope of making him feel more a part of the facility. After a period of four weeks of resident and social worker visitations, Mr. Jones was encouraged to attend a "new resident" support group intended to assist new admissions to understand and deal with the transition to long-term care. At the encouragement of the social worker, he was also assessed by a psychiatrist and placed on an anti-depressive agent.

In conjunction with these efforts, the social worker worked with the staff during the care conference to help them understand his behaviour and to develop some techniques to deal with his outbursts. A "staff buddy" system was established, which identified two direct care staff and a volunteer who were willing to work with the social worker in assisting Mr. Jones to work through his grieving.

The result of these efforts was that Mr. Jones's behaviour and emotional state became tolerable for both staff and family. A year after admission, Mr. Jones was walking again with a quad cane. His depressive episodes flared at increasingly less intervals. Even though he still had frequent periods of anger, he was able to control his outbursts. His involvement within the activities of the facility was minimal, but he would participate in a few general events. On speaking with him, he would state that he felt he could not enjoy life anymore, but it was tolerable.

Note

1. The original version of this chapter was published in M. Holosko & P. Taylor (eds.), *Social work practice in health care settings*, pp. 303–333. Toronto: Canadian Scholars' Press Inc.

References

Atchley, R.C. (2000). *Social forces and aging*. Belmont: Wadsworth.

Beaulieu, E.M. (2002) *A guide for nursing home social workers*. New York: Springer.

Becker, G. & Kaufman, S. (1988). Old age, rehabilitation and research: A review of the issues. *The Gerontologist*, 28(4).

Bennett, R. (ed). (1980). *Aging, isolation and resocialization*. Toronto: Van Nostrand Reinhold Company.

Berg, S., Branch, L.G., Doyle, A.E., & Sundstrom, G. (1988). Institutional and home-based long-term care alternatives: The 1965–1985 Swedish experience. *The Gerontologist*, 28(6).

Binstock, R.H. & L.K. George (eds.). (2001). *Handbook of aging and the social sciences*. New York: Academic Press.

Burnside, I. (1984). *Working with the elderly*. Monterey: Wadsworth Health Sciences Division.

Butler, R.N. & Lewis, M.I. (1982). *Aging and mental health*. Toronto: C.V. Mosby Company.

Chappell, N.L., Gee, E., MacDonald, L., & Stones, M. (2003). *Aging in contemporary Canada*. Toronto: Prentice-Hall Inc.

Edelson, J.S. & Lyons, W.H. (1985). *Institutional care of the mentally impaired elderly*. New York: Van Nostrand Reinhold Company.

Fabiano, L. (1987). *Supportive therapy for the mentally impaired elderly*. Seagrave: Education and Consulting Service.

Fabiano, L. (1989). *Working with the frail elderly*. Seagrave: Education and Consulting Service.

Grossman, H.D. & Weiner, A.S. (1988). Quality of life: The institutional culture defined by administrative and resident values. *Journal of Applied Gerontology*, 7(3).

Hansen, S.S., Patterson, M.A., & Wilson, R.W. (1988). Family involvement on a dementia unit: The resident enrichment and activity program. *The Gerontologist*, 28(4).

Henderson, N.J. & Vesperi, M.D. (1995). The culture of care in a nursing home: Effects of a medicalized model of long-term care. In *The culture of long-term care*, pp. 37–54. Westport: Bergin & Garvey.

Kane, R.L. & Kane, R.A. (2000). *Assessing older persons: Measures, meaning and practical implications*. Toronto: Oxford University Press.

Karuza, J., Calkins, E., Duffey, J., & Feather, J. (1988). Networking in aging: A challenge, model and evaluation. *The Gerontologist*, 28(2).

Keith, J. (1982). *Old people as people*. Toronto: Little Brown and Company.

Lasoski, M.C. & Thelen, M.H. (1987). Attitudes of older and middle-aged persons toward mental health intervention. *The Gerontologist*, 20(3).

Marshall, V.W. (ed). (1987). *Aging in Canada: Social perspectives*, 2nd ed. Markham: Fitzhenry & Whiteside.

McPherson, B. (1983). *Aging as a social process*. Toronto: Butterworths.

Moss, M.S. & Pfohl, D.C. (1988). New friendships: Staff as visitors of nursing home residents. *The Gerontologist*, 28(2).

Novak, M. (1985). *Successful aging*. Markham: Penguin Books.

Scharlach, A.E. (1988). Peer counselor training for nursing home residents. *The Gerontologist*, 28(6).

Shulman, M.D. & Mandel, E. (1988). Communication training of relatives and friends of institutionalized elderly persons. *The Gerontologist*, 28(6).

Statistics Canada. (2003). A portrait of seniors in Canada. Ottawa: Statistics Canada. Retrieved September 12, 2003, from Statistics Canada website: http://www.statcan.ca/english/ads/89-519-XPE/index.htm.

Washburn, A.M., Sands, L.P., & Walton, P.J. (2003). Assessment of social cognition in frail older adults and its association with social functioning in the nursing home. *The Gerontologist*, 43(2).

Internet Resources

Health Canada for Seniors
Canadian government Web site for seniors providing guidance to
services and suppliers on key issues facing seniors
http://www.hc-sc.gc.ca/english/for_you/seniors.html
Haworth Press Inc.
Listing of texts on aging, including social work references and free e-
mail alert option
http://www.hawpressinc.com/focus/aging/
Suite101.com
Listing of texts and courses available, in various topics, including
seniors and social work
http://www.suite101.com/article.cfm/elderly_caregiving/50804
Seniors Canada On-line
Ontario government site for seniors, listing key services and links to
applicable service agencies and services
http://www.seniors.gc.ca/index.jsp
U.K.-based site with worldwide references on seniors from a social
perspective
http://www.lancs.ac.uk/users/apsocsci/swr/older/text2.htm

Additional Readings

Beckman, B. & Harootyan, L. (eds.). (2003). *Social work and health care in an
aging society: Education, policy, practice and research.* New York: Springer
Publishing Company.

Cavanaugh, J.C. & Whitbourne, S.K. (eds.). (1999). *Gerontology: An
interdisciplinary approach.* New York: Oxford University Press.

Friedrich, D.D. (2001). *Successful aging: Integrating contemporary ideas, research
findings and intervention strategies.* Springfield: Charles C. Thomas
Publisher, Ltd.

Hill, R.D., Thorn, B.L., Bowling, J., & Morrison, A. (eds.). (2002). *Geriatric
residential care.* Mahwah: Lawrence Erlbaum Associates.

Lui, W.T. & Kendig, H. (eds.). (2000). *Who should care for the elderly? An East-
West value divide.* New Brunswick: Singapore University Press.

Namazi, K.H. & Chafetz, P.K. (eds.). (2001). *Assisted living: Current issues in
facility management and residential care.* Westport: Auburn House.

Zarit, S.H., Pearlin, L.I., & Shaie, K.W. (eds.). (2003). *Personal control in social
life course contexts.* New York: Springer.

CHAPTER 16

SOCIAL WORK PRACTICE IN NURSING HOMES

LISA S. PATCHNER AND

MICHAEL A. PATCHNER

Despite the focus on the physical health care needs of elderly people entering nursing homes, social work plays an integral role in this overall care. As a member of an interdisciplinary team, the social worker is responsible for attending to the psychosocial and familial needs of the elderly. These include: admissions, conducting psychosocial assessments; providing intake services; discharge planning; providing information and referral services; facilitating the resident's adjustment; facilitating resident councils; assisting in effecting treatment plans; and conducting in-service programs. Certainly tasks and functions vary from nursing home to nursing home; however, the importance of social work to nursing home care cannot be questioned. The future holds unlimited potential for role development in this area of practice.

Social work is probably the least understood profession in nursing homes that care for the elderly. Nurses care for the medical needs of residents, physical therapists rehabilitate, dieticians plan menus, administrators manage, recreation therapists plan and implement activity programs, but the role of social workers is often as varied as are the facilities in which they work. Yet the role of social workers is as vital to the health and well-being of a nursing home resident as any of these other professionals. Indeed, social work is an essential component of long-term care from the time a plan is being made for a person's admission into a facility until the person is discharged or expires.

I.　The Clientele

The 2000 United States Census reported that 1.4 million elderly, or approximately 4 percent of those over the age of 65, resided in nursing homes (U.S. Bureau of Census, 2000). This statistic can be misleading and at one level implies that there is a 4 percent chance of an older person going into a nursing home. However, research has shown that approximately 20–25 percent of the elderly will spend some time in a nursing home (Candy & Kastenbaum, 1973; Palmore, 1976). It is a fact that the older a person becomes, the greater the likelihood of nursing home placement. With the longevity of the population and the ability to manage chronic illnesses, it is estimated that as many as 43 percent of all individuals who turn 65 years of age after 1990 will at some point in their lives require nursing home care during some part of their aging years (Kisor & Stahlman, 2000). In 1994, 91 percent of all nursing home residents were age 65 years and older (U.S. Dept. of Health and Human Services, 2000).

Based upon type of sponsorship, nursing homes fall into three categories: proprietary, non-profit, and governmental. Proprietary homes, owned by corporations or private individuals, are in the nursing home business to make a profit. Non-profit homes are typically operated by religious or fraternal groups and are primarily intended for use by members of those groups. Governmental nursing homes are those run by federal, state, or local governments (e.g., county nursing homes and those operated by the Veterans Administration). According to the U.S. government, there are 16,995 nursing homes in the United States. Of these, 66 percent are proprietary, 27 percent are non-profit, and the remaining 7 percent are governmental (U.S. Dept. of Health and Human Services, 1997).

Depending on the type of care provided, American nursing homes that receive Medicare and Medicaid funds are certified as skilled-nursing facilities (SNFs) or intermediate-care facilities (ICFs). SNFs provide continuous nursing care on a 24-hour basis. Registered nurses, licensed practical nurses, and nurse aides provide services prescribed by the patient's physician. Emphasis is placed on medical nursing care with restorative, physical, occupational, and other therapies also provided (American Health Care Association, 1981). Patients receiving skilled nursing care generally experience serious medical illness or disability. ICFs provide regular medical, nursing, social, and rehabilitative services in addition to room and board for people not capable of independent living (American Health Care Association,

1981). According to a national survey of nursing homes in the United States, 8 percent of reimbursement was by Medicare, 68 percent of reimbursement by Medicaid, and 23 percent of reimbursement by private pay (U.S. Dept. of Health and Human Services, 1997).

Not only do nursing homes vary according to their type of sponsorship and certification, but they also vary according to size. With respect to bed size, 33 percent of nursing homes have less than 50 beds, 33 percent have 50 to 99 beds, 28 percent have 100 to 199 beds, and 6 percent have 200 beds or more (Strahan, 1987). Generally, government and non-profit facilities tend to be larger than proprietary nursing homes.

On average, nursing homes have 53 direct care staff, including 35 certified nurse assistants, 11 licensed practical nurses, and 6 registered nurses (Health and Human Services, 1997). In general, SNFs have more employees per resident than ICFs. Nearly half of all nursing home staff are nurse's aides (Beaver & Miller, 1985) and they provide 80–90 percent of the direct patient care. Further, one in ten employees is a nurse (RN or LPN) and about 5 percent are other professionals such as administrators, activity directors, social workers, physical therapists, and occupational therapists (Beaver & Miller, 1985).

Persons enter nursing homes for a variety of reasons. Ten out of every 13 residents are admitted for reasons related to poor physical health. Of the remaining three persons, two are admitted because of mental or behavioural problems and one for reasons not related to health, usually due to lack of alternative community services more appropriate to the person's need or due to family abandonment (American Health Care Association, 1981).

In 1999, more than 75 percent of nursing home residents were female (U.S. Dept. of Health and Human Services, 2002). Women outnumbered men in nursing homes not only because there are a disproportionate number of elderly women than men, but because in general women live longer than men and a greater proportion of elderly men tend to be married as compared to elderly women.

Further, non-whites comprise approximately 8 percent of the institutionalized elderly population (Kart et al., 1988). However, between the mid-1970s and 1999, nursing home utilization rates increased proportionately for the black population and decreased for the white population (U.S. Dept. of Health and Human Services, 2002). One may speculate that this low utilization of nursing homes by the non-white populations occurred because elderly non-whites lived in states that have relatively low rates of institutionalization.

Further, non-whites may not have access to nursing home care or were being institutionalized in other types of facilities, and socioeconomic economic factors, such as the ability to pay for nursing home care, influenced this statistic (Kart et al., 1988).

Most nursing home residents are functionally impaired and elderly. Only 7 percent can independently perform the activities necessary for daily living (ADLs) (i.e., eating, dressing, bathing, grooming, ambulating, and toileting) (Hing, 1981). Among adults age 65 years of age and older who require long-term care assistance, 31 percent require assistance with one or two ADLs, and 56 percent with three to six ADLs (U.S. Dept. of Health and Human Services, 2000). For the past 20 or so years, the typical nursing home resident is an "82-year old widowed female suffering from an average of four illnesses" (American Health Care Association, 1981). In 1999, the leading causes of death among persons 65 years of age and over were (U.S. Dept. of Health and Human Services, 2002):

- 33.8 percent heart disease,
- 21.7 percent cancer,
- 8.3 percent stroke,
- 6.0 percent chronic lower respiratory diseases,
- 3.2 percent influenza and pneumonia and
- 27.0 percent "other" causes.

The nursing home has been historically stereotyped as a place to go when persons could no longer take care of themselves and their families were unable to care for them. Often it was seen as a place to go and wait to die. However, the median length of stay in a nursing home in 1985 was 614 days. For a 12-month period spanning portions of 1984 and 1985, there were an estimated 1,223,500 discharges, of which 72 percent were live discharges (Sekscenski, 1987). Today's nursing homes are also for convalescents who expect to receive restorative treatment and they often recover. The emphasis is on living and helping a person to be as independent and functional as possible in order to return to one's own home or community whenever feasible.

II.   Practice Roles and Responsibilities

Nursing home services are directed at promoting, restoring, and facilitating the independent functioning of each resident and assuring that quality care is being provided. Social workers, as part of an interdisciplinary team that addresses a resident's physical, medical, psychological, and social needs, have a unique role in the nursing home even though their tasks and activities may vary from one facility to another. A number of authors have written about social work practice in long-term care facilities and have described the role and functions of social workers in these settings (Brody, 1976; Conger & Moore, 1981; Getzel & Mellor, 1982; Jorgensen & Kane, 1976; Peckham & Peckham, 1985). Although varied, the social worker's role is essential and will most often include the following tasks.

Social workers in nursing homes spend much time working directly with the residents and their families. From admission to discharge, the social worker is involved in making assessments, counselling, conducting psychosocial evaluations, and carrying out care plans. Social workers often have the first contact with the resident and their families at the time of admission. If a nursing home is small and does not have a director of admissions, it is often the responsibility of the social worker to admit persons and facilitate their transition into the nursing home. Entering a nursing home can be traumatic for some residents and their families. Families often feel very guilty about not being able to care for the person at home and having to make a nursing home placement decision. The residents, too, make numerous adjustments. Having to deal with loss of health and independence and being removed from their own familiar home is very stressful. No one ever wants to go to a nursing home as a patient, but often has to out of necessity. The social worker, therefore, has to be particularly sensitive to the feelings of the resident, his or her family, and the dynamics among them. It is the social worker's responsibility to help make the transition to the nursing home as smooth as possible by being in tune with the fears, expectations, and anxieties of all concerned and addressing the particular needs of the person and his or her family. Social workers help facilitate the admission process by showing the resident, when possible, and the family around the facility; introducing the resident to staff, other residents, and the roommate; and explaining schedules and policies (e.g., meals, bath times, laundry, smoking regulations, etc.). The idea is to acquaint the resident and family with the facility without overwhelming them, and make the new resident feel as comfortable as possible.

There are a number of documents that a social worker must complete at the time of admission, which include the admissions form, psychosocial section of the Minimum Data Set (U.S.), social history, a contract, and patients' rights form. The admission form is designed to provide some pertinent data that will be helpful to all staff. It acquaints the professional staff with many particulars about the new resident. It includes information such as the resident's preferred name or nickname, age, gender, next of kin, name of physician, medical diagnosis, religious affiliation, funeral home preferred (if needed), guardianship status or power of attorney, financial information, etc. The admission form provides information that is read by nursing, dietary, and other departments before they conduct their assessments of the resident.

The Minimum Data Set (MDS) is a computerized assessment completed on all nursing home residents in Medicare- and Medicaid-certified facilities in the United States. The MDS tracking form assesses the physical, social, and mental health of each resident and generates the initiation of the care-planning document for each resident. The care-planning document assists the multidisciplinary care team to identify resident health problems and treatment strategies to restore and/or maximize the functional capability of the resident. The MDS is also used as a prospective payment mechanism for governmental and private insurance purposes.

The social history, which can be completed on a form or done as a narrative, includes general demographic information (e.g., birthdate, birthplace, ethnic background, education, etc.), family composition, legal information (e.g., responsible person for the resident, if any; power of attorney, etc.), a general medical profile (e.g., previous hospitalizations and nursing home placements, use of appliances, eyeglasses, dentures, hearing aid, etc.), pre-admission data (e.g., prior living arrangements, incidents and conditions leading to admission, etc.), involvement in the community and religious organizations, psychosocial functioning, personal likes and dislikes, reactions to nursing home admission, and discharge potential. The social history is used to provide staff with the background and special characteristics of a resident and it allows staff to see the resident as a unique person with a particular history and not just as another patient. The contract is a signed document that states the general services provided by the nursing home and the charges for these services. It makes the resident and/or a family member responsible for paying the bills unless third-party payment is appropriate. Also, at the time of admission, residents' rights are read and residents are asked to sign the document acknowledging that they are aware of their rights as nursing home residents. If residents are unable to understand their rights as "nursing home patients," then the social worker makes sure that an immediate family member or appointed Health Care Representative is informed of them. The appended endnote is a condensed summary of residents' rights in the state of Illinois.[1]

These residents' rights are not only intended to outline the specific entitlement of the residents, but they also identify the facilities' responsibilities and obligations to each resident. It is the social worker's function to inform the residents and their families of these rights, make sure that they understand them, and assure that the residents' rights are protected. The social worker must serve as an advocate of the resident if his or her rights are violated and if there is any indication of abuse, neglect, or poor-quality care.

Once the resident is admitted to the facility, the social worker has the responsibility for facilitating the resident's adjustment. Although a few residents welcome being admitted to a nursing home because they soon find that they generally get acceptable care, good food, and can interact with staff and other residents, most residents take several weeks or longer to adjust to their new living arrangements. Social workers help residents adjust by frequently visiting with them during this period and by allowing them to express their fears, anxieties, and feelings of loss. The social worker may introduce the resident to other residents to try to facilitate some socialization and friendships. During this adjustment period, the social worker may also accompany the resident to some of the activity programs. The social worker also works closely with the family at this time. Indeed, the family, too, is adjusting, and the social worker listens to their concerns and may provide some counselling to them.

Social workers are also responsible for addressing the psychosocial problems of the residents. For example, if a resident is confused and cannot find his or her room, if a resident is lonely and feels like dying, or if a resident is bedridden or isolates himself or herself, it is the social worker's task to address these problems. These kinds of psychosocial adjustment problems are identified by conducting an assessment of each resident. This is a psychosocial assessment and it evaluates such things as a resident's orientation, memory, attention, self-image, sociability, initiative, relationships with family, staff, and other residents, etc. Problems in these areas can be addressed by working with the residents either individually, often referred to in a nursing home as working "one-on-one" or "one-to-one," or by working with residents in groups. Common types of groups used by social workers to address particular psychosocial problems include reality orientation, validation therapy, reminiscence groups, and socialization groups. Depending on the type of psychosocial problem a resident has, one-to-one interventions can include counselling, sensory stimulation, reality orientation, or just friendly visiting. Having one-to-one and group interventions with residents require good generic casework and counselling skills and often require the social worker to work with other departments within the nursing home to help coordinate the logistics of the interventions and also to have all departments follow through with the approaches being utilized by the social worker. This requires the social worker to train other staff to monitor a resident's psychosocial functioning and to intervene as appropriate when necessary.

Providing information and referral services is another important social work function in a nursing home. Specifically, the social worker informs residents and their families of particular services that they may be eligible for and links them to these services. For example, if a resident is developmentally disabled, the social worker can refer them to a sheltered workshop; if they have low incomes, the social worker can make sure that they are aware of any financial assistance they may be eligible for; if a resident desires spiritual guidance, the social worker can get them connected to a minister, priest, or rabbi; or if residents need to obtain new eyeglasses, hearing aids, or have dental work done, the social worker can arrange for these services. The social worker generally takes a very active role in providing information and referral services to the nursing home resident because the residents are often dependent and require assistance in obtaining immediate and needed services. Thus, the social worker will not only have to provide information, but most of the time will have to make appointments, arrange transportation, and either personally accompany the resident to an appointment or arrange for the resident to have an escort and often help the resident complete any paper work prior to the appointment.

Social workers may also be involved in resolving conflicts that may occur with residents. A resident can have a conflict with another resident, a staff person, or with a family member, and the social worker generally has the task of trying to remedy such situations. Indeed, interpersonal conflicts between residents are not uncommon in nursing homes. More specifically, most conflicts between residents occur between roommates. Sometimes the personalities of roommates are incompatible and the social worker intervenes to resolve such disputes. When such conflicts cannot be resolved, the social worker will usually arrange for a room change. When conflicts arise between a resident and staff member, the social worker provides suggestions to both the resident and staff member about ways of eliminating such conflicts. For example, if a resident does not want to take a shower and [constantly] argues with a nurse's aide about having the shower, the social worker may instruct the aide on appropriate ways of approaching the resident at bathing time. The social worker can also work with the resident to understand the resistance and to alleviate the resident's fears and concerns about taking a shower. Most staff members involved in resident-staff conflicts are the aides because they provide between 80 to 90 percent of the direct care in a nursing home and generally they are not trained to handle such situations. The social worker may also be involved in conflict resolution between a resident and her family. For example, if a resident resents her family because she was placed in a nursing home and makes her family feel guilty about the placement, the social worker usually intervenes. In such instances, the social worker can work individually with the resident and the family members involved or the social worker can work with them as a group. In resolving such conflicts, the social worker needs to have good listening, counselling, and crisis intervention skills, and the social worker needs to be aware that many conflicts are not easily resolved.

If a resident is not a permanent resident and will be discharged, it is the responsibility of the social worker to plan for this discharge. Discharge planning is defined as "the process of activities that involve the patient and a team of individuals from various disciplines working together to facilitate the transition of that patient from one environment to another" (McKeehan, 1981, p. 3). The social worker coordinates a resident's discharge by working with the resident, family, physician, nursing home personnel (i.e., nurses, physical therapists, dietician, activity director, etc.), and care plan team and assures that proper services will be in place to permit the resident to make the transition from being in the nursing home to having other living arrangements. If residents are being discharged to their home, to live with their family, or to another independent living situation in the community, the social worker makes sure that all necessary and appropriate services will be provided. For example, a resident might need Meals-on-Wheels; a visiting nurse or therapist; assistance with housework, shopping, and laundry; and transportation for physician visits.

Sometimes residents are discharged to another nursing home or other type of facility. In these cases, the social worker assures that all the necessary information is passed along to the other facility and that the needed services will be offered to the resident. Regardless of where residents will be living once they leave the nursing home, the social worker makes arrangements so that appropriate services from all available resources will be provided. Even though a resident leaves the nursing home, the social worker's responsibilities do not end. The social worker follows up to assure that all of the services that were arranged for are being delivered and the social worker evaluates if there are any further needs that are not being met.

Every resident in a nursing home has a care plan that specifies particular treatment and care to be given to each resident. This plan identifies resident strengths and problems, specifies approaches to address the problems, and establishes goals for residents to achieve. In the U.S. the care plan is generated by a computerized system called the Minimum Data Set (MDS). For example, if a resident had a stroke and is learning to walk again, a portion of the care plan would address this problem. The plan would state that a resident is unable to walk without assistance. The approach for staff to address this particular problem would be for the resident to walk with the assistance of a walker, be accompanied by an aide when walking, and receive physical therapy daily. The goal could be for the resident to walk 25 feet with a walker by the next care plan review (usually done every 90 days or less). This would be just one problem addressed in the care plan; others may include that the resident is depressed because of having had the stroke, not able to speak or eat properly, etc. The purpose of care planning is to provide the best possible care for each resident, care that will address each resident's specific needs and maximize his or her rehabilitative potential.

The care planning process involves systematic, coordinated, and planned procedures for the development and delivery of necessary care (Balgopal & Patchner, 1987). Care planning is an interdisciplinary process that staff from all departments within the nursing home meet to discuss and plan the care to be given. All residents are invited to attend their care plan meeting. Sometimes family, friends, and other service providers attend these meetings as well. Within seven days of being admitted to a nursing home, a care plan is generated for the resident based on the information entered into the MDS. Care plans are then re-evaluated and revised every 60 to 90 days or whenever a resident's condition changes. A social worker is intimately involved in this process by identifying a resident's particular psychosocial problems and assessing resident strengths and potential (on the MDS) and developing a plan of care to address the psychological and social needs of each of the residents. Although most nursing homes have a nurse as the coordinator of the care planning process, it is not uncommon for a social worker to be assigned this responsibility. As coordinator of the care plans, the social worker would then schedule all care plan meetings, ensure that all care plans were done in a timely manner, conduct the interdisciplinary care plan meeting, and ensure that all care plans were completed in such a way that they met all of the governmental and, where appropriate, corporate regulations. As one may surmise, this is a very demanding and time-consuming responsibility, but good care plans usually translate into good resident treatment and care.

As an avenue for residents to have input into the functioning of the nursing home and as a forum to air complaints, many nursing homes have a resident council. Such councils are organizations within the nursing home that are comprised of residents who can formally express their opinions on matters that affect their daily lives. Usually, officers are elected by their fellow residents and regular meetings are held. The resident council works in conjunction with the administration, staff, and families to promote better care within the facility and to better address the needs of the residents. It is often the responsibility of the social worker to organize and facilitate the resident council and work directly with its officers. Resident councils should be self-directed and as independent as possible; consequently, the social worker involved must be careful not to be too directive. Such councils work best when there is a commitment by the administration and staff to the council; regular, well-publicized meetings are held; there are written minutes of all council and committee meetings and these are made available to the residents; there is prompt attention by staff and administration to problems and suggestions voiced by the council; there is a specific meeting place; and some financial resources are available for the council.

Finally, social workers may also conduct in-service training programs to better educate the nursing home staff and volunteers for the purpose of improving the overall quality of care delivered to the residents. Nursing homes are required by federal and state regulations to have continual programs of in-service training for all staff. These can include such issues as fire safety, CPR, and proper techniques for cleaning up spills of body fluids, etc. However, the social worker also plays a role in training and is responsible for conducting in-services that address the psychological and social aspects of care. Some common topics for in-service training conducted by social workers include resident rights, confidentiality, remotivation of residents, stress management, conflict management, techniques for working with confused or disoriented residents, and handling death and dying.

Because of workers' schedules, most in-service training programs in nursing homes are rather focused and last for no more than one hour. By conducting these in-services, the social worker needs to be explicitly aware of the educational levels of the staff and care must be taken to give good practical information that can be readily utilized.

III. Potential for Role Development

It is very likely that the number of nursing home residents in North America will continue to grow very rapidly primarily because of the large increases expected in the elderly population. Social workers will have a unique role in admitting and discharging nursing home residents and developing and implementing programs and interventive methods to best address their psychosocial needs and those of their families. The greatest potential for the expanded role of social work in nursing homes will result from the growing view that a nursing home is no longer a place to die but a place to live within the health care continuum of services. Thus, social workers will be much more involved in programs that integrate the community into the nursing home and the nursing home into the community. Working more with volunteer groups; taking groups of residents into the community to volunteer, shop, dine, and be involved with various community efforts; facilitating the discharge of residents to less restrictive community care; and generally promoting the nursing home as an integral part of the community will take on increased importance in the future. Thus, the social worker will become more of an advocate for the needs of the elderly and may have to work against some deeply ingrained ageist attitudes [which unfortunately still prevail].

Another growth area for social workers will be increased efforts toward more psychosocial programming for the residents and their families. Although social workers are currently involved in these efforts, more attention will be given to these functions. In this regard, a greater portion of the social worker's time will be spent in developing and implementing more and better psychosocial programs for the residents. These programs will focus on restorative and preventive health care strategies with the goal of maximizing physical, social, and psychological health of each individual resident.

Finally, social workers in nursing homes will have to learn to deal with some younger clientele. Conditions such as HIV-AIDS, substance abuse, and traumatic brain injury will also be to be addressed. Working with diverse population groups has tremendous implications for social workers who have a part in educating all staff on multicultural sensitivity with varied populations and to develop meaningful interventive strategies for supporting and working with all residents.

The traditional functions of the social worker will continue, but there will also be many new opportunities for role expansion. As new situations present themselves, and with initiative and some creativity, social workers will inevitably expand their roles and functions within nursing homes to address the future needs of the residents. As indicated earlier, a social worker's job varies from facility to facility, and many times it is the social worker who is responsible for defining a fair portion of his or her own job description.

IV. Concluding Remark

Entering a nursing home does not alter the basic needs of an individual. Nursing homes are not only responsible for addressing the physical and medical needs of their residents, but they also have the responsibility for responding to residents' psychosocial needs. Social workers in nursing homes function as part of an interdisciplinary team and are responsible for addressing the psychosocial needs of the residents and their families. Although the social work role may vary from one nursing home to another, a social worker's duties are aimed at facilitating each resident's independence and maximizing his or her rehabilitative potential.

Social work is an essential component of the total care plan that is delivered to residents. To ensure that social work practice in nursing homes contributes to the well-being of residents and their families, the National Association of Social Workers (NASW) developed a set of standards for social workers to follow (Long-Term Care Facilities Standards Task Force of the NASW Committee on Aging, 1981). These are:

1. The long-term care facility shall maintain a written plan for providing social work services designed to assure their availability to all residents, their families, and significant others. It shall be developed by a qualified social worker experienced in long-term care.
2. The plan for social work services shall be guided by a written statement of philosophy, objectives, and policies.

3. The social work services plan shall provide for
    administrative accountability and direction by a social work
    director who is a qualified social worker responsible to the
    administrator of the long-term care facility or to the chief
    executive officer.

4. The functions of the social work program should include
    but not be limited to direct services to individuals, families,
    and significant others; health education for residents
    and families; advocacy; discharge planning; community
    liaison and services; quality assurance; development of a
    therapeutic environment in the facility; and consultation to
    other members of the long-term care team.

5. A sufficient number of appropriately trained and
    experienced social work and supportive personnel shall
    be available to plan, provide, and evaluate all social work
    services.

6. Social work personnel shall be prepared for their
    responsibilities in the provision of social work services
    through appropriate education and orientation specific to
    long-term care facilities and through education and training
    programs.

7. A written statement of the personnel policies and procedures
    of the agency, the social work program, and the *NASW Code
    of Ethics* shall be available to each staff member.

8. Adequate documentation of social work must be provided in
    the health care record. Confidentiality must be safeguarded.

9. The quality and appropriateness of social work services
    provided shall be regularly reviewed, evaluated, and
    assured through the establishment of quality control
    mechanisms.

10. There must be adequate budget, space, facilities, and
    equipment to fulfill the professional and administrative
    needs of the social work program.

Social work practice in nursing homes can make a tremendous
difference in the quality of care provided to the residents. Unfortunately,
the general public continues to have an unfavourable image of nursing
homes and many older individuals have negative feelings about nursing
home placement even when it becomes medically necessary. Yet once
admitted to a nursing home, many residents feel comfortable, safe, and

cared for. Social workers must promote their practice and continue to create an atmosphere of appropriate care and compassion.

Case Example

Helen had noticed that she was having some difficulty with walking. She had seen her doctor and was referred for some medical tests at the local hospital. It was discovered that she had had a small stroke. Nearly a year later, she had another stroke, which completely affected her left side and caused her to lose control over her left arm and leg. Her speech became slightly impaired, but she could still communicate fairly well. After being hospitalized for this second stroke, it was determined that she would receive better care in a nursing home rather than returning home. She was married and lived with her husband of 45 years, but she could not return home because her husband was in poor health and not able to properly care for her. She had four children; two lived out of state and the other two lived in the same town, but both worked and had families of their own. Consequently, her children were unavailable for home care services. Her income and medical insurance were limited and, as a result, she could not afford the home health care she required if she were to return to her own home. She could, however, qualify for short-term rehabilitative care under her governmental and private insurance policies.

The social worker at Pleasant Manor Nursing Home received a telephone call from the social worker at the local hospital who was planning Helen's discharge. The hospital social worker knew that Pleasant Manor Nursing Home had an excellent physical therapy department and hoped that Helen could be admitted. Fortunately, Pleasant Manor had a bed available. The social worker at Pleasant Manor made arrangements to visit Helen at the hospital. At the hospital, the social worker talked with the nursing staff, the hospital social worker, physical and speech therapy staff, Helen, and Helen's family. The purpose of this visit was to assess Helen's appropriateness for nursing home placement and to gather as much information as possible about Helen and her particular needs prior to admission. Upon her return to Pleasant Manor, the social worker met with the director of nursing, the administrator, and the physical therapist to inform them of Helen and her particular needs. She also met with the dietary supervisor so that Helen could start having meals upon her arrival and she informed the housekeeping department so they could be available to put Helen's clothing in the closet and prepare labels for her clothing.

Helen's family came to the nursing home and toured the facility with the social worker, who showed them the room where Helen would be staying as well as the physical therapy room with all of the specialized equipment. Later that day Helen was admitted. The social worker handled the admission and made Helen and her family feel very comfortable. The family seemed a bit overwhelmed by all the paperwork and all of the questions that were being asked. However, the social worker explained every form and why the certain questions were being asked. She took Helen, along with her family, and showed them around the nursing home and introduced them to staff. She took them to the room where Helen would be staying and introduced them to Helen's roommate. The social worker stayed for a while and got Helen settled. She then left to let the family have some time together and later checked on her several times that day. On one occasion she found Helen crying. The social worker reassured her that it was all right to feel sad about being in the nursing home and, because of the medical prognosis, gave her hope for improving.

Helen's care plan was discussed two days after her admission. A plan was developed for physical therapy, nursing care, dietary, and activities. Helen and her family were consulted regarding their desires for rehabilitation services with the ultimate goal for Helen to return home. The social worker addressed her adjustment to being in a nursing home and noted her slight depression, which could interfere with her motivation to work with physical therapy and to eventually improve. It was decided that the social worker would provide one-to-one counselling to address these problems.

After six months of paying nursing home bills, it came to the attention of the social worker that Helen and her husband's savings had been almost eliminated to pay nursing home bills not covered by the short-term insurance coverage. The cost of nursing home care at Pleasant Manor was nearly $5,000 per month. The social worker met with Helen's family about their financial situation and referred them to the state department of public assistance where they applied for Medicaid (U.S.), which would cover most of the nursing home expenses as long as Helen required intermediate nursing home care. Even though Helen was making very good progress, she was not ready to come home and her family was unable to provide the extensive care she currently required.

Finally, after a year in residence in the nursing home, Helen's physician said that she had improved enough for discharge home. She made enough progress that she would not be overly dependent on her husband and could take care of most of her activities of daily living. The social worker made plans for her to be discharged. She arranged for Meals-on-Wheels to be delivered to both Helen and her husband and a public health nurse would visit weekly to assure that the physical therapy exercises were being done properly. Helen's family would assist with grocery shopping, laundry, and transportation. Helen was intricately involved in her rehabilitation and discharge planning process, which allowed her to retain the right to self-determine her future.

Note

1. A condensed summary of nursing home residents' rights in the state of Illinois:
   - Each resident has all rights guaranteed by law, including the right to equal access to appropriate care regardless of race, religion, colour, national origin, sex, age, or handicap.
   - Each resident has the right to considerate and respectful care and to treatment with honesty and dignity without abuse or neglect.
   - Each resident has the right to respect, privacy, and confidentiality both in personal and medical affairs.
   - Each resident has the right to retain and use personal clothing and possessions as space permits.
   - Each resident shall be permitted freedom of religion.
   - No resident shall be required to perform services for the facility.
   - Each resident is permitted to retain a personal physician at the resident's expense or at the expense of any applicable third party payer.
   - Each resident is entitled to participate in planning his (her) medical treatment and to receive comprehensible information concerning his (her) condition, health needs, and the alternatives for meeting these needs.
   - Each resident has the right to refuse treatment to the extent permissible by law and to be informed of the consequences of such refusal.
   - Each resident has the right to be free from physical or chemical restraints except as authorized by the attending physician and documented in the resident's record.
   - Each resident has the right to be involved in his (her) discharge planning, including the right of self-discharge.

- Each resident has the right to the confidential handling of his (her) medical and personal records.
- Each resident has the right to manage his (her) own financial affairs.
- Each resident shall be informed, at the time of admission and during his (her) stay, of available services and the charges for these services.
- Each resident has the right to associate with any person of his (her) choice.
- A resident may meet with his (her) attorney or the representative of a public agency charged with supervising the facility or with a member of any other community organization during reasonable business hours.
- Married residents in the facility are entitled to share a room, unless none is available or it is medically contraindicated by the attending physician and so noted in the medical record.
- Each resident has the right to communicate with any person of his (her) choice.
- Each resident has the right to exercise his (her) rights and privileges as a citizen and resident of the facility.
- Each resident is entitled to information regarding policies and procedures for the initiation, review, and resolution of complaints.
- Each resident shall be fully informed of the facility's patient rights policies.

References

American Health Care Association. (1981). *Facts in brief on long-term health care*. Washington: American Health Care Association.

Balgopal, P.R. & Patchner, M.A. (1987). *The care planning process in nursing homes*. Urbana: University of Illinois at Urbana-Champaign School of Social Work.

Beaver, M.L. & Miller, D. (1985). *Clinical social work practice with the elderly*. Homewood: The Dorsey Press.

Brody, E.M. (1976). *A social work guide for long-term care facilities*, DHEW publication no. ADM 76-177. Washington: U.S. Government Printing Office.

Candy, S. & Kastenbaum, R. (1973). The 4 percent fallacy: A methodological and empirical critique of extended care facility population statistics. *International Journal of Aging and Human Development*, 4, 15–21.

Conger, S.A. & Moore, K.D. (1981). *Social work in the long-term care facility.* Boston: CBI Publishing Co.

Fox, P.D. & Clauser, S.V. (1980). Trends in nursing home expenditures: Implications for aging policy. *Health Care Finance Review,* 2(Fall), 65–70.

Getzel, G. S. & Mellor, M.J. (eds.). (1982). *Gerontological social work practice in long-term care.* New York: Haworth.

Haber, P.A.L. (1987). Nursing homes. In G.L. Maddox (ed.), *The encyclopedia of aging,* pp. 489–492. New York: Springer.

Hing, E. (1981). Characteristics of nursing home residents: Health status and care received. *Vital and health statistics,* 13(51). Rockville: National Center for Health Statistics.

Hing, E. (1987). Use of nursing homes by the elderly: Preliminary data from the 1985 national nursing home survey. *Advance data form vital and health statistics,* no. 135, DHHS publication no. PHS 87-1250. Hyattsville: Public Health service, National Center for Health Statistics.

Jorgensen, L.A. & Kane, R. (1976). Social work in the nursing home. *Social Work in Health Care,* 1(4), 471–482.

Kart, C.S., Metress, E.K., & Metress, S.P. (1988). *Aging health and society.* Boston: Jones and Bartlett Publishers.

Kisor, A.J. & Stahlman, S.D. (2000). Nursing homes. In R.L. Schneider, N.P. Kroph, & A.J. Kisor (eds.), *Gerontological social work: Knowledge, service settings, and special populations,* 2nd ed. Belmont: Wadsworth/Thomson Learning.

Long-Term Care Facilities Standards Task Force of the NASW Committee on Aging. (1981). *NASW standards for social work in long-term care facilities,* NASW policy statement 9. Washington: National Association of Social Workers.

McKeehan, K.M. (1981). Conceptual framework for discharge planning. In K.M. McKeehan (ed.), *Continuing care: A multidisciplinary approach to discharge planning.* St. Louis: The C.V. Mosby Company.

Palmore, E. (1976). Total chance of institutionalization among the elderly. *Gerontologist,* 9, 25–29.

Peckham, A.B. & Peckham, C.W. (1985). *You made my day.* Lebanon: Otterbein Home.

Sekscenski, E.S. (1987). Discharges from nursing homes: Preliminary data from the 1985 national nursing home survey. *Advance data from vital and health statistics,* no. 142, DHHS publication no. PHS 87-1250. Hyattsville: Public Health Service, National Center for Health Statistics.

Strahan, G. (1987). Nursing home characteristics: Preliminary data from the 1985 national nursing home survey. *Advance Data From Vital and Health Statistics,* no. 131, DHHS publication no. PHS 87-1250. Hyattsville: Public Health Service, National Center for Health Statistics.

U.S. Bureau of Census. (2000). *Current population reports: 2000*. Washington: U.S. Government Printing Office.

U.S. Dept. of Health and Human Services. (1997). *HCFA's online survey: Certification and reporting data*. Washington: U.S. Government Printing Office.

U.S. Dept. of Health and Human Services. (2000). *The characteristics of long-term care users*. Washington: U.S. Government Printing Office.

U.S. Dept. of Health and Human Services. (2002). *Chartbook on trends in the health of Americans: Excerpted from Health, United States, 2002*. Washington: U.S. Government Printing Office.

Internet Resources

Assisted Living Federation of America
    Dedicated to the assisted living industry and the population it serves.
    http://www.alfa.org/
Department of Health and Human Services—Administration on Aging
    The advocate agency for older persons and their concerns. Works to
    heighten awareness about older Americans and alerts the public to the
    needs of vulnerable older people.
    http://www.aoa.dhhs.gov/
Global Action on Aging
    Reports on older people's needs and potential within the globalized
    world economy.
    http://www.globalaging.org/
Institute for Independent Living
    Offers resources for persons with extensive disabilities and develops
    consumer-driven policies for self-determination, self-respect, and
    dignity.
    http://www.independentliving.org/
National Family Caregivers Association
    Exists to support family caregivers and to speak out publicly for
    caregivers' needs.
    http://www.nfcacares.org/

Additional Readings

Burack, O., Bogin, S., & Chichin, E. (2002). Certified nursing assistants' knowledge and attitudes about end-of-life ethics: Implications for social workers. *The Social Work Forum, 35*, 87–102.

Croxton, T., Jayaratne, S., & Mattison, D. (2000). Social workers' religiosity and its impact on religious practice behaviors. *Advances in Social Work, 1*(1), 43–60.

Ingersoll-Dayton, B., Pryce, J., & Schroepfer, T. (1999). The effectiveness of a solution-focused approach for problem behaviors among nursing home residents. *Journal of Gerontological Social Work, 32*(3), 49–64.

Jess, C. & Klein, W. (2002). One last pleasure? Alcohol use among elderly people in nursing homes. *Health and Social Work, 27*(3), 193–203.

Kramer, B. (2000). Husbands caring for wives with dementia: A longitudinal study of continuity and change. *Health and Social Work, 25*(2), 97–108.

CHAPTER 17

SOCIAL WORK PRACTICE IN GERIATRIC ASSESSMENT UNITS IN ADULT DAYCARE

PATRICIA MACKENZIE

The gradual deterioration of function with increasing age is so widely perceived and so expected that all difficulty experienced by an elderly person tends to be attributed to age. Geriatric assessment units (GAU) are built upon the premise that it is disease, not senescence, that leads to disability in the elderly. GAU programs provide an environment where it becomes routine for an older person with problems of mobility, mental change, or functional disturbance to be assessed for disease and remedial action taken. Composed of social as well as medical and functional investigations, geriatric assessment can address the complexities that accompany many acute and chronic conditions of old age. It is within this investigative environment that social work finds a natural home and the opportunities for creative and challenging practice.

From the widowed world traveller in Nova Scotia to the 80-year-old marathon runner in Calgary and the "Raging Grannies" of the West Coast, the older population in Canada uses imagination, energy, and creativity to use retirement and aging as an opportunity to accept new challenges and master new skills. These individuals engage in such activities with a zest and passion for life that was beyond their grasp when saddled with ties to jobs, families, and the other trappings of the "productive years." There are presently more than three million Canadians over the age of 65 and there is every indication that this number will increase in the ensuing years. Projections by Health and Welfare Canada estimate that by the year 2021, Canadians in the 65-

plus age group will make up one-fifth of the total population (1988). Skelton (1986) predicts that the 65 and older age group will enlarge more rapidly than any other segment of the population and those in their ninth decade will increase by more than 200 percent in the next two decades.

Despite the *joie de vivre* and independence of the majority of aging Canadians, society as a whole tends to hold fast to negative stereotypes of the older population and to equate "old" with "debilitated." Social workers often join other helping professionals, economists, statisticians, and politicians in alarmist reactions over the doom-and-gloom predictions of the greying of our society. As a result, we tend not to see the old realistically. Part of the problem might be that the word "old" conjures up images of brittle bones, wrinkled skin, fragile health, and forgetfulness, all of which serve to obscure the strengths and abilities of the majority of aging Canadians. Seniors' advocacy groups have begun to challenge societal perceptions and acceptance of the equation that relates chronological age with infirmity and dependence. This new cohort of the aging population is beginning to question the ministrations of helping professionals while pointing out the need for a reappraisal of traditional social work practice models (Greene, 2000).

Although the trend is reversing, academics continue to obtain considerable professional mileage from the study of the aged as if this group were comprised of some strange new species of being. Recent research on the biological, health, and social correlates of aging as described by Matcha (1997) indicates that the lives of older persons are not nearly as foreboding or as unhappy as the literature may have led the public to believe. As a society, we need to redefine our perceptions of exactly what the aging of our country is all about. Indeed, McDaniels (1988, p. 9) pointed out:

> The aging of Canada is not new and alarmism about aging fails to recognize some very important points. Societal aging is the unexpected consequence of successful planned parenthood. The average age of the population has increased because of declining numbers of babies and young children. What is new will be the aging trend in the Twenty-First Century as the baby boom generation swells the ranks of the elderly.

Neugarten (1974) has distinguished the young-old from the old-old and, fortunately, gerontologists, social scientists, helping professionals, and economists have begun to listen and recognize that chronological years alone do not an old person make!

Perhaps another reason for our inability to see the elderly in a more positive and differentiated light is that the media and other interested groups limit their focus on that part of the experience of aging that results in the fiscal responsibility of providing increasingly scarce resources to this segment of the population. The sheer business of living weakens the body. As people begin to age and fail to recover quickly from the insults of illness or injury, they often present for care and treatment in a health care facility. It is this entrance into the service delivery system that requires expenditure of public funds and this financial burden seems to be the issue that causes great distress for policy-makers, economists, politicians, and health/social service agency personnel. As a society, we worry about the *raging geriatric tide*, which supposedly threatens to bankrupt the health care system. Hayes and Hertzman (1985) question this fear and confront a number of popular misconceptions about the social and economic impact of an aging population.

Caring professionals seldom give credit for the benefits this group has conferred upon society and need to adopt a critical review, not only of some of the negative stereotypes of aging but also of the pessimistic predictions regarding the costs of caring for an elderly population. Negative stereotyping of the elderly must be eliminated and education and experience can serve as effective means to that end. Gaitz (1974) pointed out the necessity of relieving ourselves of repressive attitudes toward the aged when he stated:

> If one mistakenly assumes that psychiatric disorders of the aged are beyond treatment, then neglect of elderly persons with remediable conditions may occur. If one assumes that an elderly person is only waiting for death to relieve him, his family, and society of a burden, a practitioner may become the instrument of implementing the unwitting inadequate treatment plans of a society unwilling to invest the time, energy, and money to obtain the best resources available to all citizens. (p. 74)

I.   The Clientele

One of the great economic and social frailties of the present health care system is a failure to respond in such a way as to provide services tailored to meet the specific needs of the elderly. Levenson and Rathbone-McCuan (1977) have suggested that our society has been ineffective in generating strategies for providing preventive or restorative health care to the elderly. When an older person is thought to be coping poorly, there is a tendency to focus on appropriate facility-based care rather than on creative alternatives and helping strategies. As Watson (1984) stated, "too often, the individual is made to fit the system, rather than the system being adapted or modified to meet the needs of the person" (p. 659). It is, therefore, essential that before any action is taken, every frail elderly person has a proper assessment and review of potential resources and coping strategies.

A. Assessment

This assessment process is described by Kane et al. (1982) as one that "can lead to the discovery of new important and treatable problems, simplification of overly complex drug regimes, arrangements for needed rehabilitation and development or remediation of a supportive physical and social living environment to enhance patient functioning" (p. 519). The goal of any assessment procedure is to maximize the abilities and minimize the dysfunction that might result from an insult to an elderly person's vitality.

Therefore, when health crises strike, it is important that the elderly person has available to her or him a continuum of care, which includes programs designed to treat the treatable, reverse the reversible, and maintain a state of physical, functional, and psychosocial well-being. Novak (1988) suggests this continuum should range from programs that have maximal institutional support, such as hospitals and long-term care facilities, to those with little such support as exemplified by adult day programs, seniors' centres, etc.

This goal of maintaining, enhancing, and restoring both the physical and psychosocial vitality of the elderly receives little real criticism from any sector. The challenge, however, involves the actual development of creative and broad-based care delivery systems that can provide the care continuum required. A difficulty inherent in this task is described by Skelton (1986) when he cautions that:

> The present strain the elderly impose on the health and welfare services will not be relieved simply by the provision of more beds. Too frequently the problem is addressed by hasty and thoughtless provision of larger and more expensive long-term care institutions,

or by suggestions that favour rationing health and welfare services to the elderly. Better basic planning and the development of integrated and comprehensive geriatric services offer the only viable long-term solutions. (p. 21)

B. Geriatric Assessment Units

One of the components of this integrated and comprehensive geriatric service delivery system involves formal geriatric assessment programs and, before one can successfully examine the clientele, it is necessary to describe the parameters of these particular practice settings.

Geriatrics is that branch of gerontology that studies pathology, treatment, and prevention of disease among the elderly. Specialized geriatric assessment units (GAUs) have been established in major urban centres across Canada, patterning trends established in the UK, the USA, and Europe. These programs have developed in response to the growing recognition of the many unmet needs of the frail elderly and are motivated by the conviction that GAUs can have major beneficial impacts on the health and well-being of elderly patients. GAU programs trace their origins to Great Britain and were pioneered by the work of several people, including Dr. Marjory Warren and Sir Ferguson Anderson. Geared to specific local needs and available resources, these programs vary in many of their structural and functional components, including how the program is financed, institutional affiliation, which types of patients are accepted, staffing composition, etc.

Rubenstein (1987) defined geriatric assessment as a "multi-dimensional and interdisciplinary diagnostic process designed to quantify an elderly individual's medical, psychosocial, and functional capabilities and problems with the intention of arriving at a comprehensive plan for intervention and follow-up"(p. 109). Kane (1987) reviews the growing body of literature that outlines the different types and purposes of GAU programs and also describes the positive health care outcomes of GAU intervention. MacKenzie et al. (1987) point out the need for more cautious and inclusive program evaluations when measuring program effectiveness, arguing that:

Successful treatment of severe cardiac congestive failure in an 85-year-old woman which leads to successful discharge home may lead to frustration for all if the presence or absence of family or other care giving support, the possibility of drug compliance, or the suitability of the patient's housing are not taken into account. (p. 121)

Elderly patients typically present with complex and interrelated medical and psychosocial problems that often do not fit into a limited biomedical model of care. Medalie (1986) expanded the traditional approach of assessing the elderly, which generally focuses on the biological changes of the aging process, to include a review of the multiple interrelating factors associated with the patient, her or his intimate associates, cultural subgroups, and society.

Kane et al. (1982) identify the three major services of geriatric assessment units as assessment, interventions, and/or placement of the frail elderly patient. Studies reported by Flathman and Larsen (1976) have noted that patients involved in such programs improved their physical, mental, and social well-being. It is well known that elderly patients have more varied problems and health care needs than younger patients, although Barer et al. (1986) suggest that the reason for the increased utilization of health care resources by the elderly has less to do with the intensity or frequency of disease and more to do with the way the health care system responds. Schumann (1984) also identified the challenge of designing new interventions to meet these needs.

Central to GAU program philosophy is the belief that careful assessment of frail elderly patients can often reveal remediable conditions and help to better match services with needs. The GAU social worker, therefore, finds it possible to follow the principal social work objective described by Rosenfeld (1983): "the aim of social work is to match resources with needs and increase the *goodness of fit*' between them by harnessing potential provider systems to perform this function" (p. 189). It is within the GAU environment, then, that social work can find a natural home as this setting offers the opportunity to participate in a system of care that is congruent with the commitment of the profession to person-in-environment interactions. The subsequent intervention strategies (possible in a social model of health care delivery) involve efforts to keep people in their own homes when appropriate.

Since no single professional group is capable of meeting all of the elderly patient's needs, teamwork is essential (Berkman et al., 1999). Interdisciplinary GAU teams typically consist of geriatricians, other medical consultants, nurses, social workers, occupational therapists, physiotherapists, speech therapists, dietitians, and psychologists. Each team member is responsible for patient assessments in her or his field of expertise. Usually the entire team monitors patient progress and continually plans and re-evaluates therapeutic goals for individual patients. Social work is comfortable with Brill's (1976) definition of the team approach to patient care, which suggests that:

> There needs to be a mix of professions each of whom possess particular expertise; each of whom is responsible for making individual decisions; who together hold a common purpose; who meet formally and informally to communicate, to collaborate, and to consolidate knowledge from which plans are made, actions determined and future decisions influenced. (p. 42)

II.   Practice Roles and Responsibilities

As Greene (2000) outlines in her article, shifts in the age of a client group do not require the abandonment of all generic or specialized social work skills but do require that those skills be tailored to a new client group whose needs and resources may have special features. This is most certainly the case for the social worker employed in a GAU. For example, it is essential that the social worker acquire a familiarity with medical terminology enabling her or him to understand the common physical ailments and medical interventions performed with this population.

While it is true that social work alone cannot begin to harness all the resources needed by the frail elderly GAU patient, it remains that the principle feature of social work practice in this setting requires the worker to meet the objectives of social work practice outlined by other authors. The required "tailoring of skills" can be demonstrated by taking the liberty of inserting the appropriate adjectives into Hepworth and Larsen's (1986) stated *Objectives for Social Work Practice*. This process helps to lend additional relevance to this practice setting, allowing one to rewrite that GAU social workers:

1. Help (frail elderly people) enlarge their competence and increase their problem solving and coping abilities;
2. Help the (elderly patient) obtain resources;
3. Make health care and other social service organizations responsive to (frail elderly people);
4. Facilitate interactions between (older individuals) and others in their environments;
5. Influence interactions between organizations and institutions that serve (elderly people); and,

6. Influence social and environmental policy to respond to the health and social needs of the (older person).

Social work practice in GAUs can be described by using the concepts of primary, secondary, and tertiary intervention as outlined by Beaver and Miller (1985). A discussion of the application of these concepts to GAU social work practice follows.

A. *Intervention*

Primary intervention suggests that it is best to try and identify problems before full manifestation occurs and to design strategies to either eliminate or minimize the potential harmful effects. Primary intervention, therefore, leads the GAU social worker into a role of both consultant-educator and advocate. As such, energy is focused on a review of the conditions necessary for healthy and satisfactory lifestyles of all citizens, including the elderly person. The social worker is also responsible for identifying harmful influences and scarcity of resources in the physical and social environment that may have deleterious effects on the clientele served.

This practice role is easily adhered to in GAU settings as the social worker strives to provide early education of patients/families about the resources available to enhance coping. In the combined consultant-educator role, the GAU social worker is called upon to interpret agency/ hospital rules and regulations and to teach or transmit information about a host of services to patients, families, and other caregivers.

The social worker in a GAU must also act as consultant/collaborator with other health care professionals, both within and without the GAU, to design effective care plans for individual patients and thereby ensure quality service to the clientele. Virtually all types of GAU programs have some interrelationship with community services. As Williams (1987) points out, "it is obvious that, if the geriatric assessment is to contribute to the further care of the patient, its results and recommendations must reach the appropriate community services" (p. 68). Maintaining this community communication network is often the responsibility of the GAU social worker.

GAU social workers in the advocate role are usually "client-focused." Not only does the advocacy role of social work direct the worker to help patients cut through bureaucratic red tape and other systems related problems, but it has expanded to encompass a conscious movement on the part of the worker to address inequities in social and health policy decisions that adversely impact upon clients. For GAU social workers, then, advocacy is an inherent feature of practice as efforts are made to challenge, among other things, ageist discrimination, limited or rationed health and social services, and the assumption that to be old is to be sick and that sickness is to be expected and beyond treatment.

The main emphasis in secondary intervention is on early diagnosis and treatment and it is at this level that the bulk of direct practice responsibilities are found. The GAU practice setting offers opportunity to participate in strategies that are designed to improve and enhance the older person's well-being. In order to bring about a resolution of the patient's problems, or to prevent exacerbation of same, intervention is offered in the form of standard clinical casework. The goal of such intervention includes patient recovery and restoration of the previous level of social functioning. This involves the social worker and patient in problem assessment and problem-solving exercises, all of which are designed to enhance coping abilities.

As social workers assess the presenting problems of geriatric patients, it is helpful to reflect on a modified version of the psychosocial systems perspective as outlined by Beaver and Miller (1985). This approach offers a set of generic guidelines for the following: engaging the client; conducting the assessment; formulating the intervention plan; and, finally, evaluating outcomes. These concepts can be easily transcribed to GAU social work practice and offer a broad overview of the total physical-psychological-social functioning of the patient. Another assessment tool that the reader may find helpful and which can be readily adapted to GAU social work practice is the 4 Rs of medical-social diagnosis as described by Doremus (1976).

Yet another way to assess areas of the patient's life that may have been affected by current difficulties involves a review of several key "arenas" or "spheres of influence" that describe aspects of healthy, productive human functioning. These have been described by Gilmore (1973) as vitality, community, identity, accountability, activity, and frivolity. An adaptation of these ideas provides a conceptual framework for understanding the depth and breadth required for a complete gerontological social work assessment. It is reasonable, for instance, to suggest that any depletion of the patient's vitality will have an impact upon how capable she or he is of continuing her or his level of involvement in her or his social world or community (Barrett & Soltys, 2002). As well, a limitation in the activity of the patient may change that for which the individual patient is accountable, i.e., that which gives her or him identity and a sense of frivolity (defined as accomplishment/ purpose in life). This situation may hasten feelings of loss of self-worth, self-doubt, and depression. The following case example illustrates the interconnectedness of the spheres of influence concepts.

Mrs. B was referred to the GAU for consultation after a recent mild CVA [cardiovascular accident] and subsequent problems with erratic blood pressure. The GP and visiting Home Care nurse were concerned about Mrs. B's apparent total disregard for her medication regime/diet. She was described by the family physician as mentally intact but depressed. While talking with Mrs. B during the home visit, the social worker discovered that her husband had died just one month previous. Her only child, a daughter in Toronto, had made a quick trip to Victoria after her father's death and found her mother "incapacitated with grief." The daughter made all the arrangements for her father's funeral, saw to the details of the estate, and, just before returning to Toronto, convinced Mrs. B to put the large home she and Mr. B built 15 years ago up for sale. Arrangements were also made by the daughter for Mrs. B to visit a new seniors' condominium complex and put a deposit on the purchase of a suite. She also contacted the lawyer to draw up power of attorney forms for her mother to execute in her daughter's favour. Mrs. B mentioned to the daughter just after the funeral that she was feeling apprehensive about learning to manage the family finances as that was "always your father's responsibility." With that information, the daughter contacted an accountant and made arrangements for all cheques and other finances to be managed by his firm with consultation from Mrs. B.

The tragedy in this case study involves the well-intentioned but misdirected effort of a concerned daughter to make major decisions on mother's behalf and "in her best interests," which had serious negative impacts on her mother's feelings of self-worth, control, and competence. By making the assumption that mother was either not capable of or interested in learning how to manage money and other business dealings, the daughter did her mother a great disservice.

By applying the spheres of influence concepts, the social worker recognized that Mrs. B had a recent insult to her physical vitality (mild stroke with complications) that compromised her ability to cope with some of the social problems of a recently bereaved widow. The resources in the environmental system, i.e., the daughter, failed to recognize the importance for Mrs. B of maintaining a sense of identity, accountability, community, activity, and frivolity. Time and a system of instruction and support were required to help her learn or relearn to perform the activities that enabled her to continue to function in the mainstream of life, meeting the usual opportunities for success or failure present for all.

Fortunately, Mrs. B recovered well from her bereavement and stroke episode and, through counselling by the social worker and other members of the GAU team, recognized that many of the arrangements made by her daughter were unnecessary. A team meeting with the daughter on her next visit West helped to clarify and allay some of her very real fears ("Mother is all alone and I'm so far away") and when she was able to understand that her mother was in fact capable of continuing to make decisions and call for help from various sectors when required, the situation for both mother and daughter was much more relaxed.

Social workers must expand their perception of the nature of the patient's clinical condition to include a view of the person as being in transaction with their environment. It is this ability to bring an ecological perspective to GAU settings that provides social work with an important and distinct role in these particular practice settings. Social workers with their training in interpersonal relationships, group work, and interdisciplinary team skills play a vital role in the developing and functioning of the GAU (Mellor & Lindemen, 1998).

B. A GAU Example

It was the author's experience and good fortune to be employed as a social worker in a geriatric assessment unit in Victoria B.C. This GAU operates adjacent to both an acute-care hospital and a long-term care facility. Funding for the unit is from the continuing care branch of the Ministry of Health. MacKenzie et al. (1987) list the main purposes of the program as: (1) to diagnose and treat those elderly who were failing at home for uncertain cause; (2) to diagnose and treat those elderly at home or in long-term care facilities who manifested behaviourial problems based on the well-recognized premise that much disturbed behaviour has a basis in physical disease; and later (3) to admit from the acute hospital, including the emergency department, those elderly presenting with multiple diagnoses who had been admitted for an acute illness. This latter group of patients was accepted in recognition of the fact that elderly patients frequently remain in hospital longer than is optimal and develop conditions that make their discharge difficult.

Most referrals are telephoned into the unit medical director and an initial screening process occurs to determine which particular area of the GAU service would best meet the needs of the patient in question. This GAU offers service to patients in three main areas: a 50-space geriatric day hospital, a 28-bed in-patient unit and an out-patient/ domiciliary visit service. Social work service is available to patients in all three service areas via a blanket referral system. It is important to note that this particular GAU functions as a whole with interrelated components. This structure was developed with the conviction that only with a broad range of flexible services, available at the moment of referral, can the patient be helped to reach his or her best level rapidly and cost effectively. Patients are often admitted to one particular branch of the program and later transferred for treatment to other branches as their care needs change.

In this particular program, the medical director conducts a preliminary review of the patient's condition to assess the acuity/ urgency of the referral. On occasion, requests are made by the referring agent to admit patients to the inpatient unit when it is clear that their needs are chronic in nature and would best be met by either expanded home supports or admission to some form of long-term care facility. Continued vigilance has to be maintained to ensure that only those patients with some remedial condition are admitted to the in-patient unit. An active community education program by the GAU staff aids in the clarification of objectives and purposes of the GAU for physicians and other community caregivers, i.e., the assessment and treatment of episodes of recent and reversible illness.

MacKenzie (1982) confirms that all provinces and territories in Canada now have some type of home care nursing and community support service. British Columbia began a comprehensive long-term care program in 1978, which has expanded to coordinate both home help/nursing service and the waiting list for all government-funded long-term care [LTC] facilities in the province. Before any individual can be placed in a government-funded LTC facility, she or he must have her or his physical and psychosocial care needs reviewed by a staff member from the local LTC office. Needless to say, many patients referred to the GAU require either a complete redirection to the local LTC office for service and direction or a consultation by the GAU social work staff and LTC about the types of community or facility supports that can be offered to the patient while she or he is rehabilitated or treated through the efforts of the GAU program. This liaison work between the GAU and the local long-term care office is a principal and vital role of the GAU social worker.

Although there may be variations in the practice styles, modalities, and procedures to be found in GAU social work departments, most casework intervention in these settings begins with a review of what is known about a patient. Since most GAUs operate on a referral basis, information is provided to the unit by the attending physician or other referring agent. Equipped with this knowledge, members of the GAU team are invited by the unit director to become involved with the process of helping the patient regain or compensate for what was lost.

Considerable emphasis is placed on maintaining the elderly person in her or his home environment. To this end, the majority of the patients seen in this GAU service become patients in the day hospital branch of this GAU service. As reported by MacKenzie et al. (1987), the majority of patients referred to this program (> 95 percent) are usually seen at home by the social worker. The remainder comprise a patient group whose physical needs are sufficiently acute to require an urgent house call by the geriatrician, usually followed by a direct admission of the patient to the geriatric inpatient ward or transfer to the acute-care hospital.

C. Social Work Assessment

For the majority of the patients referred, the social work assessment process begins with the practitioner visiting the patient in her or his own environment. This makes it possible to truly begin where the client is at. A relationship is established with the patient on the patient's home turf and is facilitated by the social work practitioner demonstrating an interest and desire to understand the nature of the patient's present difficulties, as well as her or his interests, goals, and strengths. All of this is done in the reflective light of the patient's personal, family, and community support systems.

D. Home Visits

Mary Richmond (1917) summed up this aspect of practice well when she observed that we make home visits not to "find our clients out but rather to find out how to help them better" (p. 24). Home visits afford the opportunity for the GAU social worker to perform three very important but often-overlooked duties. The first involves preparing patients for GAU intervention by outlining the nature and the types of services offered. It is sad fact that many elderly patients are referred for various health treatments/interventions, but are seldom prepared for the rigours of these encounters. Not surprisingly, these processes are met with anxiety and reluctance by many individuals. Just as is the case for the younger patient, an elderly patient also needs to know what the helping process will contain, what will be required of her or him, and receive answers to more practical questions such as cost, transportation, etc. Provision of clear and concise information about the complexities of the process will assist in reducing anxiety and potential feelings of powerlessness.

A second essential duty of the social worker conducting the home visit is the review of the patient's presenting problem. Although the social worker has had some idea of the reasons for the GAU referral, often this information has come via the attending GP and/or family and other caregivers. Although this information is valuable, it requires supplementation by the patient. There are instances, of course, where the very nature of the patient's difficulties may preclude her or him from having the ability to communicate about problems effectively i.e., speech difficulty, cognitive failure, or denial/resistance, but it remains that engaging the patient in a discourse about her or his perceptions of the problem(s), thereby coming to an understanding of what the problems *mean* to the patient, is an essential element of good social work practice!

The third duty involves an analysis of the personal and environmental resources available to the patient. The availability of intrapersonal, interpersonal, and environmental resources is a significant part of any social work assessment. It is important to try and obtain a perception of what the personal coping strategies of each individual patient are, including a review of personal strengths such as the motivation for getting well.

The role that formal and informal caregivers play in the ability of the older patient to mobilize the appropriate resources to regain independence is also extremely important and must be included in the social work assessment. Considerable literature is available outlining some of the special roles and characteristics of formal and informal caregivers of elderly patients (see Blandford et al., 1986; Fengler & Goodrich, 1979; Snider, 1981).

E. Assessment Stages

In the beginning stages of geriatric assessment, the social worker may find it helpful to reflect on the eclectic theoretical orientation of crisis intervention as described by Golan (1986). Patients who are seen for geriatric assessment are usually responding to the impact of internal stressors such as injury or illness and/or the external stressors of recent intra- or interpersonal losses. This can create disruptions in the person's equilibrium or homeostatic balance and often thrusts the patient into a state of crisis. The significance of these events for social work practice is that when problems occur and the physical and psychosocial resources of this clientele cannot return them to a state of equilibrium, functioning may become more impaired. Such setbacks result in the elderly person developing feelings of loss of control or purpose, which may lead to depression, increased dependency, lack of motivation for getting better, and followed perhaps by the need for institutional care.

After the home visit, the social work case notes are shared with the medical director and other members of the interdisciplinary team as all prepare to admit the patient to the program. Thus, the information collected by the social worker during this pre-admission home visit provides a solid baseline from which to begin to plan therapeutic interventions with the individual patient. An example of GAU social work intervention is outlined in the case study presentation at the end of the chapter.

Upon admission of a patient, the social worker continues to maintain contact with both the patient and her or his caregiving constellation by providing the social casework services identified earlier i.e., patient and/or family counselling, liaison and referral to community resources, participation in case conferences with other members of the GAU team, etc.

Interventions at the tertiary level stress prevention or delaying the possible consequences of illness or other dysfunctional processes that may already be occurring. Aging is often accompanied by decline and threats to vitality have consequences that impact negatively on all aspects of an elderly person's personal and social world. The preventive efforts of the GAU team encourage early diagnosis and, hopefully, treatment that will remedy some of the acute problems and chronic conditions of age. This can lead to renewed interests, new hope, and a revitalized lifestyle for the elderly patient. Typical preventive intervention strategies offered to patients in GAUs are expanded beyond the treatment of the presenting problem to include suggestions for improved diet, home renovations leading to increased safety, access to expanded home or community supports such as adult daycare and medical alert systems, programs to improve medication compliance, individual and family counselling, etc.

The very essence of a discussion about prevention needs to go beyond superficial strategies, however. For preventive or restorative efforts to be successful, it is necessary to know the root cause of certain functional or social problems. This requires a diligent examination of many factors. As Hepworth and Larsen (1986) point out, "direct social workers should not limit themselves to remedial activities but should also seek to discover environmental and other causes of problems and sponsor or support efforts aimed at enhancing the environments of people" (p. 89). For example, the difficulty of getting patients and their families to admit that they have some unresolved interpersonal problems, and then believe that these can be resolved with professional guidance and support, presents an interesting, exhilarating, but occasionally frustrating challenge for social work practitioners and other team members. As well, depression is too frequent a diagnosis in the elderly and requires careful assessment and creative treatment approaches. The availability of psychological and geriatric psychiatry services to patients of GAUs is extremely important but often not available, although research findings document that elderly couples and family units frequently need and can benefit from individual, marital, sex, and family therapy (see Butler, 1975; Sander, 1976; Toseland, 1977). Social work needs to advocate for the expansion of these and other services and make continued efforts to streamline out-patient assessment programs for this populations (Saltz et al., 1998).

III.   Potential for Role Development

As the provision of health care moves into the community and away from the constraints of institutional medical care, the role of the social worker may become less tied to institutional demands, thereby freeing the profession to respond to the broad range of social factors that shape the health of individuals, family, and communities. Social work must be prepared to assume this responsibility as both direct practitioners and as health and social service policy planners/analysts.

At the same time, however, caution must be used not to embrace the concept of community care so tightly as to restrict access to diagnostic and treatment services, which will continue to be offered in institutional settings. Rather than designing the service delivery system based on concerns over cost or program ideology and then trying to fit the target population into the system, social workers and other service providers need to ensure that all health agencies continue to identify and respond to the needs of the population to be served.

Opportunities for creative and rewarding social work involvement with the frail elderly population should exist in every component of the health care continuum—from the acute-care hospital to early rehabilitation and convalescent care centres such as geriatric inpatient units, to ambulatory care programs such as geriatric day hospitals, to community support programs, i.e., adult daycares, home help agencies, seniors' centres, etc., and to long-term care facilities. These practice opportunities have become more available within the last decade and will grow as the country continues to respond creatively to the challenge of caring for our aging citizens. Social workers need to educate themselves to the particular needs of the frail elderly and focus on ways to empower this population to use its strengths and resources in mastering the difficulties associated with illness and disability.

The ideal service delivery system of the future will acknowledge that the accumulated impairments and chronic conditions of the older patient should be seen comprehensively and attention must be given to the structure or flavour of the helping agency or institution. Hospitals take great pride in becoming centres of excellence for neonatology, pediatrics, cardiology, etc. Social workers should encourage hospitals and health care centres to recognize the need to elevate the care of the elderly person to the level where we can also identify this population as deserving care from such centres of excellence, which would guarantee a program of care offered to every elderly patient rather than labelling this entire population of health care consumers as "bed blockers"!

As the health care system becomes more responsive to the needs of the elderly patient, a focus on more comprehensive models of health care will help to redefine and refocus energies and resources away from institutional, disease-related concepts of health and illness to more community-based services that stress the social and health promotion models of health care service. Social work has much to contribute to this movement and can be on the leading edge of program and policy initiatives, which will help to make health care organizations more responsive to the people.

The relatively recent development of geriatric assessment programs in this country makes it difficult to cite examples of research about the efficacy and health/social benefits to patients reviewed. Follow-up studies would provide much information relevant to social work practice with this population and would also provide support and direction to those individuals currently involved with the design and operation of GAUs. Obviously, a tremendous practice opportunity exists for social work research and publication in this "new" field.

IV. Concluding Remarks

As life is a progression of events that requires individuals to make transitions, there is no better way to perceive of old age than to think about continuing change. GAU social workers, as "agents of change," find the frail elderly struggling to adapt rapidly to change with diminished personal and environmental resources. The recognition of multiple disabilities, particularly psychosocial disability, is of particular interest to social work in this practice setting. The social work practitioner in these programs has much to offer as efforts are made to understand the interrelationship of all factors that lead to dysfunctional change and then to design interventions to return the elderly patient to good health and as much independent function as is possible or desired.

Since reversible health problems and individual problems in social functioning may incorrectly be attributed to the infirmities of age, continued efforts must be made by social workers to ensure that stereotypical perceptions of elderly persons do not distort assessments, limit goals, nor restrict interventions. Unless such efforts are made, the elderly of today, and we as the elders of tomorrow, will have to endure the final years of life with services that are designed to provide less-than-adequate support and opportunities to compensate for human frailties.

Case Example

Pre-admission visit: Mr. Joe Bloggs
Mr. Bloggs is an 83-year-old gentleman who was visited today in his home on Main Street where he lives with his well and active 81-year-old wife. He has been referred to the GAU by his attending physician at the urging of his son, George. George lives in Calgary, but manages to visit his parents every three to four months. On a visit last weekend, he was alarmed to note a rapid deterioration in his father's physical and mental functioning. He is concerned that his mother is becoming exhausted with caring for Mr. Bloggs and "wants something done."

Mental Function and Mood
Mr. Bloggs appeared listless and depressed during the home visit. Efforts to engage him in conversation were difficult and most questions were answered by his wife before he had an opportunity to respond. A gentle direction was given to Mrs. Bloggs to allow Mr. Bloggs to respond in order to allow an assessment of how well he was processing information. On further questioning, Mr. Bloggs appeared oriented to person and place, but disoriented to time, but his poor response may be related more to his feelings of poor physical health than a dementing process.

Ambulation
Mrs. Bloggs reports that her husband has been having difficulty walking lately and has had many falls. He gets up often at night to use the bathroom and frequently stumbles en route. His most recent fall was four days ago when he suffered a severe bump on the head from the edge of the bathtub. She feels his condition has become worse since then.

Medical Background
Appendectomy—1923, prostatectomy—1987, hiatal hernia, borderline diabetes, hypertension, and recent falls.

Medications
Tagamet 300 mg. tid, Dalmane 30 mg. @ hs, Diabeta 0.5 mg. OD, Moduret 25 mg. bid

Social History
Mr. Bloggs is a retired accountant who moved to Victoria from Calgary with his wife 11 years ago. He is described by his family as a shy and quiet gentleman who kept to himself and had few interests outside the home, save his woodworking hobby. Even though Mr. Bloggs has a fully equipped workshop in the basement of their home, it seems he lost interest in this pastime some six to seven months ago. He takes great pride in his business competence, but had his ego sorely bruised last spring when he made a number of errors in preparing the tax returns of several friends from their bridge club. Mrs. Bloggs reports that he has appeared depressed and withdrawn since that time and rarely responds positively to social invitations with the individuals he feels he wronged.

Patient/Family Perception of the Presenting Problem
Mrs. Bloggs appears to be very perplexed by her husband's behaviour and confided that she really does believe that he has the beginnings of senility. She states that she is desperate for some assistance or will have to make arrangements to place her husband in a long-term care facility.

Social Work Impression and Plan
It appears this gentleman was having some problems with depression over the past several months, but was otherwise functioning relatively well. His behaviour has changed significantly in the past week. His wife is his primary caregiver and is quickly becoming exhausted. The nature of the geriatric assessment program was explained to both Mr. and Mrs. Bloggs and after some gentle persuasion and coaxing by his wife, Mr. Bloggs agreed and arrangements were made for him to be seen in the geriatric day hospital in two days' time.

Social Work Case Notes: Mr. Joe Bloggs
Mr. Bloggs was seen in the geriatric day hospital in December, 1988. The geriatrician noted a number of neurological deficits during his physical examination and arranged for an immediate CT scan after learning of Mr. Bloggs's recent fall and head injury. The CT scan showed a subdural hemotoma. Mr. Bloggs was admitted to the geriatric inpatient unit for further observation and transferred the next day to the acute-care hospital for surgery to release the intracranial pressure from the hemotoma. He returned to the geriatric in-patient unit after a six-day stay on the acute-care ward for further investigation of some other physical problems (borderline diabetes, urinary tract infection) and where his medication regime was restructured (including an anti-depressant) and a physiotherapy program begun to restrengthen him. Both Mr. and Mrs. Bloggs were seen by the nutritionist for counselling for his diabetic condition. The social worker arranged to have the local long-term care office send homemaker help once per week to help Mrs. Bloggs with the heavy cleaning. Both Mr. and Mrs. Bloggs rejected the idea of any home help coming to assist in the personal care needs of Mr. Bloggs, such as assistance with bathing. The occupational therapist arranged to visit the Bloggs at home to install railings around the bathtub and a raised toilet seat. Mr. Bloggs responded well to the music program while on the in-patient ward and was encouraged by the OT to return to his long-neglected hobby of restoring musical instruments. The staff reported at case conference that he was thinking

more clearly, although his mood remained somewhat depressed. Mr. Bloggs remained on the in-patient ward for three weeks and was then discharged home to the care of his wife with the understanding that he would continue his rehabilitation by attending the geriatric day hospital program of the GAU three days each week. His attendance at the GDH program was somewhat sporadic as he often would find excuses not to be ready when the GDH bus came to call for him. The social worker made subsequent house calls to follow up on the concerns of the geriatrician and other members of the team that Mr. Bloggs continued to be depressed and unmotivated.

With some reluctance Mr. Bloggs began to discuss his feelings of apprehension, despair, and uselessness. He stated that he felt ridiculous having to depend on his wife for assistance with his personal care as he had been rarely ill and needy of this type of care before. He was very fearful that he might become ill again and that caring for him would be too much for his wife. A subsequent exploration of the sense of failure he experienced when making errors on the tax forms for his friends was structured around helping him to modify his negative self-thoughts and subsequent sense of embarrassment and frustration. Further sessions with both the social worker and the visiting psychiatrist allowed Mr. Bloggs to ventilate some of these feelings and come to some resolution over disappointments he had experienced both in the past and recently. Mr. Bloggs also responded well in group settings with the social worker and other patients of the GAU. He admitted coming to the realization that many other older people like himself struggled with similar feelings of depression over the dependency sometimes associated with ill health. Mrs. Bloggs was seen both separately and conjointly with her husband as the team attempted to help her understand her husband's care needs as well as recognize her need for support in dealing with the situation. Mrs. Bloggs was initially very resistive of the idea of accepting home help as she was very proud of her own homemaking abilities. After some discussion with Mr. Bloggs, the son, and the GAU team, Mrs. Bloggs recognized that relinquishing some of the more mundane and exhausting household duties would free her time and energies to allow more opportunities for Mr. and Mrs. Bloggs to become re-involved in a social world they had neglected for some time. The Bloggs were referred to a local seniors' activity centre and encouraged to participate in the organization as one way of redeveloping a sense of activity, community, and frivolity. Mr. Bloggs was encouraged to redefine his sense of identity, which to this point had always told him that he "must be in control at all times." Mrs. Bloggs and the son, George, had a tendency to mistakenly assume that Mr. Bloggs would not recover from his recent illness and were about to make arrangements with the bank and the accountant to take over their financial affairs. Fortunately, staff were able to convince Mrs. Bloggs and the son that this potential insult to Mr. Bloggs's sense of accountability and identity was not necessary as his vitality returned.

Mr. Bloggs was discharged from the geriatric day hospital program of the GAU after an eight-week stay.

Discharge Note: Six Month Follow-up
The Bloggs were contacted by the social worker for follow-up information. Mr. Bloggs recovered well from his numerous physical problems, although he continues to struggle with feelings of depression. He is seen monthly by his family physician for re-evaluation of his anti-depressant medication. Mrs. Bloggs reports that they have taken a number of short day trips with a group from the seniors' centre and hope to participate in a six-day tour of the Southern United States next month. Mrs. Bloggs cancelled the homemaker help as she found she had plenty of free time since Mr. Bloggs had returned to his woodworking hobby.

Note

1. The original version of this chapter was published in M. Holosko & P. Taylor (eds.), *Social work practice in health care settings*, pp. 353–381. Toronto: Canadian Scholars' Press Inc., 1989.

References

Abrass, I., Kane, R.L., & Rubenstein, L.Z. (1981). Improved care for patients on a new geriatric evaluation unit. *Journal of the American Geriatrics Society, 29*, 531–536.

Barer, M.L., Evans, R.B., Hertman, C., & Lomas, J. (1986). Toward efficient aging: Rhetoric and evidence. Paper presented at the Third Canadian Conference on Health Economics, Winnipeg, Manitoba.

Barrett, K. & Soltys, F. (2002) Geriatric social work: Supporting the patients' search for meaning. *Topics in Geriatric Rehabilitation, 17*(4), 53–64.

Beatty, P. (1989). Notes from an address to the Canadian Club. Ottawa.

Beaver, M.L. & Miller, D. (1985). *Clinical social work practice with the elderly.* Homewood: The Dorsey Press.

Berkman, B., Bonander, E., Chauncey, S., Daniels, A., Holmes, W., Robinson, M., & Sampson, S. (1999). Standardized screening of elderly patients needs for social work assessment in primary care. *Health and Social Work*, 24(1), 9–16.

Blandford, A., Chappell, N.L., & Strain, L. (1986). *Aging and health care*. Toronto: Holt, Rinehart & Winston of Canada Ltd.

Brill, N.I. (1976). *Team work: Working together in the human services*. Philadelphia: W.B. Saunders Co.

Butler, R. (1975). *Why survive? Being old in America*. New York: Harper & Row.

Calkins, E., Davis, P., & Ford, A. (1986). *The practice of geriatrics*. Philadelphia: W.B. Saunders Co.

Doremus, B. (1976). The four R's of medical social diagnosis. *Health and Social Work*, 1(4), 120–139.

Fengler A.P. & Goodrich, N. (1979). Wives of elderly disabled men: The hidden patients. *Gerontologist*, 19, 175–183.

Flathman, D.P. & Larsen, D.E. (1976). An evaluation of three geriatric day hospitals in Alberta. Calgary, Alberta. Unpublished report, Division of Community Health Services, Faculty of Medicine, University of Calgary.

Gaitz, C.M. (1974). Barriers to the delivery of psychiatric services to the elderly. *Gerontologist*, 14, 210–214.

Germain, C.B. (1973). An ecological perspective in casework practice. *Social Casework*, 54, 323–330.

Gilmore, S.K. (1973). *Counselor-in-training*. Englewood Cliffs: Prentice-Hall.

Golan, N. (1986). Crisis theory. In F.J. Turner (ed.), *Social work treatment: Interlocking theoretical approaches*, 3rd ed. New York: The Free Press.

Hayes, M. & Hertzman, C. (1985). Will the elderly really bankrupt us with increased health care costs? *Canadian Journal of Public Health*, 76, 373–377.

Health and Welfare Canada. (1988). *Health Promotion Directorate, Health Service and Promotion Branch*, 27(2).

Hepworth, D.H. & Larsen, J.A. (1986). *Direct social work practice: Theory and skills*, 2nd ed. Chicago: The Dorsey Press.

Hooyman, N.R. & Kiyak, A. (1988). The importance of social supports: Family, friends and neighbours. In *Social gerontology: A multi-disciplinary perspective*. Boston: Allyn & Bacon.

Kane, R. (1987). Contrasting models: Reflections on the pattern of geriatric evaluation unit care. In L.Z. Rubenstein, L.J. Campbell, & R.L. Kane (eds.), *Clinics in geriatric medicine*. Philadelphia: W.B. Saunders Co.

Kane, R.L., Rhee, L., & Rubenstein, L.Z. (1982). The role of geriatric assessment units in caring for the elderly: An analytic review. *Journal of Gerontology*, 37, 513–521.

Levenson, J. & Rathbone-McCuan, E. (1977). Geriatric day care: A community approach to geriatric health care. *Journal of Gerontological Nursing*, 3(4), 43–46.

Lindeman, D. & Mellor, M.J. (1998). The role of the social worker in interdisciplinary geriatric teams. *Journal of Gerontological Social Work*, 30(3/4).

MacKenzie, J.A. (1982). Aging in Canadian society. *Issues in Canadian social policy: A reader, II*. Ottawa: Canadian Council on Social Development.

MacKenzie, P., Parker, G., & Wooldridge, D.B. (1987). An acute inpatient geriatric assessment and treatment unit. In L.Z. Rubenstein, L.J. Campbell, & R.L. Kane (eds.), *Clinics in geriatric medicine*. Philadelphia: W.B. Saunders Co.

Matcha, D. (1997). Aging and health care. In D. Matcha (ed.), *The sociology of aging: A social problems perspective*, pp. 131–151. Boston: Allyn & Bacon.

McDaniels, S.A. (1988). Prospects for an aging Canada: Gloom or hope? *Transition*, 9–11.

Medalie, J.H. (1986). An approach to common problems in the elderly. In E. Calkins and A. Ford (eds.), *The practice of geriatrics*. Philadelphia: W.B. Saunders Co.

Mellor, J.M. & Lindeman, David. (1998). The role of the social worker in interdisciplinary geriatric teams. *Journal of Gerontological Social Work*, 30, 3–4, 3–7.

Neugarten, B. (1974). Age groups in American society and the rise of the young-old. In *Political consequences of aging*, The Annals of the American Academy of Political and Social Science, 415, 187–198.

Novak, M. (1988). *Aging and society*. Scarborough: Nelson Canada.

Richmond, M. (1917). *Social diagnosis*. New York: The Russell Sage Foundation.

Rosenfeld, J. (1983). The domain and expertise of social work: A conceptualization. *Social Work*, 28, 186–191.

Rubenstein, L.Z. (1987). Geriatric assessment: An overview of its impacts. In L.Z. Rubenstein, L.J. Campbell, & R.L. Kane (eds.), *Clinics in geriatric medicine*. Philadelphia: W.B. Saunders Co.

Sander, F. (1976). Aspects of sexual counselling with the aged. *Social Casework*, 58, 504–510.

Skelton, D. (1986). The future of geriatric medicine in Canada. *Gerontion: A Canadian Review of Geriatric Care*, 1, 19–23.

Schumann, J.Z. (1984). Maintaining ability in the elderly. *Canadian Family Physician*, 30, 607–610.

Snider, E.L. (1981). The role of kin in meeting health care needs of the elderly. *Canadian Journal of Sociology*, 6, 325–336.

Toseland, R. (1977). A problem-solving group workshop for older persons. *Social Work*, 22, 325–326.

Watson, M. (1984). Alternatives to institutionalizing the elderly. *Canadian Family Physician*, 30, 655–660.

Westberg, S. (1986). An aging population: Implications for social workers in acute hospitals. *The Social Worker — Journal of the Canadian Association of Social Workers*, 107–109.

Williams, T.F. (1987). Integration of geriatric assessment into the community. In L.Z. Rubenstein, L.J. Campbell, & R.L. Kane (eds.), *Clinics in geriatric medicine*. Philadelphia: W.B. Saunders Co.

Internet Resources

A Social Gerontology Index
    Resources in Social Gerontology.
    http://www.trinity.edu/mkearl/geron.html
Primary Care Internet Guide
    Geriatrics resource guide.
    http://www.uib.no/isf/guide/geri.htm

Additional Readings

Berkman, B. & Harootyan, L.K. (eds.). (2003). *Social work and health care in an aging society: Education, policy, practice, and research*. New York: Springer.

Berkman, B., Silverstone, B., Simmons, W.J., Volland, P.J., & Howe, J.L. (2000). Social work gerontological practice: the need for faculty development in the new millennium. *Journal of Gerontological Social Work*, 34(1), 5–23.

Gleason-Wynn, P. (2002). Teaching geriatric assessment: a hands-on educational experience. *Journal of Gerontological Social Work*, 39(1–2), 195–202

Greene, R. (2000). Serving the aged and their families in the 21st century using a revised practice model. *Journal of Gerontological Social Work 2000*, 34(1), 43–62.

Howe, J.L., Hyer, K., Mellor, J., Lindeman, D., & Luptak, M. (2001). Educational approaches for preparing social work students for interdisciplinary teamwork on geriatric health care teams. *Social Work in Health Care*, 32(4), 19–42.

Kivnick, H.Q., Murray, S.V. (2001). Life strengths interview guide: Assessing elder clients' strengths. *Journal of Gerontological Social Work,* 34(4), 7–32.

Naleppa-Matthias, J. & Reid-William, J. (2003). *Gerontological social work: A task-centered approach.* New York: Columbia University Press.

Naleppa, M.J. & Reid, W.J. (2002). Integrating case management and brief-treatment strategies: A hospital-based geriatric program. *Social Work in Health Care,* 31(4), 1–23.

Saltz, C., Shaefer, T., & Weinreich, D. (1998). Streamlining outpatient geriatric assessment: Essential social, environmental and economic variables. *Social Work in Health Care,* 27(1), 1–14.

CHAPTER 18

SOCIAL WORK PRACTICE WITH THE ELDERLY IN AN INTEGRATED ADULT DAY CENTRE PROGRAM

FRAN KLEINER, RHODA KOPSTEIN,

JOYCE LAGUNOFF, AND SORELE URMAN

This chapter describes social work practice within a unique non-medical, community-based service designed to meet the differential psychosocial needs of the elderly. The goal of this service is to help older persons stay in control of their situation by using basic contracting principles with them and their family care system. The functions of social worker both as case manager and group worker are described. The main assumption put forward is that by acknowledging dependency and focusing on strengths, older adults may be helped to achieve their potential.

The National Institute of Adult Day Care (NIAD), established in the United States in 1979, defined adult daycare as "a community-based program that is a structured, comprehensive program that provides a variety of health, social and related support services in a protective setting during any part of a day but less than 24 hour care. Individuals who participate in adult daycare attend on a planned basis during specified hours. Adult daycare assists its participants to remain in the community, enabling families and other caregivers to continue caring at home for a family member...." (p. 42). This definition embraces all adult day programs whether they serve the frail elderly, the cognitively impaired elderly and/or employ a social work model, a health-based model, or a combination of both (Weissert, 1989).

I.   The Clientele

The Day Centre (DCP) at Baycrest Centre for Geriatric Care in Toronto, Ontario, is a non-sectarian program that uses a unique social work model for serving a community-based population of approximately 175 registered elderly people, with an average age of 87. It was founded in 1959, and has the distinction of being the oldest adult day program in Ontario [and possibly all of Canada].

The primary goals and objectives of the Baycrest Community Day Centre for Seniors program are:

- addressing the diverse needs of an aging population;
- enabling individuals to realize their maximum physical, psychosocial, and spiritual well-being;
- striving for excellence in the services through the integration of care, research, and education;
- maintaining and improving the current level of functioning of the participants, whenever possible;
- expanding the social network of the members by creating a sense of belonging to a community;
- providing respite for caregivers; and
- helping prevent unnecessary or premature institutionalization.

"Some day programs are designed for people with mild to moderate cognitive impairment due to Alzheimer's disease or another type of dementing illness" (Gordon & Michaels, 2001). The DCP is made up of three clubs and refers to clients as members. The Parkland Club serves the well elderly and physically frail. Oceanside Club's activities are geared to meet the needs of the mildly cognitively impaired elderly. The Samuel Lunenfeld Mountainview Club (MVC) serves the moderately to severely cognitively impaired elderly within a safe and secure environment, and is provided for those who may wander. The Parkland and Oceanside Clubs (POC) share another physical space nearby. The environment for all three clubs has been structured to promote socialization, with common lobby areas and adjustable activity space that are walker/wheelchair user-friendly. POC can accommodate up to 55 people daily; MVC can accommodate up to 32 people daily, and a waitlist is established when this number is exceeded. All members have access to other out-patient/in-patient Baycrest services housed on site, thus offering a "campus of care" for the older person.

In the professionally staffed DCP, virtually all of the participants are vulnerable and struggling with one or more of the following areas: physical, emotional, social, or cognitive, i.e., some mild forgetfulness or dementia diagnosis. Applications to the DCP are accelerated by a specific crisis in an older person's life. Such crises have a mixture of losses of spouse, physical vitality, friendships, employment, family roles, income, and /or familiar environment. Regardless of what combination of such losses are experienced, the results are usually the following: (1) feelings of uselessness because of a lack of meaningful socially based roles; (2) feelings of loss of control, engendering fear, anger, and various forms of defensive behaviour; and/or (3) severe lowering of self-esteem. Since most participants are in their 80s or 90s, their family caregivers are usually in their 50s or 60s. As a result, respite for caregivers is part of the mandate of the program (Miller, 1989). Research among the family caregivers of persons with dementia consistently reveals that respite ranks among the most urgently desired community services. The fact that respite services occupy a prominent place in government long-term or continuing care plans testifies to the recognition among policy-makers of the sustained energy and commitment that are called for by the caregiving role (Gottlieb & Johnson, 2000).

The combined deficits usually experienced by this population are reflected by its auspices, that of a home for the aged and an adjacent hospital. DCPs in free-standing facilities may have fewer physically handicapped elderly than in a facility connected to a hospital such as this program (Weissert, 1989). However, DCPs in general are experiencing an increase in a more frail clientele as their population "ages in place" and the median age increases.

The litany of losses and deficits of program members are balanced by the strengths that such people retain. For instance, most have lived very full and long lives and take much pride in their families and social networks. Further, many come with obvious or latent skills in such activities as crafts, creative writing, or drama. All have lived through momentous events and usually have both decided opinions about issues such as religion, family, and politics and emotional memories of their past experiences. As well, some have other skills in making and keeping friends and many are blessed with a sense of humour (Miller & Solomon, 1980).

Meeting the psychosocial needs of this clientele for a regained sense of community, relationships, new experiences, self-esteem, and control over decisions that affect their lives is the primary responsibility of the social work staff. Thus, the social worker relates to the elderly person's strengths and builds supports into the program to acknowledge and compensate for their existing deficits (Miller & Solomon, 1980). Further, arrangements to meet health care needs and other case management issues such as help to the families in supporting their relatives are important social work responsibilities, which attempt to provide service to the whole person.

The concern of some is that the concept of a day program may serve to reinforce non-functional dependency. However, what may appear as dependency "may be a reaction to the actual absence of needed supports, and when these are in fact provided, dependency decreases rather than increases" (Miller & Solomon, 1980, p. 76). When non-functional dependency occurs, it is explored and dealt with by staff.

All of the DCP members live in the adjacent community in their own residence with a paid caregiver, or with their families, or in group homes. Each participant retains his or her own personal physician in the community and is required to have a medical examination every year. Referral by the DCP member's physician to out-patient clinics in Baycrest Centre is facilitated by the DCP social worker.

DCP social workers assist individuals and their families to enter into the program. Each participant is assigned to a social worker who carries a caseload of up to 35 individuals and their families, in addition to leading groups, supervising volunteers, educational supervision of students in practicum, program development, as well as attending to some of the management tasks of the DCP. In addition, case management and complex discharge planning involving the family are important aspects of the job (Burack-Weiss, 1988). Integral to the provision of optimal service are: (1) a director, social workers, nurse clinicians, certified health care aides, therapeutic recreationists, and clerical staff; (2) volunteers and a part-time creative arts specialist who enrich the service and who are supervised by DCP social workers; (3) a reliable escorted door-to-door transportation system within a large catchment area; (4) a diet-controlled, full-course hot lunches and snacks prepared and served daily by the food services staff of Baycrest Centre; (5) an activity schedule geared to adults that permits individualized choice and is changed a minimum of four times a year; (6) access to a beauty and barber shop, numerous outpatient clinics, and consultants; (7) the use of F.M. hearing-assistive devices for discussion groups; and (8) health care promotion, emergency care, and first-aid provided by the nurse clinicians.

II. Practice Roles and Responsibilities

A. Intake, Admission, and Contracting Functions

In order for the program to meet the psychosocial needs of the individual, s/he must participate in the decision-making process. For instance, even if a professional (e.g., doctor, social worker, public health nurse, etc.) determines that the program would be good for them, if the elderly persons do not agree or is not facilitated in helping overcome their fears of participation, they will not enter the program. It should be noted that in the Mountainview Club there is a shift in the decision-making process of admissions. This function rests primarily with the caregiver or substitute decision maker due to the clients' cognitive impairment.

1. Steps in Intake
The intake process requires full family participation, both together with and separate from the applicant.

1. *Enquiry:* Initially a client, family member or a referring agency calls Baycrest Seniors Counselling and Referral or personally comes in to discuss the need for this service. Subsequently, an enquiry is written up by the social worker on duty. Information and support is provided if the service is not deemed appropriate and/or there is a crisis requiring immediate attention.
2. *Initial Screening:* The enquiry is passed on to the DCP director, who then assigns it to the appropriate DCP social worker for processing.
3. *Assessment and Orientation:* This includes at least one formally structured interview with the client and his or her family jointly to establish the needs of the client and determine whether the service is suitable. Basic information about the DCP is given to the client and family on the understanding that neither the DCP nor the client/family are making a commitment that the client will enter the DCP. The purpose here is to: (1) ensure that the person does not feel s/he is being rushed into something; (2) that s/he still retains control over the situation; (3) assure the client that s/he will have adequate opportunity to test out the program before making a decision.

The purposes of the assessment are: (1) to contract with the applicant/family for a mutually agreed-upon number of trial visits (using the guideline of one half-day visit and one full-day visit); and (2) to contract about mutually agreed-upon expectations that the applicant may have of the DCP and expectations that the program will have of him or her.

4. *Admissions and Contracting:* The contract interview is essentially where the program's purpose and the applicant's needs come together (Gitterman & Shulman, 1986; Schwartz & Zalba, 1971). The idea that there will be expectations of her or him is both thrilling and fear inducing for the individual. Thus, most applicants need reassurance that the social worker will be available to help them.

    Elements of the contracting interview (not necessarily in order) include:

    - A statement of the purpose of the meeting.
    - Reaching for feedback of applicant's overall understanding and clarifying the agenda for the meeting.
    - Conveying that the applicant is in charge of the decision after the agreed-upon number of trial visits.
    - Encouraging the applicant to describe her or his own need for the program and expectations of it. In this context, respond honestly as to which expectations can be met by the program and also those that cannot be met.
    - Describing the expectations that the DCP has, i.e., to learn to accept help in the beginning; to help others when s/he is comfortable; to try to connect with other members with whom she or he might like to become friends; to attend the daily morning meeting group with the DCP social worker.
    - Describing the initial supports and ongoing assistance that s/he will receive from the day centre social worker. For instance, the social worker will meet her or him when s/he first arrives and make sure that s/he attends the early morning activities and the morning meeting; the DCP social worker will ensure the client is seated at a compatible table in the dining room. Also, the client will

be reminded of the activities available and receive help to access them.

- Negotiating the days s/he will attend (minimum two days per week) and discuss transportation arrangements.
- Reassuring the client that s/he will not have to remember everything as staff will write information down and "help remember for her or him."
- Acknowledging the help the client has been given by his or her family in attending the meeting. Encouraging the client, if it seems appropriate, to express feeling to those members of his or her family who are present re: the support they have provided.
- Describing to family members their responsibilities, i.e., picking up their relative if s/he becomes ill during the program. Families are also given information about the programs that they will be invited to such as family meetings, family education, and support groups, etc. Families are assured that they will continue to receive counselling or help if they require it. Developing family education/training programs sponsored by respite programs is an important activity for social workers (Monahan, 1993).
- Discharge planning is first discussed at intake with a review of the *Limits of Care* of the DCP. The applicant/ family are also given a typed copy of the *Limits of Care* to take home.
- Providing information about fees for the visits and program, which are shared with the person(s) responsible. A copy of the fee schedule is given.

5. *Initial Visit:* Once the DCP social worker establishes with the client and the family the elderly person's need for and readiness to become involved, the social worker arranges for the client to visit individual programs. Scheduled times and transportation must also be arranged with the applicant and family as DCP transportation is not used until later in the process when the client becomes a member. The focus is to help the client feel that s/he has potential for self-determinism and can cope with the pending situation. For instance, if the client knows s/he has the capacity and desire to participate in the program after the first visit, a further

orientation is usually arranged, e.g., s/he may then stay for the morning. If all goes well during this visit, the applicant moves on immediately to the next stage, which is a full-day visit.

a)   For the full day visit, the applicant obtains formal medical clearance for the program from one's physician, and meets with the DCP nurse clinician who reviews the medical, completes a functional assessment, and makes health promotion recommendations. The client/family then formally completes a DCP membership form. Payment for services is discussed with applicants and family and, if need be, their children are asked to fill out a financial form if their help is needed and if they (the clients) are unable to pay the full program costs. If a subsidy is requested, the centre's financial officer determines with the client and family the amount of the payment and the method of payment of fees.

b)   The social worker prepares a summary outlining what s/he knows about the applicant's characteristics and needs, information about past and present social relationships, occupational information, and family background data. This information is shared with the DCP multidisciplinary staff team in order to help integrate the applicant into the program.

If the applicant decides, after the contracted number of visits, to remain in the program, the transition to membership is formally completed. A meeting is held with the DCP program co-ordinator to complete an individualized program participation plan. A joint welcome letter from the DCP director and social worker is sent to the new member and a designated family member. The new member also receives a DCP handbook/calendar for future reference, program schedule, and the most recent Day Centre newsletter.

This type of systematized contracting with the individual who has identified her or his own needs, who has a beginning understanding of the service and what s/he can get from it, and what s/he can give to it is a powerful incentive to many, and enables many individuals to stay in control of their program participation every step of the way. Social work's role in contracting and recontracting as such facilitates both individualized programming and safeguards the overall self-determinism of clients in the Parkland/Oceanside Clubs.

B. Activity Planning and Management Function

The DCP activity schedule is designed, continuously evaluated, and redesigned four to five times a year by social work and program staff with input from members. The schedule is very structured, offering a minimum of three activity choices during each program time slot. Offering choices as such is necessary not only to take into account varied interests and abilities but also to help people retain their uniqueness and dignity through having personal choices. Activities are designed to highlight members' strengths and offer the needed supports in order for members with cognitive impairment to participate at their optimum level in appropriate groups. As well, the structured schedule helps members to stay oriented to time.

The various small group activities offered provide opportunities for mutual aid and the development of friendships. Some mass activities are also held, which provide for welcome anonymity, e.g., concerts, bingos, etc. The activity schedule is routinely evaluated as to whether it contains the right mix of physical fitness, active games, music, discussion groups, structured time to gain new knowledge and other intellectual challenges, and experiences that promote personal growth and self-expression. Inherent in such activities are the opportunities for development of social relationships and self-esteem building.

The so-called management tasks include providing support so that people can meaningfully participate. That is, making arrangements for hearing-assistive devices, which assist the hearing impaired stay connected in discussion groups; arranging for people to be taken in wheelchairs to the dining room for those who find it too exhausting to walk there; and staff providing program promotion reminders to help individuals get to programs they have previously selected. Adult day programs provide supervised individual programming in a group setting to help adults achieve and maintain their maximum level of functioning to avoid premature and inappropriate institutionalization, and to provide respite and information for caregivers (Government of Ontario, 2003).

C. Group Work

The task of each social worker is to assist in establishing a culture of a community of mutual aid and support (Gitterman, 1989; Miller & Solomon, 1980). In the Parkland/Oceanside DCP, this culture is operationalized by each of the staff with members of their own caseloads in a meeting called "the morning meeting group." While this morning meeting group has seemingly loose cohesion, its boundaries are very clear. Specifically, everyone in the DCP belongs to a morning meeting group led by a social worker and is entitled and expected to attend. The introduction of a new member to the group is the beginning of the socialization process to the culture of the therapeutic community.

As with traditional groups, the morning meeting group has certain rituals, e.g., taking attendance and reporting by the staff and members on absent members, plans for contacting people who are ill, opportunities for members to acknowledge one another's life cycle events, i.e., birth of a new great-grandchild, etc. In these groups, which also include persons with short-term memory problems or beginning Alzheimer's, the worker announces the day, date, and time and orients members to the season/upcoming holidays.

Day centre social workers also lead groups for members who may not be on their caseloads. In discussion groups, such as reminiscence programs and current events, frequent synopses of content by the group leader compensates for short-term memory loss by some members and for those who are hearing impaired. In all of the groups a strong leadership role is played by the social worker. This is usually different from group work done with other age groups where the worker normally acts a resource person and, through process, the group develops ownership of itself (Schwartz & Weisman, 1989). Acknowledgement of dependency of older adults by the worker pays homage to the principle of beginning where people are at (Miller & Solomon, 1980).

D. Supervision

Not all the activities of the DCP require leadership by a social worker. Some activities are more suitable for recreation workers, adult educators, and specialists in areas such as creative arts, horticulture, music, etc. (Briggs et al., 1973). The role of the social worker in supervising specialists and group leaders then becomes: (1) to act as resource person; (2) to provide them with materials that they need to carry out the program; (3) to establish expectations of involving everyone in the group; and (4) to ensure that they use appropriate supports so that members can have a sense of achievement and purpose that they value. All group leaders [as well as bus drivers] are expected to report any changes they may see in participants, and to alert social workers and staff who may need to discuss such concerns with staff and family members.

E. Casework and Case Management

The social worker provides support to members/families who are experiencing problems coping with illness, loneliness/isolation, long-term placement, caregiving needs, and/or family conflict. All participants in the Parkland/Oceanside DCP require "private time" with their social worker to discuss concerns and issues that have arisen in their lives. For some people, the providing of individual attention is enough. Often, however, a counselling relationship is required whereby the social worker may assist clients, for example, to come to grips with attitudes and behaviours that may be preventing them from finding acceptance or friends in the DCP (Gitterman & Shulman, 1986). As well, frail and mildly cognitively impaired adults in the program may be concerned about their future living arrangements and may require help in planning for institutionalization.

The role of the social worker is to help sort out immediate needs with the individual, his or her family, and to enable the family to provide additional supports for the individual team when needed. Thus, the social worker deals with differences and conflicts within the family, ambivalence (around plans), and generally helps the individual and family sort out together what their next steps will be. As such, the social worker provides casework for the individual and family within the context of the DCP.

As a case manager, the social worker ensures that the living arrangements for the individual are satisfactory and that the client has the financial resources to live with dignity. Some individuals may have case managers in other agencies and this then involves the day centre social worker in periodic interagency consultations. By referring members to other services in the community as such, the social worker acts as an advocate for the client. Case management is a social work intervention that could be used to help families identify community resources, and may be particularly effective for employed caregivers (Monahan, 1993).

The above steps in this process are depicted in Figure 18.1, which describes the admission flowchart and the time frames involved.

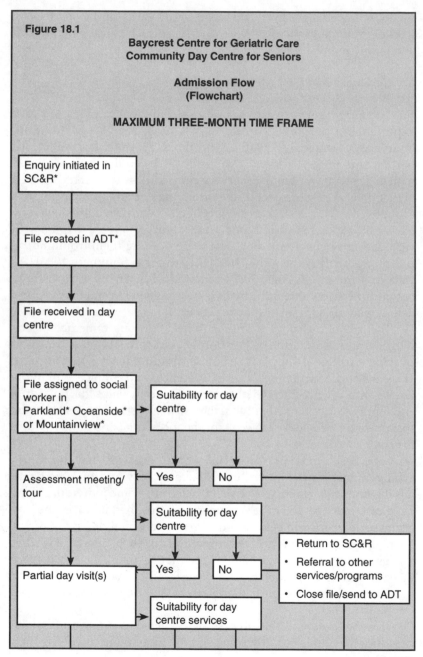

Figure 18.1

Baycrest Centre for Geriatric Care
Community Day Centre for Seniors

Admission Flow
(Flowchart)

MAXIMUM THREE-MONTH TIME FRAME

Enquiry initiated in SC&R*

File created in ADT*

File received in day centre

File assigned to social worker in Parkland* Oceanside* or Mountainview*

Suitability for day centre

Assessment meeting/tour

Yes

No

Suitability for day centre

Partial day visit(s)

Yes

No

- Return to SC&R
- Referral to other services/programs
- Close file/send to ADT

Suitability for day centre services

con't

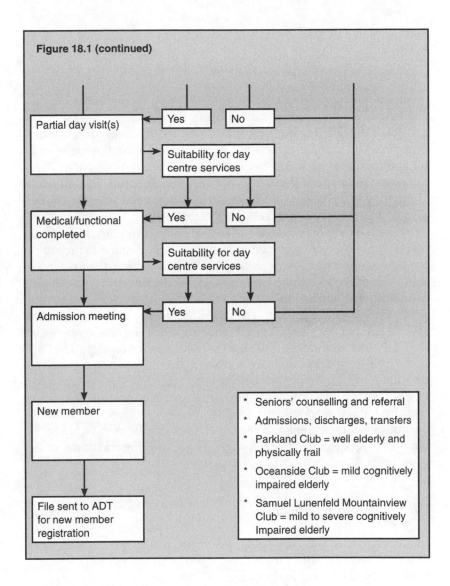

Figure 18.1 (continued)

III. Potential for Role Development

An increasingly frail and medically unstable clientele has inevitably involved the DCP in providing some nursing services. Presently, members attend certain out-patient clinics at the Baycrest Centre, focused on health promotion, referred to by their personal physicians and facilitated by their social worker. The trend toward meeting both health and social needs of older adults will require social workers in this setting to become skilled in interdisciplinary and holistic treatment, which is needs driven. It sounds simple, but it is not, as both the service delivery system and changing client needs present enormous challenges to social workers attempting to provide the best services possible. As well, it is our perception that the demand for adult day programs will increase as there is a strong preference in the community for community-based care over institutional care (Wood, 1989). There are many indications that adult daycare centres are a cost-effective alternative in the health care continuum and provide a nontraditional area of practice for nurses (Fettig & Reigel, 1998).

Finally, one of the objectives of any adult day program is to provide respite for families. Respite services are generally defined as providing temporary opportunities for caregivers to get away from their eldercare duties in order to reduce caregiver stress and to delay or prevent nursing home admission. For a variety of reasons, working adults, both middle-aged and older, are carrying a heavy load in their work and caregiving responsibilities (Monahan, 1993). Families report that the DCP does provide some respite for them, but not enough. The DCP as a whole does not provide for weekend, evening, or holiday care, or provide a bed for a member who needs care while the caregiver has to go to the hospital or would like a much-needed vacation. It appears then that social workers will need to conduct more research on the optimum hours needed and other types of respite care required by families in an age when many caregivers are working and under stress (Capitman, 1989).

IV.   Concluding Remarks

In working with the "very old," the roles, functions, and activities of a social worker differ from those used with younger age groups. Specifically, the salient features are:

- A longer pre-affiliation process with "mini-contracts" with the worker and assurance of retaining control over the decision (on behalf of the client).
- Full and active involvement of the family in the process.
- A structured program.

- Proactive involvement of the worker in providing support for participants to use the program and interact with one another.

It is universally found in adult daycare centres that programs are strengthened and services improved when the participants' needs take precedence over rigid or artificial lines of responsibility. Because the program is client-centred and since the participants' needs are complex and interrelated, staff interaction and collaboration are needed to respond to those needs. The unique blend of characteristics of the adult daycare centre as a mode of service delivery includes: a primary focus on the holistic needs of the participant, the individualized plan of care for each participant, the significance of the family or caregiver and consideration of their needs, and the importance of the sense of community—the sense of belonging that alleviates the isolation caused by the severe impairments experienced by the participants (National Institute on Adult Daycare, 1990).

The challenges and opportunities for social work in this field are many and varied and require a social worker who has a humanistic touch and competent skills. Only then can the rewards in working in this field be truly realized.

Case Example of a Parkland Club Applicant

Respecting the client's right to make her or his own decision often produces serious problems for families who must also be helped to trust the process and allow for the careful working through of the decision. "Day care administrators and social workers can make a huge difference to first-time caregiving adult children and spouses who are unaware of how to handle all the eldercare issues they face. They are usually in a crisis, trying to manage it all ..."(Marcell, 2002). This example illustrates this point.

Mrs. Smith was referred by the social service department of a local hospital where she had been briefly hospitalized. The family had been referred by her physician because of their concern about the mother living alone and their frustration in dealing with her. An overweight, alert, and strong-willed person, Mrs. Smith had been insistent on living alone, even though she was unable to cope in many areas of functioning and was increasingly dependent upon her four children, especially her two daughters. At the same time she was becoming increasingly more resistive to her children's suggestions and directions about her life situation.

The family eagerly accepted referral to the Baycrest Community Day Centre for Seniors. It took a concentrated period of very careful work with the family, and between the hospital worker and the DCP, and with Mrs. Smith to get her into the office for an appointment.

Fearful of engagement, she contended, against all evidence, that she could manage well on her own in her one-bedroom apartment. She also indicated that she was not isolated or lacking the company of friends or relatives. She even claimed her children told her that she did not need a day centre program, much to her children's consternation. One by one we began to deal with Mrs. Smith's many fears. She believed agreeing to the day centre program was consenting to the first step in a dreaded admission to the home for the aged, which she could correctly sense her children wanted. Thus, we initially needed to help the children realize that admission to the home was not needed and to assure their mother that they were not making any arrangements for her "behind her back." Mrs. Smith also seemed surprised to learn that over 50 percent of the members in the DCP at that time were not applicants and did not want the home, nor were we [the program] interested in either their business or hers. Many elderly are struggling to stay out of nursing homes and hospitals, and may require only minimal assistance. Many live alone or a distance from family members and prefer not to impose on family for such care (Fettig & Reigel, 1998).

We then began to systematically confront some of Mrs. Smith's distorted ideas about the people who attended the DCP. In her mind, they were all old and "senile." In reality, very frightened by her obvious decreasing ability to function, she tried to cope by denying this both to herself and her family. This, of course, would provoke her children into furious and frustrating arguments with her. Attacking this defence only made her more unreasonable and suspicious of their efforts. On their part, they thought she was becoming "senile," making her feel that they regarded her as childish and incompetent. In helping the children to realize that their mother was frightened and comforting herself by her pretence, the children were able to back off. They did not necessarily change their minds about what was good for her, but they were able to simply give their opinions and leave their mother room and time to think through and decide what she wanted to do. As well, they were instructed not to attempt to answer her questions or criticisms about the DCP, but to refer them to us directly.

At the same time, Mrs. Smith was encouraged to come and see for herself what the DCP was and then make up her own mind about the program. The fact that coming to the office for an appointment did not obligate her to the program was an important component in this early process.

Subsequently, she did come in to discuss and then to see part of the program, being constantly assured that she would not be pushed into doing or deciding anything until she was ready. She was, however, challenged to see and to test out some of the activities. Thus, she went to a concert, tried crafts, an indoor gardening group, and a current events discussion group on a trial basis.

Alert, intelligent, and very able to socialize, she met people she knew and made friends in the program, agreeing that she enjoyed it. It took almost three months from the time the hospital first called us until Mrs. Smith began to come regularly to the DCP. She needed to have private time with her social worker, although not frequently. Periodically she questioned whether she needed the day program or whether physically it was too much for her or whether it wasn't a step into the home after all.

Her relationship with her children and, in particular, with her two daughters, improved greatly. Mrs. Smith was no longer angry with them and they were relaxed and more comfortable with her. She now has a part of her life that is under her control and that she can talk about with her children when they visit. Everyone seems satisfied leaving her living situation as it presently is.

Group Orientation
Mrs. Smith came into my morning meeting on her first full-day visit. I settled the other members (of the program) into the circle and proceeded with the taking of attendance. I placed Mrs. James beside me because she appreciates it when I cue her when she is wandering off topic. This is an arrangement that she and I have because she finds it embarrassing, but sometimes can't help herself.

Mrs. Deven said, "I know there is going to be a new tax and they are even going to be taxing funerals." Everyone in the room gasped. Mr. Goldberg said, "You don't have to worry about it right away, they're not putting the tax on until next year. If you die this year, you don't have to pay it." Mrs Deven said, "That's good, if we don't want to pay the tax, we will either have to live forever or die this year." Everybody laughed and I was delighted to see that Mrs. Smith "got the joke" and was looking with interest at Mrs. Deven, who did not fit Mrs. Smith's image of a "senile" day centre member at all.

At this time I said I wanted to introduce the new visitor to the members. I introduced Mrs. Smith, as a first-time full-day visitor to our morning meeting group. The members immediately responded by applauding, with some smiling and nodding their heads in welcome.

Since this was Mrs. Smith's first full day, I asked the group if they would help her understand what the day program was all about. Several of the members talked about their favourite activities. Mrs. Ray told Mrs. Smith that the DCP was important because some people needed help, and she could help them by showing them where creative arts was when they couldn't remember, or by walking alongside somebody when he or she felt tired. This was an important statement for Mrs. Ray who, in making it, reaffirmed her contract with the day centre. Everybody joined in and as the discussion warmed up, several people stated that they found it very lonely at home. Many said that coming to the day centre was wonderful because they made friends here and felt they were with their "family."

Mrs. Smith appeared to feel a response was expected of her at this time. She said that she had a wonderful family, but they were pushing her to come to the DCP and she was sure that they were trying in this way to get her into the home for the aged. Mr. Kane hadn't quite grasped what Mrs. Smith had said, so I repeated it. Mr. Kane laughed. He said, "Listen, I have been waiting to get into the Home for nearly two years, it's not so easy to get in and they aren't going to take you if you don't want to go, so don't worry."

Mrs. Deven asked, "What's it like for you at home anyway? You've got lots of company and you are busy all day?" Mrs. Smith's eyes filled and she said, "No, it really is very lonely." She had promised her family that she would try the day centre. The members rushed in their eagerness to assure her that she would love the day program. After all, she would be in their group with their social worker, Jane, who was "wonderful and helps us, so you don't have to worry." I assured Mrs. Smith that I was there to assist her, but that was only part of what happens in the day centre. I turned to the group and said, "Please explain to Mrs. Smith how you help each other." Mrs. Berman said, "We support each other by listening to people who are feeling depressed," looking pointedly at Mrs. Lee, who said, "Yes, Mrs. Berman listens to me when I'm not feeling well and it makes me feel better." Mr. Goldberg said, "Jane can't do everything. We come to the day centre to help each other. I myself try to be helpful to everybody and I have met some nice people here." Mrs. Davis, eager to be included among the supportive, said, "I phoned Mrs. Simpson and she was happy to hear from me. She sends everybody regards." I intervened at this point and said, "Mrs. Smith, you hear what the members are saying. I am here to help you, but they are explaining what the DCP is all about supporting one another within our community. If you decide to become a member, you will want to help others and welcome their assistance when you need it." Mrs. Smith nodded and said, "You know, it would be nice maybe to have a life of my own, away from my kids, and it may be good to do something for somebody else and feel like a person again, but I don't know anybody here really, and everything seems so strange." I turned to the group and asked them to think back to their first full day in the program. The members started to compete with each other about who felt worse on their first day. "Mrs. Smith, when you get to know us," said Mrs. Gould, "you will want to become a member." I said we all hoped she would join the program and that she would be in charge of that decision herself.

I told Mrs. Smith that she would be seated at the same dining table with Mrs. Deven and Mrs. Lee, and I wondered if the ladies would like to show her where the table was. I also explained that she would be at that table every time she came to the program if she liked it. Mrs. Smith said, "I'm still not sure, but I am going to try it anyway."

In summary, the two-sided struggle (for Mrs. Smith) involved in both owning her need and risking the pursuit of help if necessary to enter the increasingly more demanding "mini-contracts" used for interviews and for program visits. Specifically, owning one's needs and "risking trying" are necessary preconditions if the applicant is to derive the ego-supportive social experiences she or he requires from the program. As indicated many times in this chapter, our goal is to empower the client and her or his family system to achieve a more complete balance in their lives.

References

Briggs, T.L. et al. (1973). An overview of social work teams, the team model of social work practice. *Manpower Monograph*, 5. Syracuse: Syracuse University, School of Social Work.

Burack-Weiss, A. (1988). Clinical aspects of case management. *Generations*, 12(5), 23–25.

Capitman, J.A. (1989). Policy and program options in community-oriented long-term care. *Annual review of gerontology and geriatrics*, 9, 357–388. New York: Springer.

Fettig, E. & Riegel, D. (1998, July–August). Adult daycare: An entrepreneurial opportunity for nursing. *Nursing Economics*, 16(4), 189.

Gitterman, A. (1989). Building mutual support groups. *Social Work with Groups*, 12(2).

Gitterman A. & Shulman, L. (1986). *The skills of helping individuals and groups*, 2nd ed. Itasca: F.E. Peacock Publishers Inc.

Gordon, M. & Michaels, E. (2001). *The encyclopedia of health and aging: A complete guide to health and well-being in your later years*. Toronto: Key Porter Books Ltd.

Gottlieb, B.H. & Johnson, J. (2000). Respite programs for caregivers of persons with dementia: A review with practice implications. *Aging & Mental Health 2000*, 4(2), 119–129.

Government of Ontario. (2003). *A Guide to Programs and Services for Seniors in Ontario*. (2003). Toronto: Government of Ontario.

Marcell, J. (2002, March). Helping families get loved ones to daycare. *Contemporary Long-Term Care*.

Miller, B. (1989). Adult children's perceptions of caregiver stress and satisfaction. *Journal of Applied Gerontology*, 8(3).

Miller, I., & Solomon, R. (1980). Development of group services for the elderly. *Journal of Gerontological Social Work*, 2(3), 241–257.

Monahan, D. (1993). Utilization of dementia-specific respite day care for clients and their caregivers in a social model program. *Journal of Gerontological Social Work*, 20(3/4).

National Institute on Adult Daycare. (1990). *Standards and guidelines for adult day care*. Washington: National Council on the Aging.

Schwartz, P. & Weisman, C.B. (1989). Worker expectations in group work with the frail elderly: Modifying the models for a better fit. *Social Work with Groups*, 12(3), 47–55.

Schwartz, W. & Zalba, S. (eds.). *The practice of group work*. New York: Columbia University Press.

Weissert, W.G. (1989). Models of adult day care: Findings from a national survey. *Gerontologist*, 29(5), 640–649.

Wood, J.B. (1989). Emergence of adult day care centers as post-acute care agencies. *Journal of Aging and Health*, 1(4), 521–539.

Wood, J. (1989). The emergence of adult day centers as post-acute care agencies. *Journal of Aging and Health*, 1(4).

Internet Resources

A Respite Resource for Caregiving Adult Day-care Programs
    http://www.bigtreemurphy.com
Adult Day Care
    http://www.gwbweb.wustl.edu/users/gfi/adc.html
Adult Day Care Programs
    http://www.pmhs.org/crs/sha/sha/adaycare.htm
National Respite Network and Resource Centre
    Adult Day Care: One form of Respite for Older Adults
    http://www.archrespite.org/archfs54.htm

Additional Readings

Gallagher, B.J., III (2002). *The sociology of mental illness,* 4th ed. Upper Saddle
    River: Practice-Hall Inc.
Haber, D. (2003). *Health promotion and aging: practical application for health
    professionals,* 3rd ed. New York: Springer.
Hooyman, N. & Nourjah, P. (1999). *Social gerontology,* 5th ed. Boston: Allyn &
    Bacon.
Thorson, J. (2000). *Aging in a changing society.* New York: Taylor & Francis.
Wilson, R. et al. (2002). Participation in cognitively stimulating activities and
    risk and incident of Alzheimer's disease. *Journal of the American Medical
    Association,* 287, 742–748.

CHAPTER 19

SOCIAL WORK PRACTICE WITH FAMILY CAREGIVERS OF FRAIL OLDER PERSONS

RONALD W. TOSELAND, TAMARA L. SMITH,

AND MICHELE ZINOMAN

This chapter begins with a review of the major issues and concerns facing family caregivers of frail older persons. Described next are generic social work roles and responsibilities, as well as consultation, coordination, and management, three specific social work roles that are commonly used in work with family caregivers and frail older persons. Opportunities for social workers in outreach, supervision, coordination, and delivery of services, particularly as they relate to the needs of underserved family caregivers, are also described. The chapter ends with three case examples illustrating the three previously discussed social work practice roles.

I.   Introduction

Family caregivers play a vital role in maintaining the health and independence of frail older persons. It has been estimated, for example, that the national economic value of informal family caregiving is almost 200 billion dollars per year, which is about 18 percent of total national health care spending (Arno et al., 1999). National surveys indicate that one in four households in the United States have spent some time in the previous 12-month period providing care for a frail older person (National Alliance for Caregiving & AARP, 1997; MetLife, 1997), and caregivers spend an average of about eight years in the caregiving role (MetLife, 1999). The role that family caregivers play in helping to maintain frail older persons in community settings will become even more important as the percentage of the population that are elderly increases in the next several decades (Coleman & Pandya, 2000; McCallion et al., 2001).

II.   The Clientele

Close family members, particularly spouses and adult daughters, are the most likely to assist frail elderly with physical and emotional needs. Shanas (1968) suggested that the decision about who will provide care follows a "principle of substitution." If a spouse is available, he or she is most likely to provide care. If a spouse is unavailable, an adult daughter is most likely to become the primary caregiver. In the absence of adult daughters, daughter-in-laws, sons, son-in-laws or other relatives, neighbours, or friends are most likely to provide care.

The Family Caregiver Alliance (2001) has provided helpful data about family caregivers. Approximately 22.4 million households (1/4 of households in the US) provide care to persons over the age of 50. Most of these caregivers (75 percent) are female and their average age is 46 (National Alliance for Caregiving & AARP, 1997). The relationship between caregivers and care recipients is most likely to be familial. Spouses account for 23.4 percent of all caregivers to older persons, and adult children provide 41.3 percent of the care (Spector et al., 2000). Ethnic differences exist in rates of caregiving. Whereas 24 percent of Whites aged 18 and over provide care for someone 50 years or older, 29 percent of African Americans, 27 percent of Hispanics, and 32 percent of Asian Americans are caregivers (National Alliance for Caregiving & AARP, 1997). Most caregivers are engaged in paid employment. Over half are employed full-time, and two-thirds are employed full-time or part-time (National Alliance for Caregiving & AARP, 1997). Caregiving for the elderly is an intensive task: the average caregiver spends 20 hours per week caring for individuals over the age of 65 (Health and Human Services, 1998). The role of being a caregiver is all encompassing, and often produces anxiety, mental stress, and poor health for caregivers.

A.   The Effects of Caregiving

The impact of caregiving has both positive and negative aspects. Practitioners should recognize that even though caregiving is often demanding and stressful, it is frequently perceived as a rewarding experience. Rewards of caregiving include: (1) feeling useful, needed, and engaged in a meaningful role that really makes a difference in the life of the care recipient; (2) feeling a sense of accomplishment and competence because one is better able than anyone else to manage complex caregiving tasks and to provide high-quality care in difficult caregiving situations; (3) having the opportunity to express feelings of empathy, intimacy, and love to the care recipient; (4) experiencing satisfaction that one has fulfilled one's responsibility and paid the care recipient back for all that he or she has done for the caregiver in the past; (5) feeling appreciated by family members and friends for all that one has done for the care recipient; and (6) self-respect and altruistic feelings that one has done all that one can for the care recipient without being asked (Bass, 1990; Bengtson et al., 1990; Aneschel et al., 1996). The entire family can also experience rewards, including feeling secure in a strong kinship system, learning more about aging and late life development, attaining a better understanding of each other's needs, and gaining greater tolerance for other people's problems (Bass, 1990; Beach, 1997).

Although caregivers may not experience all of these rewards, or they may complain that they do not get the credit they deserve from the care recipient or from family members and friends, it is important for practitioners to encourage caregivers, and to acknowledge, recognize, and articulate the important role that they play in the lives of their frail loved ones. Finding meaning and reward in the caregiving situation has been shown to be associated with reduced perceptions of burden and stress and with better health outcomes (Kramer, 1997; Noonan & Tennstedt, 1997). Therefore, recognizing the important role that caregivers play can help them to cope more effectively with the demands of caregiving.

Despite the rewards of caregiving, education, support, and training programs are important because a great deal of evidence has accumulated over the past 20 years indicating that caregiving can have a negative impact on the health and well-being of the caregiver. Physical problems such as exhaustion and fatigue result from providing constant and seemingly never-ending attention to the care recipient's needs. These problems may also be exacerbated by the caregiver's own health problems. Physical exhaustion and deteriorating caregiver health often contribute to the development of psychological problems such as depression and anxiety.

Social isolation may occur because the long duration of many chronic illnesses and disabilities can lead to a restriction of caregivers' contacts with friends, neighbours, and other social contacts in the community. The revival or exacerbation of sibling or parental conflicts, and the frustrations and misunderstandings endemic to providing care for someone on a 24-hour on-call basis can also lead to interpersonal conflict with the care recipient and with other family members. Caregivers can become stressed by such tasks as: (1) maintaining family communication and the exchange of information; (2) balancing the needs of the care recipient with the needs of other family members; (3) managing feelings toward family members who do not help; (4) maintaining the family as an effective decision-making group over the long term; and (5) asking for help from other family members when necessary.

Caregiving can also place families at risk financially. Medical, pharmaceutical, therapeutic, and equipment costs are often not covered by insurance, or only partially covered. An increased use of utilities (e.g., washer and dryer due to incontinence), special diets, and clothing, etc., can place household budgets in jeopardy. At the same time, caregiving frequently results in reduced employment or unemployment, thus making it especially difficult to meet the increased expenses of caregiving (MetLife, 1999; MetLife, 1997; National Alliance for Caregiving & AARP, 1997; Cafferata et al., 1987).

Emotional health is the one aspect of primary caregivers' lives that is most affected by caring for a frail elderly family member. Some of the problems that family caregivers find especially difficult to cope with emotionally include: (1) loss of control over one's time; (2) constant demands to do things for care recipients or for the household that care recipients could previously do for themselves; (3) guilt about whether one is doing all that is possible for the care receiver or other family members or about negative feelings that one might have; (4) loss of privacy; (5) grief over the care receiver's decline; (6) feelings of anger about the care receiver's behaviour or physical disabilities, and about unfulfilled relationship expectations during the retirement years. As compared to the general population, primary caregivers are frequently more depressed and anxious, are more likely to use psychotropic medications, and have more symptoms of psychological distress (see, for reviews, Neundorfer, 1991; Schulz, 2000; Bookwala et al., 1995; Schulz & Williamson, 1994). Among all of the adverse emotional outcomes that are possible, depression represents the greatest risk. It has been estimated that between 20 to 50 percent of caregivers report depressive disorders or symptoms (Bookwala et al., 1995; Schulz, 2000).

Practitioners should pay particular attention to the emotional health of caregivers of persons with dementia and stroke because they are at the highest risk for depression. These caregivers have to adjust to cognitive and behavioural symptoms as well as the physical impairments of the care recipient, which can increase anxiety and depression. At the same time, those in the aging network should also be aware that much of the research on caregivers' emotional health does not adequately account for the great diversity of the resilience and other personal characteristics of caregivers and the nature and severity of the care recipients' disability (Bloch et al., 1997; Quittner & Schulz, 1998). Because the vast majority of researchers have focused on caregivers of persons with Alzheimer's disease and other dementias, less is known about the emotional impact of caregiving for those with other disorders such as heart disease or cancer. Still, given the available evidence, it is important for practitioners to assess all caregivers for symptoms of depression and anxiety.

The risks of family caregiving extend well beyond the primary caregiver to encompass the entire family system. Strawbridge and Wallhagan (1991), for example, reported that as many as 40 percent of the caregiving families they surveyed had experienced family conflict. Strain on the entire family system may result from such issues as conflict between caregiving obligations and other family tasks, disagreements among family members about the form or amount of caregiving, readjustments in family roles, the emotional impact of caregiving on all involved family members, and feelings of family stigma (Bass, 1990; Bengtson et al., 1990). Families with the greatest risk for negative outcomes are those having poor communication skills, limited resources, many demands on their time and resources, suppressed or open conflicts, poor parent-child relationships, and high resistance to change (see McCallion et al., 2001 for a more complete discussion of the impact of caregiving on the family system). It is important for practitioners, therefore, to assess family functioning, and to encourage family meetings where all those in primary and secondary caregiving roles have a chance to express their feelings about the best care practices for their situation. Family meetings provide and important opportunity to reduce conflict and to develop coordinated care plans among formal and informal caregivers.

III. Practice Roles and Responsibilities

Social work practice roles and responsibilities with caregivers are similar to those engaged in with other client groups. For example, social workers establish therapeutic relationships, assess needs, and plan, implement, and monitor intervention plans as they would with other client groups (McInnis-Dittrich, 2002; McCallion et al., 2001). However, specific adaptations in these roles and responsibilities are needed when serving caregivers.

A. *Engaging the client*

Making initial contact with caregivers is sometimes difficult. Caregivers are often reluctant to ask for help. Some believe it is their responsibility to provide care and that relinquishing that responsibility would be like abandoning the person for whom they are caring. This is particularly true in certain ethnic groups where family bonds are strong and normative expectations prescribe family caregiving as a duty. Caregivers may never have had to ask for help before and pride may become an obstacle. In other situations, it is the frail older person who resists or refuses "outside help."

For all these reasons, it is important for social workers to engage in active outreach efforts that make information about services and resources for family caregivers available throughout the community. In-person telephone contacts with health, social service, religious, and civic organizations; press releases; newspaper stories; appearances on talk shows; public service announcements on radio and television; and educational forums and workshops sponsored by community planning agencies are all useful ways to reach out to caregivers (Corcoran et al., 2003; Jones et al., 2003).

Social workers must be particularly careful in designing outreach strategies for particular groups of caregivers. For example, black and Hispanic caregivers rarely respond to traditional avenues of publicity used in recruiting participants (Aranda et al., 2003; Biegel & Song, 1995). Extensive personal contacts through established and trusted religious and service organizations in the community are a much better approach to engaging this client group (Aranda et al., 2003; Coogle, 2002).

Male caregivers are also difficult to reach. Studies indicate that that even though men from a larger caregiver program request smaller, male-only support groups, these men were only willing to participate when they were told that the group was part of a pilot program to test a new intervention. They were unwilling to join the group for the sole purpose of gaining help for themselves as caregivers (Kaye, 2002; McFarland & Sanders, 2000).

B. Establishing a Relationship

Once initial contact has been made, the primary job of the social worker is to develop a trusting and supportive relationship with the caregiver. Research suggests that many caregivers are reluctant to admit to difficulties with caregiving, even though they may be nearly overwhelmed by them (Bauer et al., 2001). We have interviewed caregivers who break down and cry during interviews and say they have not slept well in weeks. Yet when asked about their stress levels, these same caregivers say they experience "a little" stress. Many caregivers would rather bear their burdens in silence than risk being seen as complaining or uncaring. To make it possible for caregivers to acknowledge and accept their thoughts and feelings about the caregiving situation, social workers should be attentive and empathic listeners.

Caregivers have a strong tendency to believe that those who have never been in their situation cannot possibly understand what they are going through. If the worker has had direct experience with caregiving, appropriately timed self-disclosures can be helpful for universalizing the experience and for increasing trust and promoting client self-disclosure.

In addition to providing an opportunity for ventilation, the worker should be a supporter and an enabler. As a supporter, the worker provides encouragement and validation. Many caregivers are unnecessarily critical of themselves. They believe that they are not doing all they could do in the caregiving role. They also tend not to take as good care of themselves as they could, foregoing their own needs for those of the care receiver and other family members. As a supporter, the worker applauds any indication that the caregiver is taking better care of herself or feeling better about how well she is providing care. The worker also validates and elucidates more fully the caregiver's experiences so that the caregiver can better accept negative feelings such as anger or frustration with the care receiver.

As an enabler, the worker encourages change by helping the caregiver to become motivated to mobilize social resources to improve a problematic situation. To function effectively as an enabler, the worker must be aware of available community services that caregivers and care receivers are likely to need. The worker should also be aware of eligibility requirements and other difficulties in accessing services. The worker may help a client complete necessary paperwork to obtain services or go to an agency with the client to provide support and assistance during the application process. In some situations, the worker may also act as an advocate for the client, helping her to obtain services that are not readily available.

C. Assessing the Situation

As the caregiver discloses information about herself and her situation, the worker assesses her needs. Assessment of the caregiving situation includes not only understanding the caregiver and the care receiver but also their relationship to each other, to other family members, and to the larger society. Ideally, social work assessments should include a thorough examination of the current physical, psychological, emotional, social, financial, and environmental status of the caregiver and the care receiver and their life situation. Any pertinent historical data bearing on the current situation should also be ascertained (Kuerbis & Levine, 2003).

In many health care settings, it is important for social workers to coordinate their assessments with allied health personnel. For example, important information about the course of a specific illness, the effects of medications, and the physical limitations and abilities of the care receiver may be provided by doctors, nurses, and physical therapists. For this reason, comprehensive assessments of the caregiving situation are sometimes best made by a health care team.

As team members, social workers may be expected to focus their assessment on certain dimensions of the caregiver or care receiver functioning. For example, the social worker may be the member of a team who is responsible for gathering pertinent data about the caregiver's social support networks. To gather such data, the social worker might inquire about the individuals who comprise the caregiver's support network and the quality of existing relationships with these individuals. The social worker might also assess the extent to which the caregiver is satisfied with existing informal social supports and whether the caregiver is motivated to reach out for additional support. The social worker uses this information, with information obtained from other team members, in the development of a comprehensive assessment of a caregiver's situation.

D. Developing an Action Plan

Based on the needs and desires of the caregiver and the care receiver, an intervention plan is developed. A major decision in developing an action plan is what mode of intervention would be most beneficial. For caregivers with very high levels of psychological stress, those with very personal issues, or those who are not ready to share their experiences with a group, individual counselling may be most appropriate. In contrast, family or couple counselling may be most appropriate in situations where interpersonal tensions and conflicts predominate (McCallion et al., 2001). Recent research indicates that support groups may be particularly useful for reducing feelings of loneliness and isolation and for increasing social support (Bergeron & Gray, 2003; Kaye, 2002). Participation in a support group helps caregivers to feel understood and supported by others in similar situations.

Another important decision when developing an action plan is determining the most appropriate role to take in a particular situation. A social worker may play three primary roles: consultant, coordinator, and manager. Each of these roles requires different actions and responsibilities on the part of the caregiver and the worker, which are summarized in Table 19.1.

Table 19.1 was developed to distinguish and highlight the differences in the three roles. In actual practice, in many health care settings social workers are expected to move comfortably from one role to another depending on the changing needs and evolving health status. At one point in time, the worker may act as a consultant. Later, the worker may act as a manager. With some family caregivers, the social worker may actually play different roles with the same person. For a particular concern, a family caregiver may need only consultation to be able to cope with or resolve a problem. However, for another concern, the caregiver may need the social worker to act as a coordinator.

E. Consultant Role

The social worker should consider adopting the consultant role in situations where the caregiver is an independent, responsible, dedicated person who: (1) prefers to take primary responsibility for the care receiver's needs without deferring to outside help; (2) is coping effectively; and (3) has been assessed by the social worker as in need of relatively little assistance. When deciding on whether the consultant

Table 19.1: Social Worker Roles and Responsibilities When Working with Family Caregivers

Selected Decision Criteria	Consultation	Coordination	Management
Type of caregiver	An independent, responsible, dedicated, informed caregiver with time, energy, and competence to cope with the situation and to meet the care receiver's needs	A competent caregiver seeking assistance because she is becoming overwhelmed with duties and responsibilities and needs help on a regular basis	Unable to fulfill many caregiving duties, e.g., caregiver is out of town and unable to take care of many of the day-to-day needs of the care receiver
Need for outreach	Greatest	Intermediate	Least
Responsibility for care	Primarily with caregiver	Shared between caregiver and social worker	Primarily with social worker
Assessment	Caregiver plays a major role by providing information about the care receiver's condition	Social worker and caregiver jointly assess situation	Social worker plays a major role in determining accuracy of information
Development of action plan	Caregiver in consultation with social worker	Social worker in consultation and collaboration with the caregiver	Social worker responsibility in consultation with caregiver and care receiver

con't

Table 19.1 (continued)

Implementation of action plan	Social worker maintains occasional contact on an "as needed" basis	Social worker providers some services and helps caregiver and care receiver to utilize other community services as needed	Social worker delivers or arranges for the delivery of services to the care receiver
Monitoring action plan	Caregiver monitors situation and requests support, information, and help gaining access to services as needed	Caregiver monitors care plan day to day, social worker maintains regular contact monitoring situation and the delivery of services	Social worker monitors day-to-day situation of care receiver, coordinates services, and arranges for services as needed

role is most appropriate, the social worker assesses caregiver capacities and abilities, as well as his or her current level of functioning. The social worker should also assess the client's willingness to ask for help when needed. Because of heavy caseloads, social workers may not be able to contact the client very frequently Therefore, before assuming a consultant role, social workers should assess whether or not they can rely or the client to acknowledge a need and request appropriate help.

The worker must also consider the ethical issue involved in deciding whether to adopt the consultant role or a more active role. Ethical issues often arise when, in the worker's judgment, clients could benefit from more help than they think they need. A general practice principle that applies in this situation is that unless caregivers or care receivers are in jeopardy of endangering themselves or some other third party, the client's request for autonomy should be respected. The worker should also guard against adopting a consultant role because of caseload considerations.

Because caregivers who are independent and competent feel the least need for assistance, active outreach is often needed to inform them about community resources and services that may be helpful to them in their current situation or in the future. But no matter how this group of caregivers comes into contact with social workers, Table 19.1 clearly indicates that the responsibility for providing care and ensuring the well-being of the care receiver remains primarily with the caregiver.

When social workers adopt a consultant role, the caregiver is expected to play a major role in the assessment process. The worker recognizes that the caregiver is intimately familiar with the situation and can provide information about the care receiver's functioning in a variety of areas. Because caregivers in this category are responsible and competent, they are relatively reliable and accurate sources of information on which the social worker heavily depends.

As a consultant, the social worker may be asked to help the caregiver and the care receiver with a wide variety of environmental, social, behavioural, and emotional problems. Research indicates that some of the more frequent are helping with: (1) the nursing home placement decisions; (2) adjustments in living status such as when a frail older person moves from her own home to her daughter's home; (3) behavioural and emotional problems; (4) resistance to some aspect of what the caregiver believes is in the best interest of the care receiver; (5) alcoholism; and (6) mental impairments such as Alzheimer's disease (Ferry & O'Toole, 2002; Jess & Klein, 2002).

When developing and implementing action plans, social workers who are acting as consultants rely heavily on caregivers' input. For example, a caregiver requests information about a day care centre that the worker had mentioned during a previous contact. When the worker provides the information, the caregiver indicates that she will contact the centre and enroll her mother. As consultant, the social worker supports the caregiver and informs her that she is available should any obstacles be encountered when attempting to obtain the service.

Social workers may adopt a consulting role following a period of more active intervention. In the consultant role, social workers sometimes maintain occasional contact to assure that the situation remains stable, to offer information and advice, or to help the caregiver connect with needed services. At other times, workers respond on an "as needed" basis with information, advice, and other help that is requested by the caregiver.

F. Coordinator Role

Because of the care receiver's situation or the caregiver's ability or willingness, more assistance may be needed than can be provided by a consultant. Some caregivers have provided care for many years without the need for the assistance of a coordinator, but then become overwhelmed by their duties and responsibilities. The care receiver's physical or mental condition may deteriorate or the caregiver's abilities may become diminished by health problems or increased responsibilities at work or at home. For caregivers who are overburdened and finding it difficult to cope with increasing stress, the social worker should consider adopting the role of coordinator.

Table 19.1 indicates that outreach efforts can be a little less active with this group of caregivers than with those who can benefit from consultant services only. Stress resulting from feeling overburdened is more likely to motivate caregivers in this group to seek services for the care receiver or for themselves. Another reason why outreach does not have to be as active with this group of caregivers is that they are more likely to be receiving services, and referrals from health care and social service providers are likely to be more frequent.

In the coordinator role, the worker and the caregiver share responsibility for ensuring that the care receiver is receiving needed services in a well-planned fashion. In assessing the situation, social workers should gather as much data from the caregiver as possible. However, they are more likely when acting as a consultant to make independent assessments of caregivers' and care receivers' abilities.

In the coordinator role, the social worker may provide needed services such as individual, family, or group counselling. For example, the worker might provide brief family counselling to reduce conflicts about caregiving responsibilities in the family and to develop a more complete and coordinated plan of care.

The social worker helps to arrange for whatever services the caregiver needs by being an enabler, a broker, or an advocate. The worker also helps the caregiver to arrange for services for the care receiver. This might include helping the caregiver to develop a written schedule of informal and formal services (Scott & Van Gerpen, 1997). Such a schedule could be posted on a refrigerator or a bulletin board so that appointments for different services will not be confused or improperly scheduled.

Once the services for the caregiver and the care receiver are in place, the worker generally maintains regular contact with the caregiver. However, the caregiver continues to take the day-to-day responsibility for the functioning of the care receiver and for the appropriate provision of services. As coordinator, the worker makes sure that any difficulties the caregiver is having in fulfilling these responsibilities are resolved during their regular meetings.

Because the caregivers and care receivers with whom a worker might function as a coordinator differ greatly in their levels of stress, capabilities, and needs, it is important for the worker to consider each caregiver's short- and long-term needs. For example, if the caregiver is an older person who has chronic health problems, the worker might need to maintain more frequent contact than with a caregiver in better health.

G.   *Management Role*

The management role is differentiated from the coordinator and the consultant role by the degree to which the caregiver is involved in the plan of care for the care receiver and in the implementation and monitoring of that plan. When caregivers are unable to fulfill duties and responsibilities necessary for the care of frail older persons in their family, social workers who are managers ensure that proper care is provided.

As Table 19.1 indicates, there is frequently less need for outreach with this kind of caregiver and care receiver because many are already in contact with health and social services for chronic health problem before their need for management arises. In other situations, acute medical problems bring older persons who are unable to care for themselves into contact with medical social workers.

In the management role, the worker takes primary responsibility for helping the care receiver live independently in the community. After gathering information from the caregiver and the care receiver, the worker makes independent assessments of the condition of the caregiver and the care receiver and determines what services, if any, are needed. To whatever extent possible, the practitioner involves the caregiver and care receiver in the development and implementation of the action plan. The social worker then either provides the needed services or obtains whatever services are needed and sees to it that these services are administered in a timely, efficient and effective manner.

As a manager, the social worker is expected to: (1) develop a comprehensive assessment of the client without relying solely on the judgments of a family member who may not be able to fully provide what the care receiver needs; (2) develop a comprehensive plan for the care of the frail older person whose needs cannot be fully provided for by a care receiver; (3) implement the plan by providing and coordinating health and social services to meet the needs of the caregiver and the care receiver; and (4) monitor the situation to ensure that the caregiver and the care receiver are receiving services that are appropriate (Capitman, 2003; Scott & Van Gerpen, 1997).

In the management role, workers maintain frequent and regular contact with care receivers to make sure their needs are being met. Continuous monitoring is important because, unlike in the coordinator or consultant role, the manager can't rely on a family caregiver to monitor the day-to-day situation or to take appropriate action should problems arise in the delivery of services. As manager, the worker either provides all needed services for the care receiver or ensures that they are being provided by informal caregivers or by professional health care and social service providers.

IV. Potential for Role Development

There is great potential for the development of social work with family caregivers, particularly in the following areas: (1) home health care, (2) collaborative work with peer helpers, (3) outreach, and (4) the development and management of caregiver-support programs.

The anticipated increase in the elderly population, particularly the old-old, in the next 40 years, means that there will be a greater need for home care services in the future. Social work services are an important component of comprehensive home care. Therefore, as the population ages, the social work role in home health care should increase dramatically, unless social work services are performed by other professional helpers. This is a real possibility as nurses and psychologists trained in community work are now performing many of the tasks traditionally considered to be a part of the social work domain.

Working with peer helpers is a second expanding area for social workers. There are thousands of self-help support groups for caregivers sponsored by organizations such as the Alzheimer's Disease and Related Disorders Association. Working with peer helpers requires a relationship that is based on mutual respect. Social workers can build such relationships by reaching out to peer helpers and developing a relationship with them. Ideally, these relationship should be based upon social workers' appreciation of the experience that peers can bring to the situation, the therapeutic benefit of self-help efforts for both the person giving help and the person receiving help, and a respect for the autonomy of peer helpers.

There is also a need for innovative outreach and culturally sensitive intervention programs in minority ethnic communities. Cultural differences may influence how minority caregivers respond to efforts to inform them about services and also how they respond to intervention efforts (Aranda et al., 2003; Connell & Janevic, 2001; Biegel & Song, 1995). Therefore, development of appropriate, culturally sensitive outreach and intervention programs is an important, albeit neglected, role for social workers.

Fourth, there is an expanding role for social workers in the development and management of caregiver programs. In future years, there will be an increasing recognition of the importance of family caregiver to the welfare of frail older persons. With this recognition, social workers will be called upon to develop and implement programs of support to assist caregivers. This, in turn, will require social workers to be familiar with the array of administrative, supervisory, and direct service skills that are necessary to develop and manage a social service program.

V.   Concluding Remarks

The typology of social work roles outlined in Table 19.1, and described in this chapter, is intended as a heuristic device to elucidate the range of social work practice roles in health care settings with caregiver; of frail older persons. In actual practice, the roles may not be so clearly differentiated. The changing needs of caregivers and care receivers, the availability and receptivity of different referral sources, the degree of emotional burden experienced by caregivers in relation to specific caregiving tasks and responsibilities, and a host of other factors often necessitate the use of a mix of roles and practice strategies in a particular situation. Still, the typology that has been presented should serve as a useful guide for social work practitioners deciding on the most appropriate mix of roles and strategies to employ in the caregiving situations they confront in many health care practice settings.

Case Example

Social Worker as Consultant
Marie, at 43, is energetic, capable, well educated, and in excellent health. She works as a freelance artist and has a self-defined work schedule.

Her husband, Earl, owns a small business and his responsibilities allow him to take time off from work when necessary. Since he works only five minutes from home, he is able to respond to emergencies that may arise at home.

Marie's mother, Theresa, aged 83, had lived at Marie's brother's house for seven years. While visiting Marie during her son's annual winter Florida vacation, Theresa experienced stomach pains and was taken to the nearby hospital where she was diagnosed as having cancer. Following an operation, which was not able to remove all of the cancer, she moved to Marie's home to be closer to the hospital and to the rest of her family. The immediate family was highly supportive. Marie's older brother and sister lived approximately one half hour away. Each volunteered to provide respite for Marie and Earl, and each visited with Theresa at least one or two half-days per week while she was in the hospital.

Prior to discharge, the hospital social worker talked with Marie, Theresa, and others about Theresa's situation. Marie's brother agreed to look after the paperwork, which Theresa had difficulty doing, regarding medical insurance and hospital bills. Marie agreed to have her mother continue to live with her, but enquired about a service to "look in on Theresa" should she suddenly take a turn for the worse.

With the hospital social worker's help, Marie made some phone calls and arranged for services from a local hospice program. After contacting the hospital social worker and receiving a formal referral, the hospice team initiated regular contact with Theresa. The hospice program continued to provide service to Theresa, who remained mentally alert and able to ambulate with the assistance of a cane until she died at home six months later.

Social Worker as Coordinator
Julie is an 82-year-old black woman who is in poor health. Her husband, Jim, has advanced heart disease, diabetes, hearing loss, and severe arthritis. The latter problem worries Julie, who fears that Jim will try to move about when she is not home, will fall down, and hurt himself. Julie has always taken care of Jim and would not consider placing him. Their only child died five years ago in an automobile accident and there are no other immediate family members who live close enough to provide care for Jim. However, Julie has a close friend, Ann, who sometimes watches Jim and is a source of emotional support.

Julie was brought to the social worker's attention by Ann. When Julie refused to go to the community senior centre for their weekly card game, Ann went anyway. She mentioned that Julie seemed as if she was having an increasingly difficult time caring for Jim to a social worker who worked for an affiliated community health centre, which was located directly across the street. The worker contacted Julie, who said she was not feeling well and didn't think she had the strength to leave the house. However, because she knew the worker from previous visits to the centre, she agreed to a home visit. During several home visits over the course of a month, the worker concluded that Julie could use some help in caring for Jim. Julie reluctantly agreed to some help as long as she could remain in charge of Jim's care.

In assessing the situation, the worker determined that Jim's increasing deafness was an important problem. The worker consulted a non-profit agency for the deaf and through them arranged for Julie and Jim to acquire a telephone amplifier, a device to allow them to see captioning on television and a light hook-up on the doorbell so that Jim could see that someone was at the door when Julie was not at home.

The couple's financial situation was also problematic. Recently, they had incurred non-reimbursable medical expenses, which their pension and social security checks did not cover adequately. Accepting any financial assistance was difficult for Julie, who had been brought up to believe that a person should avoid being "on welfare" at all costs. The worker explained to Julie that the taxes she had paid over the years entitled her to financial assistance now that she needed it. With the worker's help, Julie was able to reframe her situation and realize that to refuse assistance might result in a deterioration of her own health condition or that of her husband's. This, in turn, might cost society even more money in the long term. Therefore, she reluctantly decided to accept the worker's assistance and applied for food stamps and Meals-on-Wheels.

Convincing Julie to get out of the house and remain active was another issue that needed to be addressed. Julie's main concern was that Jim would fall down and hurt himself while she was out. The social worker recommended that Julie enroll in Lifeline, a program sponsored by a local hospital. They fitted Jim with a special device that hung around his neck and connected to the telephone so that he could signal for help at any time.

Julie was also somewhat depressed about her situation. The worker, concluding that Julie was suffering from a mild reactive depression, helped Julie and her friend Ann, who was also a caregiver, to enroll in a support group program for caregivers sponsored by a nearby family service agency. These sessions, and the other services that were arranged, proved to be very helpful, and soon Julie began going to the senior centre again. The social worker continued to monitor the situation by meeting with Julie at the senior centre on a regular basis, but provided no other active support for the three years she remained working for the agency.

Social Worker as Manager

Mary, aged 79, began living independently again after 32 years of hospitalization with a DSM-5 diagnosis of bipolar disorder, depressed. In the early 1970s she was given a trial of lithium, which stabilized her mood swings.

Sarah, Mary's social worker from a social health maintenance organization (SHMO), first met Mary while she was an in-patient. Together with the discharge planning team in the hospital, a small one-bedroom apartment was located for Mary with a landlord who had previously rented to former psychiatric patients and was tolerant, if not sympathetic, to their plight.

Sarah helped Mary to contact her niece, Gwen, who lived about a mile away and who had not seen Mary in about 13 years. Gwen offered to assist Mary in any way possible, although it was clear that Gwen, who worked part-time and had her own family, would not be able to provide a great deal of assistance.

Sarah helped Mary to pay bills and deal with other paperwork, which Mary was not familiar with because she had lived so long as an in-patient. Gradually, Mary learned to handle most other own affairs, except for complicated paperwork that she sometimes encountered when applying for or receiving health and social services.

Sarah encouraged Mary to enroll in a seniors-only day treatment program at the health centre. She also helped to arrange for transportation to and from the program. This arrangement worked quite well.

Mary did not experience any difficulty until about 18 months after leaving the hospital. She stopped taking her lithium and soon became quite depressed. Sarah, who had continued to see Mary on a monthly basis after setting up the day treatment program, went to see Mary in the hospital and arranged a plan with Mary and Gwen to keep Mary's apartment for one month until she could be stabilized and returned to the community.

Once Mary returned home, Gwen agreed to monitor Mary's medication. Every other day Gwen stopped by to see Mary. She watched while Mary took her medication and she checked on the remaining pills to make sure that Mary was taking the correct dosage when she was not present.

Sarah arranged for Mary to have more frequent checkups to monitor her lithium blood level. She also arranged for Mary to attend the day treatment program again. As Mary's needs change, with Gwen's help, Sarah will continue to help Mary live independently.

References

Aneschel, F., Mullan, J., Pearlin, L., & Whitlach, C. (1996). Caregiving and its social support. In R.H. Binstock and L.K. George (eds.), *Handbook of aging and the social sciences*, 4ᵗʰ ed., pp. 283–302. New York: Academic Press.

Aranda, M., Ramirez, R., Ranney, M., Trejo, L., & Villa, V. (2003). El Portal Latino Alzheimer's project: Model program for Latino caregivers of Alzheimer's disease-affected people. *Social Work*, 48(2), 259–272.

Arno, P., Levine, C., & Memmott, M. (1999). The economic value of informal caregiving. *Health Affairs*, 18(2), 182–188.

Bass, D.S. (1990). *Caring families: Supports and intervention.* Silver Spring: NASW Press.

Bauer, M., Burns, T., Kirk, L., Kuskowski, M., & Maddox, M. (2001). Progressive dementia: Personal and relational impact on caregiving wives. *American Journal of Alzheimer's Disease and Other Dementias*, 16(6), 329–334.

Beach, D. (1997). Family caregiving: The positive impact on adolescent relationships. *The Gerontologist*, 37, 233–238.

Bengtson, V., Blum, M., & Gatz, M. (1990). Caregiving families. In J.E. Birren & K.W. Schaie (eds.), *Handbook of the psychology of aging*, 3ʳᵈ ed., pp. 404–426. San Diego: Academic Press.

Bergeron, L. & Gray, B. (2003). Ethical dilemmas of reporting suspected elder abuse. *Social Work*, 48(1), 96–105.

Biegel, D. & Song, L. (1995). Facilitators and barriers to caregiver support group participation. *Journal of Case Management*, 4(4), 164–172.

Bloch, S., Herman, H.E., Murphy, B., Schofield, H.L., & Singh, B. (1997). Family caregiving: Measurement of emotional well-being and various aspects of the caregiving role. *Psychological Medicine*, 27, 647–657.

Bookwala, J., Fleissner, K., O'Brien, A., & Schulz, R. (1995). Psychiatric and physical morbidity effects of dementia caregiving: Prevalence, correlates, and causes. *The Gerontologist*, 35, 771–791.

Cafferata, G.S., Sangl, J., & Stone, R. (1987). Caregivers of the frail elderly: A national profile. *Clinical Gerontologist*, 1(1), 87–95.

Capitman, J. (2003). Effective coordination of medical and supportive services. *Journal of Aging and Health*, 15(1), 124–164.

Carter, G.W., & Steinberg, R.M. (1983). *Case management and the elderly*. Lexington: D.C. Heath.

Coleman, B., & Pandya, S. (2000). *Caregiving and long-term care*, Fact Sheet #82. Washington: Public Policy Institute.

Connell, C. & Janevic, M. (2001). Racial, ethnic, and cultural differences in the dementia caregiving experience: Recent findings. *Gerontologist*, 41(3), 334–347.

Coogle, C. (2002). The families who care project: Meeting the educational needs of African American and rural family caregivers dealing with dementia. *Educational Gerontology*, 28, 59–71.

Corcoran, M., Dennis, M., Gitlin, L., Hauck, W., Schinfeld, S., & Winter, L. (2003). Effects of the home environmental skill-building program on the caregiver-care recipient dyad: 6-month outcomes from the Philadelphia REACH initiative. *Gerontologist*, 43(4), 532–546.

Family Caregiver Alliance. (2001). *Fact sheet: Selected caregiver statistics* (no page numbers). Retrieved September 11, 2003, from http://www.caregiver.org/factsheets/selected_caregiver_statistics.html

Ferry, J. & O'Toole, R. (2002). Geriatric care managers: A collaborative resource to the physician practice. *Journal of Medical Practice Management*, 18(3), 129–132.

Health and Human Services. (1998, June). *Informal caregiving: Compassion in action*. Washington: Department of Health and Human Services.

Jess, C. & Klein, W. (2002). One last pleasure? Alcohol use among elderly people in nursing homes. *Health & Social Work*, 27(3), 193–201.

Jones, R., Mahoney, D., & Tarlow, B. (2003). Effects of an automated telephone support system on caregiver burden and anxiety: Findings from the REACH for TLC study. *Gerontologist*, 43(4), 556–567.

Kaye, L. (2002). Service utilization and support provision of caregiving men. In B. Kramer & E. Thompson (eds.), *Men as caregivers: Theory, research, and service implication*, pp. 359–378. New York: Springer.

Kramer, B. (1997). Gain in the caregiving experience: Where are we? What next? *The Gerontologist*, 37(2), 218–232.

Levine, C. & Kuerbis, A. (2002). Building alliances between social workers and family caregivers. *Journal of Social Work in Long-term Care*, 1(4), 3–17.

McCallion, P., Smith, G., & Toseland, R.W. (2001). Helping family caregivers. In A. Gitterman (ed.), *Handbook of social work practice with vulnerable and resilient populations*, 2nd ed., pp. 548–581. New York: Columbia University Press.

McFarland, P. & Sanders, S. (2000). Educational support groups for male caregivers of individuals with Alzheimer's disease. *American Journal of Alzheimer's Disease*, 15(6), 367–373.

McInnis-Dittrich, K. (2002). *Social work with elders: A biopsychosocial approach to assessment and intervention*. Boston: Allyn & Bacon.

MetLife. (1997). *The MetLife study of employer costs for working caregivers*. Westport: Metropolitan Life Insurance Company.

MetLife. (1999). *The MetLife juggling act study: Balancing caregiving with work and the costs involved*. Westport: Metropolitan Life Insurance Company.

National Alliance for Caregiving & AARP. (1997). *Family caregiving in the United States: Findings from a national study*. Washington: American Association of Retired Persons.

Neundorfer, M.M. (1991). Family caregivers of the frail elderly: Impact of caregiving on their health and implications for interventions. *Community Health*, 14, 48–58.

Noonan, A.E. & Tennstedt, S.L. (1997). Meaning in caregiving and its contribution to caregiver well-being. *The Gerontologist*, 37, 785–794.

Quittner, A.E. & Schulz, R. (1998). Caregiving for children and adults with chronic conditions: Introduction to the special issue. *Health Psychology*, 17, 107–111.

Schulz, R. (2000). *Handbook on dementia caregiving, Evidence-based interventions for family caregivers*. New York: Springer.

Schulz, R. & Williamson, G.M. (1994). Health effects of caregiving: Prevalence of mental and physical illness in Alzheimer's caregivers. In E. Light, G. Niederehe, & B. Lebowitz (eds.), *Stress effects on family caregivers of Alzheimer's patients: Research and interventions*, pp. 38–63. New York: Springer.

Scott, C. & Van Gerpen, B. (1997). Home care: What is it? *Journal of the Medical Association of Georgia*, 86(2), 119–120.

Shanas, E. (1968). *Old people in three industrial societies*. New York: Atherton Press.

Spector, W.D. et al. (2000, September). *The characteristics of long-term care users*, AHRQ Publication No. 00-0049. Rockville: Agency for Healthcare Research and Policy.

Steinberg, R.M. (1985). Access assistance and case management. In A. Monk (ed.), *Handbook of gerontological services*, pp. 211–239. New York: Van Nostrand.

Strawbridge, W. & Wallhagen, M. (1991). Impact of family conflict on adult child caregivers. *The Gerontologist*, 31, 770–777.

Internet Resources

American Association of Geriatric Psychiatry
   Site with information for both caregivers and care recipients; includes depression and dementia fact sheets, resources for caregivers, and the latest caregiver research.
   http://www.aagpgpa.org
Children of Aging Parents
   A non-profit organization website that provides information and support to caregivers of older people.
   http://www.careguide.com/
Family Caregiver Alliance Resource Center
   This site provides information on variety of caregiving resources.
   http://www.caregiver.org/
National Alliance for Caregiving
   This site provides tips for caregivers, links to other caregiving resources, and a comprehensive database of books and websites.
   http://www.caregiving.org/
Oregon Department of Human Services
   Offers communication tips for interactions between caregivers and physicians, caregivers and care receivers, and caregivers and family members.
   http://www.oregoncares.org/

Additional Readings

Brandt, A. (1997). *Caregiver's reprieve: A guide to emotional survival when you're caring for someone you love*. Atascadero: Impact Publishers, Inc.
Caroll, D.L. (1990). *When your loved one has Alzheimer's: A caregiver's guide*, rev. ed. New York: Harper & Row.
Carter, R. (1994). *Helping yourself help others: A book for caregivers*. New York: Times Books.
Gray-Davidson, F. (1996). *The Alzheimer's sourcebook for caregivers: A practical guide for getting through the day*, rev. ed. Boston: Lowell House.
Mace, N. & Rabins, P. (2001). *The 36-hour day*, rev. ed. New York: Warner Books.

Morris, V. & Butler, R. (1996). *How to care for aging parents.* New York: Workman Publishing.

Pennsylvania Department of Aging. (no date). *A guide for family caregivers of older Pennsylvanians.*

CHAPTER 20

SOCIAL WORK PRACTICE WITH THE RURAL ELDERLY WITH MENTAL RETARDATION

BARBARA A. DICKS AND

VINCENT J. VENTURINI

The rural elderly with mental retardation represent a microcosm of the rapidly increasing aged population in the United States. This subgroup has received very limited attention in social work literature. The subgroup has a dual stigma barrier to deal with — one being mental illness, the other being rural elderly. With the projected escalation of the aged over the next decade, increased emphasis is needed on service delivery, programming, and recruitment and training of social workers to meet the needs of this age cohort. Practice roles with this unique subpopulation discussed in this chapter include social broker, enabler, teacher, mediator, and advocate. A case study illustration of one southern rural retardation centre's approach to service delivery with elderly persons with mental retardation is presented.

I. Introduction

Elderly persons with mental retardation are a group that has been relatively obscure in social work literature. Furthermore, there are debates over rudimentary issues such as the size of the population and use of a standard of chronological age to classify as elderly (Cotten & Sison; 1989; Drew & Hardman, 2002; DeWeaver et al., 1989; Seltzer & Seltzer, 1985). Mellor (2000) described challenges and implications for social work education in the next decade in responding to the needs for the escalating group of special older populations around such issues as dual stigma, varying definitions of elderly, caregiving stressors and needs, differential treatment needs, and limited knowledge of service providers. These concerns are especially prominent with rural social workers as a wave of elderly migration to rural areas has been noted.

Recent literature has reviewed the tasks facing social workers and other mental retardation professionals in helping prepare this population for later life. Goatcher and Mahon (1999) examined the effects of a "leisure education-based later-life planning model" on older adults with mental retardation. They discovered that training participants were better able to make decisions concerning leisure activities and showed higher levels of life satisfaction. Heller, Hsieh, Miller, and Sterns (2000) investigated the role of later-life training with older adults carrying a diagnosis of mental retardation. Their findings indicated that those who received such training were better able to make individual choices as to retirement and leisure activities than the control group.

Given the nature of limited availability and accessibility to social service programs in rural areas, rural values such as self-reliance and extensive use of informal systems (Johnson, 1980), and stereotypes regarding persons who are mentally retarded, the profession has a mammoth task of educating the community and other professionals to the needs of this special population. The purpose of this chapter is to describe social work interventions with such persons.

II.   The Clientele

The specific population discussed here are elderly clients served by Boswell Regional Center, in Sanatorium, Mississippi. The authors focus on social work practice roles employed with this population, including particular tasks central to each role. Before beginning the discussion, it is important that the reader have an understanding of mental retardation.

In the new definition by the American Association on Mental Retardation (AAMR), an individual is considered to have mental retardation based on the following three criteria: intellectual functioning level (IQ) is below 70–75; significant limitation exists in two or more adaptive skill areas; and the condition manifests before the age of 18 (American Association for Mental Retardation, 2000a). Adaptive skill areas are those daily living skills needed to live, work, and play in the community. This definition includes 10 adaptive skills: communication, self-care, home living, social skills, leisure, health and safety, self-direction, functional academics, community use, and work. Adaptive skills are assessed in a person's typical environment across all aspects of an individual's life. A person with limits in intellectual functioning who does not have limits in adaptive skill areas may not be diagnosed as having mental retardation.

Historically, persons have been assigned to categories of mental retardation based upon three factors: mental ability, adaptive behaviour, and physical development. The American Psychiatric Association (2003) presented the following categories of mental retardation based upon the intelligence quotient (IQ): mild (IQ 50/55 to approximately 70), moderate (IQ 35/40 to 50/55), severe (IQ 20/25 to 35/40), profound (IQ below 20/25) and severity unspecified for persons unable to be tested as a result of extreme intellectual limitations. Over two decades ago Grossman (1983) described the percentage ranking for the degree of retardation in the general population: mild (89%), moderate (6%), severe (3.5%), and profound (1.5%). This has continued to hold true over the past twenty years, as today, nine out of ten persons with mental retardation are diagnosed with mild mental retardation (Portland Community College, Office for Students with Disabilities, 2000).

There are approximately 9.2 million people in the USA with mental retardation and other developmental disabilities (such as cerebral palsy, autism, and epilepsy). There are at least 560,000 persons 60 and over in this subgroup. According to the American Association for Mental Retardation (2000b), the number of elderly in this group is expected to double to over 1 million by the year 2030 as the post-World War II baby boomers will be in their sixties.

The heterogeneity of persons with mental retardation makes it difficult to assign a specific age as the beginning of elderly chronological status for this population. Some persons with mental retardation in the 30–50 age range often manifest certain physiological changes that produce functional impairments typically associated with the aging process (DeWeaver et al., 1989). As a result of the early physiological changes, age 55 best minimizes potential errors in misclassification of diverse populations of persons with mental retardation (Krauss & Seltzer, 1987). Therefore, age 55 is used in this chapter to designate Boswell Regional Center's elderly clients.

Boswell Regional Center was created by an act of Mississippi's legislature in 1976 to provide a less restrictive environment for high-functioning adults with mental retardation. The Center is located in Mississippi's rural Piney Woods region, approximately 45 miles south of the state's capitol city, Jackson. The main campus comprises 80 acres of lush green farmland with a picturesque lake in its midst. Boswell is one of the few institutions that have several staff members residing on the grounds. Most client activities take place in a nearby small town of Magee, population 3,500. While there is no mass transit system, vans are available to transfer clients to various activities in Jackson and other places.

Boswell Regional Center's three components include: (1) the Intermediate Care Facility, (2) the Independent Living Skills Training, and (3) Community Services. The Intermediate Care facility receives Medicaid funding and provides training in self-care and survival skills for clients, who generally have severe or profound levels of mental retardation, coupled with a physical disability.

The Independent Living Skills Training component serves approximately 150 clients and is a transitional program between an Intermediate Care placement and community living. Clients in the dormitory receive training in personal grooming, domestic activities, functional academic skills, yard maintenance, and vocational training. The Community Service component provides alternative living arrangements for an average of 50 clients in supervised homes, apartments, or retirement homes.

Other services provided at Boswell include specific programs related to community living, vocational training/placement and leisure education. Pre-retirement training is offered for clients who are elderly or approaching elderly status to help them prepare for changes brought on by retirement. Clients have the option of retiring from vocational programming or working fewer hours.

Clients who reside in the retirement homes have the option to spend their day engaging in leisure activities, performing domestic chores, participating in shopping trips, and/or preparing meals if they choose. Retirement home clients are also provided the options of continuing to work or participating in volunteer activities. Those who are at least 60 years of age can attend a local elderly nutrition centre for meals and socialization with senior citizens who are not mentally retarded.

Social work activities within the Intermediate Care Facility and the Interdependent Living Skills Training components of Boswell Regional Center are provided by the Social Services Department.

This department is headed by a coordinator, who holds an MSW and supervises a staff of BSW-level employees. The Community Services Program has a separate social work staff of two, one has a MSW and one a BSW. Both social workers in this unit report directly to the coordinator of Community Services, who is a psychologist. The nature of Boswell Regional Center's client community and the services offered allow for social workers employed at the centre to perform a variety of social work task, roles, and responsibilities.

III. Practice Roles and Responsibilities

Numerous authors have addressed the diverse generic roles of social work practitioners (Compton & Galaway, 1999; Germain & Gitterman, 1996; Goldberg & Middleman, 1998), but the literature is very limited regarding social work roles with older persons with a diagnosis of mental retardation. The most comprehensive typology of interventive roles with the population is presented by DeWeaver, Glicker, and Kaufman (1989). A case management model of social work practice focusing on the roles of outreach worker, advocate, teacher, therapist, enabler/facilitator, and broker/coordinator with the mentally retarded aged who are institutionalized, deinstitutionalized, or living in a family unit is outlined by DeWeaver et al. (1989). Case management activities represent the basic social work model of practice with those diagnosed with mental retardation (DeWeaver & Johnson, 1983; DeWeaver et al., 1989). Given the nature of daily activities at Boswell, discussion will centre on the following roles: social broker, enabler, teacher, mediator, and advocate.

A. Social Brokerage Role

Social brokerage is a social work function intended to assist a client system to identify, locate, and acquire resources necessary to problem solving. Social brokerage activities assist different segments of the community in the enhancement of their mutual interests by connecting them with one another (Barker, 2003; Germain & Gitterman, 1996; Goldberg & Middleman, 1998). Assisting elderly clients in acquiring transportation necessary to perform essential daily tasks or linking them with an elderly community service project are examples of social brokerage. At Boswell Regional Center, social brokerage activities may be divided into four categories: (1) community-based services, (2) placement activities, (3) employment, and (4) social interactional activities.

For clients in the institutional setting, social brokerage services are largely directed at linking them with age-specific programs and residential living arrangements. The institutional social worker is part of the interdisciplinary team, which makes decisions concerning a client's individual program plans and living arrangements.

Social brokerage activities pertinent to Boswell's Community Services clients entail linking them with necessary community-based services, including medical/dental, nutrition, religious, recreational, shopping, employment, and voluntary activities. Social brokerage undertaken to provide clients access to volunteer or employment activities are provided for elderly clients on an individual basis. Not all of the elderly clients served by the program possess the necessary cognitive or social skills to adequately perform employment or voluntary tasks in a community setting. Therefore, efforts are made to enable access for those clients capable of performing such roles in the community should they desire to do so. Other elderly clients who choose to continue working are permitted to do so in Boswell's Work Activity Center or Adult Activity Center, depending upon their individual skills levels.

Another unique and integral part of social brokerage activities at Boswell Regional Center entails providing elderly clients opportunities for social interaction with other elderly persons who are not mentally retarded. In the institutional setting, this function is largely carried out through "Adopt-a-Friend" activities. Institutional social workers coordinate activities with local churches, civic organizations, and the Retired Senior Volunteer Program to enlist an "Adopt-a-Friend" for clients who are isolated and have no family contact. "Adopt-a-Friend" activities can also include receiving letters from a community person or attending church and/or recreational programs with that individual.

Social brokerage activities with Community Services' clients focus more upon client integration into social settings. Clients are encouraged to participate in all programs offered for older persons in the community. For instance, some clients are active participants in Mississippi's Senior Olympics. Community Services Department social workers work with other staff in ensuring that their application to participate in the Senior Olympics are completed and mailed and that they are provided transportation to and receive proper supervision during the event.

Elderly clients who reside in the community are provided the option of attending church services in the community or at Boswell Regional Center's Chapel. It is an important social brokerage role to ensure that elderly clients have access to the churches of their choice and to link them with transportation services to all church activities. Case managers have also been instrumental in facilitating mid-week services in the retirement homes through volunteer efforts from local churches.

B. Enabler Role

The enabler role is utilized when social workers seek to assist clients to discover coping strengths and resources within themselves to achieve desired ends (Compton & Galaway; 1999). This definition has been expanded through identification of specific skills employed by the social worker in the execution of this role (Barker, 2003; Goldberg & Middleman, 1998). These skills include: conveying hope, reducing resistance and ambivalence, recognizing and managing feelings, identifying and supporting personal strengths and social assets, dividing problems into manageable parts to facilitate problem resolution, and maintaining a focus on goals and the means to achieving them. The social worker seeks to direct clients to accomplish positive change through their own efforts. Social work intervention utilizes the enabler role in assisting clients to effect both personal and environmental changes.

Most Boswell clients possess the cognitive skills to draw upon personal resources to accomplish a needed and desired change. While some changes sought for Boswell's elderly clients appear rudimentary, such as understanding the importance of waiting for one's turn during a conversation or learning how to offer constructive criticism to peers, they signify important social skills for persons with mental retardation, especially when they interact in the wider community. Social workers frequently utilize the enabler role in assisting clients to acquire these or similar skills.

Institutional social workers at Boswell Regional Center frequently utilize the enabler role when implementing written training programs. The social worker identifies and prioritizes the client's deficient social skills and presents them at the annual staffing on the client. The interdisciplinary team decides upon the deficient skills that should be addressed by the social worker. The enabler role is utilized by the social worker to assist clients in accomplishing objectives of the written training programs. An example is a written training program designed to reduce episodes of volatile behaviour in a client. Social work activities in this context are directed at helping the client to identify and understand the causes of his/her volatile behaviour, the consequences of such behaviour, and more appropriate responses to these causes. The social worker does not provide the client with answers, but rather guides the client in identifying and practising steps s/he can take in reducing volatile episodes. Through these activities the client is enabled to express his/her anger in more socially appropriate ways.

Social workers in the Community Service setting generally have more flexibility in designating certain areas in social functioning as problematic and implementing enabling activities with clients. Here, the social worker has the advantage of allowing clients to practise appropriate responses in a "real world" social setting. It should also be noted that elderly clients residing in a community setting often have greater personal and environmental resources available.

Employing enabling activities with elderly clients is more difficult in the area of effecting environmental changes. An example of enabling activities directed at altering the environment may include steps undertaken to assist elderly clients who reside in the community and attend an elderly nutrition centre in understanding the reluctance of other elderly persons to interact with them. Once a client can recognize environmental cues that influence his social interaction with non-mentally retarded elderly persons, s/he can identify positive actions that may facilitate enhanced social interactional opportunities with other elderly persons in the community. In short, the client can be enabled to communicate her own personal worth to "normal" elderly persons and allow them to recognize that a person with mental retardation possesses unique qualities and experiences to share in social interaction. The performance of volunteer tasks by elderly persons with mental retardation is an important function relative to engendering environmental changes. It informs community citizens that elderly persons with mental retardation can be providers as well as receivers of vital services. This, in turn, enables elderly persons with mental retardation to acquire a fuller partnership in community affairs that affect them, and hence it enhances self-esteem.

On an individual level, social work enabling activities with Boswell's elderly clients are employed to assist clients to verbalize their problems, vent their frustrations, and arrive at appropriate, workable resolutions. It is sometimes necessary for the social worker to take a directive role in identifying problems or stressing the need for change with this population; efforts are still undertaken to assist the client in fostering change as much as possible.

The enabler role demands the social worker's primary focus and interaction with the client rather than with external systems (Compton & Galaway, 1999). Persons with mental retardation have often led cloistered lives, whether in an institutional setting or in family systems. Their reduced abilities to understand and manipulate the rules of external systems minimize their potential for acquiring maximum benefits available in the systems. In such instances, the enabling role must be modified to allow the social worker to act on behalf of the client in effecting environmental changes. When vested interests are discovered in the environment that are hostile to client interests, the social worker must intervene and make decisions regarding the course of action to be taken.

C. The Teacher Role

The teaching role entails providing the client with information essential for accomplishing desired objectives. Social work teaching activities can also be directed at assisting clients to gain new skills or to replace negative behavioural patterns with more positive ones (Germain & Gitterman, 1996; Goldberg & Middleman, 1998). A primary teaching activity employed with clients who have mental retardation is the Written Training Program. Traditionally, this has been known as the habilitation plan or individual program plan. The Written Training Program is a task-oriented active treatment module implemented to impart new skills to the client. It entails teaching the client to perform desired tasks independently via incremental steps. Social work written training programs most often involve teaching social skills or assisting the client in learning how to appropriately utilize social skills in public settings.

Elderly clients who reside in the community may have greater interactional opportunities with non-mentally retarded persons in the community than other Boswell clients through various Council on Aging Programs. It is important that they acquire skills on how to conduct themselves, which will facilitate psychosocial integration. The social worker directs activities intended to assist the client in acquiring appropriate behavioural patterns within the community setting. Very often these activities are facilitated with the assistance of the home managers.

Boswell Center's pre-retirement curriculum provides perhaps the best example of teaching activities. While this curriculum is the result of an interdisciplinary effort, social workers, including the current project director, have been instrumental in the development and coordination of this curriculum. The purpose of the pre-retirement curriculum essentially is to teach elderly persons with mental retardation what retirement is and how to retire. Learning exercises during classes are very simple by using pictures to illustrate options in a specific context. Exercises are repeated throughout two-hour-long sessions. Clients learn that retirement provides them with such options as attending an elderly nutrition centre or continuing to work part-time. This, in turn, permits them to choose whether they participate in an elderly nutrition program, continue to work part-time, or engage in various leisure pursuits.

Social workers also participate in the curriculum component involving Community Support Services. Clients are taught that they are entitled to a host of programs and benefits in the community, not necessarily because they are elderly and/or carry a mental retardation diagnosis, but because they are people and citizens. They are also taught the responsibilities those rights carry.

Community Services social workers are responsible for always ensuring that clients are aware of their legal, civil, and constitutional rights. This requires coordinating activities with home managers to ensure that clients have the opportunity to vote, attend the church of their choice, and to see that they are able to utilize public recreational facilities, the same as other persons.

One of the most important advocacy activities employed by Community Services social workers entails the acquisition of Social Security, Supplemental Security Income, or other benefits to which the client is legally entitled. The social worker makes application for these benefits for the client and represents the client's eligibility for and entitlement to these benefits to the appropriate agency. In the event a client is refused these benefits, the social worker argues the appeal in an effort to secure benefits outright for the client. Since this activity is vital to the client, the social worker as advocate must be knowledgeable of the eligibility guidelines of a host of public benefits.

IV.   Potential for Role Development

The potential for role development with this population is inherent in the broker, enabler, teacher, mediator, and advocate roles. It should be the goal in any type of social work intervention to encourage and direct the client's right to self-determination as much as possible. This relates directly to advocacy activities. Unless a protective function must be utilized, the social worker "should go no further in advocacy activities than the client wishes to go" (Hepworth & Larsen, 2002). Therefore, a social worker involved with elderly persons with mental retardation must assist clients to realize their rights and to ensure that they understand as much as possible the potential ramifications in the exercise of these rights.

Promoting self-determination requires employment of the teacher and enabler roles. It is in the capacity of teacher that the social worker imparts knowledge to the client pertinent to his/her rights in a given situation and possible consequences should the client choose to exercise these rights. In fact the teaching here should reinforce to the clients that the exercise of self-determination must involve "options" and "choices" relative to the courses of action they may wish to take.

Once the social worker has directed the client toward a greater understanding and exercise of self-determination, enhancement of the broker and mediator roles will inevitably result. The mediator role will be strengthened as a result of an increased bargaining power the social worker will acquire, since the client is more assertive in demanding certain rights and/or services. In short, the social worker would be representing the client on a higher multi-system level. Instead of taking a lead role in determining what the client's best interests are, the social worker would be representing the client's decision as to what his/her best interests are. This applies to the enhancement of the advocate role as well.

Enhancement of the social broker role should result from the client's increased assertiveness pertinent to desired services. The social worker and client can list together the various services the client wishes to receive or become involved with. It would be the social worker's primary responsibility in this phase of the activity to suggest services the client may be seeking and explain any pitfalls inherent in potential choices. Once the client has determined desired services, the social worker should assist the client in their acquisition.

The teacher and advocate roles can also be enhanced on different levels. Teaching activities have previously been discussed solely from the perspective of direct intervention with the client. These activities can also be employed with the personnel of various service agencies and with persons in the community at large. Social workers at Boswell

Regional Center have been active in recent years in presentations at conferences on the pre-retirement curriculum and retirement home clients. Many of the pervasive myths pertinent to elderly persons with mental retardation have been dispelled. More activities of this type are needed. Most importantly, social workers should endeavour to speak at civic clubs and organizations. It is crucial that community members understand that a diagnosis of mental retardation does not diminish an individual's worth as a person, or necessarily significantly decrease skills in all domains.

Through the advocacy roles, the social worker should employ and impart an awareness of the client's individuality and right to be treated with dignity regardless of mental limitations. When interacting with non-mentally retarded elderly persons in normal life circumstances, they are generally referred to by such titles as Mr., Mrs., or Ms. We generally use first names with elderly persons only when they have requested that we do so. Should social workers not do the same when speaking to an elderly client who happens to have a diagnosis of mental retardation? After all, we are attempting to advocate for their rights to be treated the same as other elderly persons. What are we communicating to non-mentally retarded persons who reside in the community if we do not accord the same deference to our elderly clients given to other elderly persons?

Case Study

Mr. J is a 64 year-old white male client of Boswell's Community Services department with a diagnosis of mild retardation of measured intelligence concurrent with mild adaptive behaviour deficits. He has a medical diagnosis of seizure disorder and has a history of alcoholism, although he has been sober for the past several years. Mr. J is ambulatory and verbal, but has limited reading, writing, and counting abilities, having completed only the fifth grade. He speaks and understands complex sentences and can integrate past and present events. He has been more successful than other elderly clients served by Boswell's Community Services department in integrating into social networks of non-retarded elderly persons in Simpson County.

Mr. J was admitted to the state hospital for alcoholism and was transferred to Boswell Regional Center due to his mental retardation. After a ten-year period, he transitioned to supervised apartment living and recently moved into a senior citizens' apartment building in the same complex. Although he was no longer a resident of the supervised apartment program, he continued to receive case management and other support services from Boswell.

Concerns were raised over the condition of Mr. J's apartment by Community Services staff. Reports were also made to the social worker by Boswell's Work Activity Center staff that Mr. J came to work with an offensive odour and apparently was neither bathing nor washing his clothes regularly. An investigation by the staff social worker uncovered several packages of green, spoiled meat in the refrigerator and mouldy loaves of bread. Mould was also discovered in the bathroom and rats had chewed a hole in a bushel bag of peanuts stored in the living room. Mr. J initially protested that he was adequately caring for himself and his apartment and accused staff and other clients of lying about him in an attempt to hurt him. When confronted by the social worker, he admitted his need for help.

Mr. J and the social worker agreed that he required assistance in the performance of domestic duties. The social worker presented this to the Community Services Coordinator, along with the contention that a significant number of professionals and other non-mentally retarded persons are poor housekeepers. Thus, the argument was made that the condition of Mr. J's apartment was not necessarily a consequence of his mental retardation diagnosis. The coordinator, social worker, and Mr. J decided that he should hire another Community Service client to clean his apartment for a fair wage. A younger client who worked domestic jobs in the community accepted Mr. J as one of her customers.

Mr. J received counselling regarding his poor grooming and hygiene skills. The social worker discussed with him the need to bathe daily with a good deodorant soap, use deodorant, brush his teeth regularly, and wear clean clothes. He was also instructed in the need to wash clothes regularly. The client was advised that since he was now in a case management program, he was responsible for performing these tasks on his own initiative. Most importantly, he was told that despite the fact that he now employed a housekeeper once a week, he was responsible for the daily maintenance of his apartment, including sanitary conditions. Mr. J was informed that this required placing dirty clothes in a hamper, throwing away spoiled food, properly storing unused food items, and taking out his garbage regularly. The social worker also emphasized that his poor hygiene habits could cause negative responses from citizens in the community toward persons with mental retardation.

Case Analysis Discussion

Mr. J's case provides a viable example of the employment of different social work practice roles and the manner in which these roles overlap in social work activities. Interventions with Mr. J employed all the roles discussed in this chapter. The broker role was employed to assist Mr. J acquire necessary services to keep his apartment clean and meet housing authority standards. Enabling activities were directed toward prompting Mr. J to utilize the skills he already possessed pertinent to his personal hygiene and domestic skills. The social worker employed the teaching role in activities designed to instruct Mr. J in appropriate shopping skills and proper food storage. The teaching role was also utilized concerning community expectations relative to personal hygiene.

Distinctions between the mediator and advocacy roles are more difficult to distinguish in this case example. The advocacy role was employed when the social worker stated the case that several non-mentally retarded older persons require assistance in keeping their homes clean and argued that Mr. J should remain in his apartment and acquire the services of a housekeeper. This entailed advocating that the same right accorded other elderly persons to remain in their homes with appropriate support services should be available to elderly persons with mental retardation. Mediation activities involved requesting that the landlord exterminate the apartment.

Brokerage activities were employed when the social worker facilitated arrangements with Mr. J and another client for Mr. J to receive housekeeping services. The two parties were assisted in agreeing on the day and time she would work and the salary she would receive. During this session, delineation of tasks specific to both Mr. J and the housekeeper were decided.

Mr. J did demonstrate some improvement in the areas of concern as a result of social work intervention utilizing the practice roles described above. His food-storage habits improved and his apartment ceased to attract rodents. He also demonstrated progress in his personal hygiene and appearance. Both his competency and self-esteem increased.

V.   Concluding Remarks

Several changes have occurred at Boswell Regional Center since the first publication of this chapter twelve years ago. Several elderly clients have died. A larger percentage of Boswell's population is now elderly, due to the confluence of the natural aging of long-term residents and the admission of older persons from other programs. Boswell's newer older clients more typically function at lower intellectual and adaptive behaviour level than in the original cohort. This is as true for the group moving into community settings as for those remaining in the institutional grounds.

There are two primary reasons for this shift in the functioning capacities of elderly persons with mental retardation. First, those persons with mental retardation who became elderly during the 1980s represented a cohort who would most likely never have been institutionalized under current standards. Many were placed in state institutions due to the inability of their parents to adequately attend to their special needs and the absence of special education programs in their local communities. Some were slow with special learning disabilities, but were not necessarily diagnosed with mental retardation. Others were diagnosed as having mild or borderline functioning levels. Such individuals were better able to adjust to community settings and were in many cases indistinguishable from other older persons. As these persons die, the cohort of elderly persons with mental retardation is becoming represented more by those who have more severe and profound levels of mental retardation.

The second reason is due to the increasing focus of placing persons with mental retardation, regardless of functioning level, in smaller, community-based facilities. Even though Mississippi has maintained a preference for the larger institutional settings, the state has opened several community-based group homes during the last decade. Larger numbers of older clients with severe and profound levels of mental retardation are now living in group homes located in rural communities. These clients require more staff assistance in using services and community resources available to older persons.

Social work practice with elderly persons with mental retardation residing in rural communities is an area that will deserve greater attention from the profession in the immediate future. In the next decade, there will be a considerable increase in elderly persons and consequently the potential for a larger subgroup of elderly individuals with mental retardation. Concerns relative to this population reflects the need for pertinent service regarding all individuals with mental retardation as they struggle for equitable treatment in a society that has difficulty accepting and tolerating differences. Elderly persons with mental retardation have dual difficulty in our society due to prejudices against the elderly as well as those with mental disabilities.

Given the nature of the varied roles undertaken by social workers to provide services to this population in rural communities, there are formidable challenges for social workers and human service providers. Schools of social work should become more active in assuring that they promote work with both the population of persons with mental retardation and other elderly persons through curriculum content and fieldwork opportunities. State institutions and local programs can begin to take a more proactive role in educating and sensitizing the public to the needs of one of our most vulnerable populations.

Finally, with the advent of the beginning of the 21st century, social work must meet the challenge of ensuring that the needs of those clients approaching the end of life who are intellectually unable to advocate for themselves in all arenas can depend on the services of a dedicated profession.

References

American Association for Mental Retardation. (2000a). Definition of mental retardation. Retrieved from http://www.aamr.org/Policies/faq_toc.shtml.

American Association for Mental Retardation. (2000b). Fact sheets. Retrieved from http://www.aamr.org/Policies/faq_sheets.shtml.

American Psychiatric Association. (2003). *DSM IV TR: Diagnostic and statistical manual of mental disorders—text revision*, 4th printing, pp. 42–43. Washington: American Psychiatric Association.

Barker, Robert L. (2003). *The social work dictionary.* Silver Spring: National Association of Social Workers.

Brody, Stanley J. & Ruff, George E. (1986). *Aging and rehabilitation 11: Advances in the state of the art.* New York: Springer Publishers.

Compton, B.R. & Galaway, B. (1999). *Social work processes,* 6th ed. Belmont: Wadsworth.

Cotten, P.D. & Sisson, G.F.P. (1989). The elderly mentally retarded person: Current perspectives and future directions. *Journal of Applied Gerontology,* 8(2), 151.

DeWeaver, K., Glicker, M., & Kaufman, A. (1989). The mentally retarded aged: Implications for social work practice. *Journal of Gerontological Social Work,* 14(1/2), 93–111.

DeWeaver, K.L. & Johnson, P.J. (1983). Case management in rural areas for the developmentally disabled. *Human Services in the Rural Environment,* 8(4), 23–31.

Drew, C. & Hardman, M. (2002). *Mental retardation: A life cycle approach*, 7th ed., pp. 325–345. Upper Saddle River: Merrill Publishers.

Germain, C.B. & Gitterman, A. (1996). *The life model of social work practice*, 2nd ed. New York: Columbia University Press.

Goatcher, S. & Mahon, M.J. (1999). Later-life planning for older adults with mental retardation: A field experiment. *Mental Retardation*, 37(5), 371–382.

Goldberg, G. & Middleman, R. (1998). *Social service delivery: A structural approach to social work practice*. New York: Columbia University Press.

Grossman, Herbert J. (1983). *Classification in mental retardation*. Washington: American Association on Mental Deficiency.

Heller, T., Hsieh, K., Miller, Alison B., & Sterns, Harvey. (2000). Later-life planning: Promoting knowledge of options and choice making. *Mental Retardation*, 38(5), 395–406.

Hepworth, D.H. & Larsen, J.A. (2002). *Direct social work practice: Theory and skills*, 6th ed. Pacific Grove: Brooks Cole Publishers.

Janicki, M.P. & Wisniewski, H.M. (1985). *Aging and developmental disabilities: Issues and approaches*. Baltimore: Paul H. Brookes Publishing Company.

Johnson, H.W. (1980). *Rural human services: A book of readings*. Itasca: F.E. Peacock Publishers.

Krauss, M.W. & Seltzer, M.M. (1987). *Aging and mental retardation: Extending the continuum*. Washington: Monographs of the American Association on Mental Retardation (9).

Mellor, M.J. (2002). Special older populations and implications for social work education. Retrieved from http://www.agesocialwork.org/fall2000feature.html.

Portland Community College, Office for Students with Disabilities. (2000). Information about mental retardation. Retrieved from http://spot.pcc.edu/osd/ddinfo.htm.

Seltzer, G.B. & Seltzer, M. (1985). The elderly mentally retarded: A group in need of service. In G.S. Getzel & M.J. Mellor (eds.), *Gerontological social work practice in the community*. New York: Haworth.

Internet Resources

Administration on Aging
    The advocate agency for older persons and their concerns. Works to heighten awareness about older Americans and alerts the public to the needs of vulnerable older people.
    http://www.aoa.gov/

Ageline
> A research resource accessed through the American Association of
> Retired Persons (AARP).
> http://research.aarp.org/ageline/access.html

Aging Statistics
> http://www.agingstats.gov

American Association for Mental Retardation
> Promotes progressive policies, sound research, effective practices, and
> universal human rights for people with intellectual disabilities.
> http://www.aamr.org

American Association of Retired Persons
> A non-profit membership organization dedicated to addressing the
> needs and interests of persons 50 and older.
> http://www.aarp.org

American Journal of Mental Retardation
> Promotes progressive policies, sound research, effective practices, and
> universal human rights for people with intellectual disabilities.
> http://aamr.allenpress.com/aamronline/?request=index-html

ARC (formerly the Association for Retarded Citizens of the United States)
> Works to include all children and adults with cognitive, intellectual, and
> developmental disabilities in every community.
> http://www.thearc.org

Association for Gerontology Education in Social Work
> Provides leadership and assistance to social work educational
> programs and professionals in order to advocate for the integration of
> gerontological content in social work education.
> http://www.agesocialwork.org

Boswell Regional Center
> Provides Mississippians with mental retardation and other
> developmental disabilities a comprehensive array of service options
> promoting independence and an optimal quality of life.
> http://www.boswell.state.ms.us/index.html

Geriatric Case Managers
> A non-profit, professional organization of practitioners whose goal is
> the advancement of dignified care for the elderly and their families.
> http://www.caremanager.org/

Gerontologist
> Archive of on-line journals.
> http://gerontologist.gerontologyjournals.org/contents-by-date.0.shtml

Haworth Press Aging and Gerontology Page
> Books on aging and gerontology.
> http://www.haworthpress.com/focus/Aging

Additional Readings

Blank, M.M., Guterbock, T., Jeanne C., & Marcus, F. (2002). Alternative mental health services: The role of the black church in the south. *The American Journal of Public Health*, 92(10), 1668–1673.

Brody, Stanley J., Gregory, & Pawlson, L. (eds.). (1990). *Aging and rehabilitation 11: The state of the practice.* New York: Springer Publishers.

Dillion, M. & Holburn, S. (2003). Preserving oral histories: Example of the institutional experience. *Mental Retardation*, 41(2), 130–132.

Rosenbaum, S. (2000, November). *Olmstead v. L.C. Implications for older persons with mental and physical disabilities.* Washington: Public Policy Institute, AARP.

Smyer, M.A. & Qualls, S.H. (1999). *Aging and mental health.* Malden: Blackwell Public Policy Institute.

Walsh, Patricia N. (2002). Ageing and mental retardation. *Current Opinion in Psychiatry*, 15(5), 509–514.

Table 20.1: Social Work Practice Roles with the Rural Elderly with Mental Retardation by Programs

Program Components

Practice Roles	Intermediate Care Facility	Independent Living Skills Training	Community Services
Social broker	• Develop written training programs • Ensure access to institutional services • Ensure appropriate client placement	• Develop written training programs • Ensure access to institutional services • Ensure appropriate client placement	• Arrange client access to local community services
Enabler	• Facilitate client development of coping skills • Identify strengths and personal assets	• Facilitate client development of coping skills • Identify strengths and personal assets	• Empower clients to overcome service barriers • Identify strength and personal asset

con't

Table 20.1 (continued)

Teacher	• Implement written training program • Assist client development of social skills	• Implement written training program • Assist client development of social skills • Prepare clients for retirement	• Assist client development of social skills • Assist client development of communication skills • Educate community about needs of MR persons
Mediator	• Assist client in resolving disputes • Arrange age-appropriate programs for client	• Assist client in resolving disputes • Arrange age-appropriate programs	• Assist client in resolving disputes • Negotiating concessions for client
Advocate	• Advise client of rights • Ensure client freedom to exercise • Promote client right to less restrictive living situation	• Advise client of rights • Ensure client freedom to exercise rights • Promote client right to less restrictive living situation	• Advise client of rights • Ensure client freedom to exercise rights • Ensure equitable rights accorded other community citizens • Promote client eligibility for needed services • Sensitize community to human qualities of clients

CHAPTER 21

SOCIAL WORK PRACTICE IN A PRIVATE RETIREMENT COMMUNITY

VIRGINIA L. FITCH, LEE R. SLIVINSKE,

AND SALLY NICHOLS

This chapter describes the practice roles and responsibilities of social workers in a private, non-profit continuing care community. Although the interventions and services offered are similar to those offered to elders in other settings, the wide range of client needs and the variety of care options available require innovative approaches to practice; the ability to work with individuals, families, groups, communities, and other agencies; and knowledge of the elderly and the relationship of staff to client in a long-term relationship. The social worker plays an integral role in helping residents adapt to the setting and achieve a quality of life that affords them satisfaction.

I. Introduction

This chapter describes the roles and activities of social workers in a continuing care retirement community. Rockynol is one of eleven facilities operated by Ohio Presbyterian Retirement Services (OPRS) in the state of Ohio, founded in 1922. OPRS is a private, non-profit organization with corporate headquarters based in Columbus. Today it is Ohio's oldest and largest not-for-profit provider of continuing care retirement communities.

Rockynol is located on 12 campus-like acres in the city of Akron and serves a total of 300 residents, most of whom are from Akron and surrounding areas or have returned to live near relatives.

Organizational governance is accomplished through structures that provide for input at many levels. Residents of each OPRS facility participate in councils that meet regularly to provide input on current operations and future plans. Their concerns are transmitted to a local advisory council composed of community leaders and a resident representative. Community members of each of the seven advisory councils are appointed to the volunteer board of trustees of OPRS. The seven resident representatives elect one among themselves to serve on this board. The procedure insures that residents have a voice in planning and policy issues concerning their community and home.

Rockynol provides long-term care. Originally, long-term care referred to a secondary, primarily custodial function of the health care system. As used today, long-term care is broad in nature and includes a range of care sources and settings (Beaver, 1983).

Rockynol has several distinguishing features. It is one of a minority of full-service continuing care retirement communities in the country accredited by the Continuing Care Accreditation Commission. The commission is sponsored by the American Association of Homes for the Aged. Second, a team from OPRS headquarters makes periodic visits throughout the year and conducts an annual quality-assurance review. The standards of the OPRS quality-assurance program are more stringent than those required by government regulations. Third, Rockynol functions as a small community within the larger urban community. It has a library, art gallery, banking system, chapel, and full-time chaplain, accommodations for visits from family and friends, beauty/barber salon, activities department, transportation, as well as a full complement of services. Forth, four levels of care are offered, including independent living, congregate living, assisted living, and intermediate/skilled nursing care.

In addition, a number of the long-term care services offered at the facility are now available to the community. A full range of skilled services, including skilled nursing, medical social work, occupational therapy, physical and speech therapies, and the like, is accessible to those who are homebound. Adult day care also is provided in two area locations. These home-based and community-based services afford seniors a level of care in their own homes that enhances their quality of life while providing a needed source of support to their caregivers (Gaugler & Zarit, 2001). [As] Keating, Otfinowski, Wenger, Fast, and Derksen (2003) point out, these informal networks may not have the resources to sustain the high levels of care needed by frail older adults with chronic health problems.

Admission is based on a formula that includes consideration of the elderly person's income and assets, past and current health, and life expectancy. The cost of residency is substantial and varies depending upon level of care. Rockynol does accept some individuals on Medicaid. In addition, OPRS maintains a policy called Life Care. Once admitted, no resident has ever had to leave due to depleted finances. The organization assumes responsibility for the resident's service and supports the Life Care plan through a separate foundation established by OPRS.

The mission of the facility is to provide older adults with caring and quality services to enhance physical, mental, and spiritual well-being. The goal is to have every resident living in the least restrictive environment at the highest level of autonomy possible consistent with individual service preference. In practice this means that a resident who could live more independently may prefer to receive help in some activities of daily living.

II.   The Clientele

Rockynol serves a predominantly upper-middle-class, white clientele. Although clients from all ethnic and racial groups are welcomed, the demographic composition seems to reflect the differential socioeconomic conditions and aging patterns that exist between groups (Jenkins, 2001).

Greater diversity in religious affiliation is found. Although the organization has historical ties with the Presbyterian Church, 15 denominations, including Protestant, Catholic, Jewish, and Orthodox are represented.

Although the residents in this facility tend to be affluent, there is still some diversity in the primary source of funding for their care. Sources of funding include Medicaid, Medicare, Life Care, and private pay.

Rockynol residents are predominantly female with an average age of 84. This places the majority in the old-old category, those aged 75 and over. Neugarten (1981) described this group as experiencing the most significant and rapid decrease in health status. They are the most frail and vulnerable and have the greatest need for a wide spectrum of services (Myers, 1989). This is an important consideration for social workers and other staff at Rockynol. With this in mind, Rockynol has developed policies and programs designed to address quality of life issues for people with these varying problems and needs. As noted in the introduction, a variety of activities and care options are available. The needs and problems of residents vary from one level of care to another and within each care option.

At present, 39 percent of Rockynol's residents are in independent living. These residents are totally autonomous and do not require assistance or supervision from staff in any way. They live in high-rise apartments, engage in all self-care, arrange all their own activities and appointments, although they are welcome to attend the activities offered by the facility. Many maintain their own cars and use public and other transportation. Their problems are primarily health-related and may include chronic heart conditions, cancer, and similar conditions. They typically require the services of a social worker for temporary crises involving their health. Some utilize walkers and other supportive devices such as a cane, brace, wheelchair, etc., but they require no staff assistance to remain independent.

Congregate living provides a level of service that allows a resident to live independently but with staff assistance with meals, housekeeping, and personal laundry. Residents in congregate living make up about 26 percent of the total community and live in one of the towers that comprise the main building. They are usually capable of independent living, but choose to have some services provided by the facility.

Many of those in independent living and congregate living are motivated to seek admission because Rockynol residents have priority access to skilled nursing care if needed. Factors precipitating admission often include chronic health conditions that make care of both home and health burdensome, a significant breakdown in the client-support system such as the death of a spouse, or pressure from adult children to move into a protected environment. Residents who are influenced by others to seek admission usually have the most difficulty adjusting to the community.

Assisted living provides licensed rest home care that is designed to provide a range of services to residents who need assistance and supervision in activities such as walking, bathing, dressing, housekeeping, transportation, and taking medications among others. These residents make up 8 percent of the retirement community. They do not require constant supervision to carry out the activities of daily living even though some may appear forgetful or confused at times. They have special activities designed to meet their needs and limitations. A health maintenance nurse and an aide are with them daily.

They and the social workers serve as their primary on-site contact. Due to their frequent interactions, the social worker is aware when problems arise that require intervention.

Skilled nursing/intermediate care is the highest level of care provided. Residents require a range of service that may include staff assistance and supervision in planning and carrying out all activities of daily living and total care in addition to full professional nursing care. As in the other levels of care, residents present a range of problems and needs. For example, they range from individuals with physically incapacitating diseases, such as rheumatoid arthritis, but who are alert and independent in other ways, to people who are bedridden, confused, and unresponsive to their surroundings. The proportion of persons with Alzheimer's and related disorders in this level of care has increased, necessitating special management and care plans.

A special care unit provides round-the-clock personal care and programming for those who are experiencing early to mid-stage Alzheimer's or related memory disorders. Through a variety of activities, residents are given opportunities for developing new interests as well as maintaining or reconnecting with their former interests. An emphasis is placed on maintaining a familiar environment by furnishing residents' rooms with personal possessions.

Admission to independent, congregate, or assisted living often includes a three-day guest visit. This gives the staff an opportunity to assess the applicant in the setting and allows the individual to make a more informed decision about entering the community. At other times circumstances require an appointment with the applicant and family in the hospital, another nursing home, or private residence.

Admission to skilled nursing/intermediate care usually is arranged by someone other than the applicant. When an opening occurs, it is filled quickly by admissions personnel unless it can be filled from within the facility. Level of care change by residents occurs frequently and often in both directions. A sudden illness may necessitate assisted living, intermediate care, or skilled nursing. After recovery, the resident may be able to return to a level offering less care. Facility policy allows the individual to retain a place on two levels of care [for] a limited time if progress is being made toward the more independent level of care. This provides an impetus to recover more quickly. Even after the designated time period, the resident is encouraged to return to a more independent level, although the original apartment may not be available. A more complicated problem results when a couple is admitted with vastly different care needs or when one spouse experiences accelerated physical or mental deterioration while the other remains physically and mentally capable. Separate care options may be necessitated.

Residents are assigned to a social worker's caseload based on their level of care or program assignment. One social worker serves residents in intermediate and skilled nursing care. Another social worker assumes primary responsibility for independent, congregate, and assisted living.

III.   Practice Roles and Responsibilities

Unlike many nursing homes and retirement communities, at Rockynol social work is in the program service department. The department has its own budget and a social worker as director. This extends the range of roles and responsibilities of social workers beyond those filled in many retirement communities. As in many agencies the social worker is a generalist who works with individuals, families, small groups, the community of residents, and the larger community context. The variety of social and personal problems and needs experienced by the elderly provide the focus for these roles. In addition, social workers perform major administrative tasks, including budgeting, planning, and policy-making. Since these may be unique to this organization, this chapter will examine only the direct service tasks, functions, duties, and responsibilities of practitioners as they are interpreted in the retirement community setting.

The social worker is involved with all residents from the time of initial contact with the agency when admission is sought and throughout the duration of their tenure in the community. Actual client admission decisions are undertaken by a separate department established for this purpose. The social worker completes a client assessment prior to admission unless client circumstances dictate otherwise. For example, if admission is arranged by a third party for a family member hospitalized out of town, the assessment process will be completed within three days after admission. The initial interview by the social worker includes both the applicant and family members. The social worker elicits their feelings and expectations about admission, their perceptions of the facility, and the quality of their relationship. Engagement of both begins at this point. As pointed out by Abramovice (1988), excluding the family unit contributes to the development of loss of status and loneliness in the elderly. Thus, efforts are made to reach out to and involve families.

The initial interview includes obtaining a social history and detailed assessment of the resident. The purpose of the assessment is to identify the person's capacity for independent living and self-care and the existence of limitations that would interfere with adjustment to the residential environment. For example, the social worker assesses the client's ability to perform the activities of daily living, including dressing, toileting, bathing, housekeeping, laundry, shopping, meal preparation, mobility, and similar concerns. Questions regarding customary behaviour patterns, mental alertness, drug usage, interpersonal relationships, communication skills, and ability to seek assistance when needed also are addressed. Areas where assistance is needed or where social work intervention is indicated are noted for immediate follow-up. Appointments for assessment by other staff are scheduled as needed.

Out of this assessment an individualized care plan is developed. A team headed by a social worker and consisting of a chaplain, dietician, nurse, and activities person meet to discuss programming needs, services, and interventions indicated by the assessment. The team identifies any early indicators of change in the client's current status. They try to anticipate whether the resident will remain at the current level, deteriorate, or improve in the next six months. Based on the team's recommendations, the social worker develops a care plan within the first five days after admission. The plan is discussed and reviewed with the client and family.

The team meets twice weekly to review and develop care plans. One meeting reviews residents in nursing and skilled care, and the other [in] congregate and assisted living. Individualized plans for health care residents must be updated every 90 days, but are reviewed more frequently when warranted by a change in the client's status. Social work progress notes are written as change occurs, but must be written at least quarterly. The nature of continuing care in a retirement community and the limited size of the client population allow social workers to become very familiar with each resident and family.

The social work practitioner works with residents and families formally in scheduled office sessions and informally in daily encounters. Clients are helped to articulate their needs, identify their problems, explore alternative approaches to problem solving, engage in decision-making, and enhance their capacity to meet their needs. Their problems may range in scope from those that are temporary to those that require long-term intervention. For example, the social worker addresses a variety of problems, including conflicts between residents, problems adjusting to the facility, unresolved grief, and physical and/or mental deterioration. Methods of intervention may include individual counselling, group treatment, family counselling, and environmental modifications among others. Clients also may be referred to external resources. A community resource file is maintained and updated regularly by the social workers. This provides prompt access to the community services needed by residents. When a resident needs service from an external source, the social worker assumes the case management role. In this role, the social worker identifies the need, contacts external resources, and coordinates services. Generally, the more independent the level of care, the less frequent the need for social work intervention.

Upon admission, the immediate responsibility of the social worker is to assist the individual in dealing with some degree of role loss. With the move into a retirement community, there is shrinkage of the range of roles played by any resident. Having many services provided for them, many experience an increase in unoccupied time and a subsequent decrease in self-esteem. The social worker helps residents identify their interests and abilities and make connections for volunteer opportunities and other activities both in and outside the retirement community.

Level of care change also is the responsibility of the social worker. Initial level of care placement decisions are made by admissions personnel in consultation with the social worker. Thereafter, placement suitability is reassessed by the social worker in the care setting on an ongoing basis. When physical or mental deterioration begins to occur, both the resident and family are involved in discussion and decision-making. The family frequently has difficulty perceiving the changes that are occurring and may resist a move from the level of care to which the resident is accustomed. The adjustment of the resident is enhanced when the family is involved and supportive of the move. The social worker tries to anticipate the need for change in advance since adjustment by both resident and family is more difficult when a sudden crisis necessitates immediate change. As part of the formal orientation procedure for new residents, the social worker conducts a seminar on level of care change. Long-time residents also are invited to reacquaint themselves with the procedure and ask questions.

The family is encouraged to maintain close involvement with the resident and to participate in the facility community. Social workers conduct formal group meetings with families and residents at least three times a year. These meetings enhance communication, educate, and provide support to families. They also serve as a forum to give and receive feedback on resident care. The social worker takes responsibility for transmitting concerns to the appropriate staff and conducts a follow-up to see that a response is made.

The social worker also is responsible for working with two resident's councils and linking them with the facility. One council, consisting of those in intermediate and skilled nursing care, requires greater assistance from the social worker in conducting meetings. The residents in more independent levels have their own constitution, elect their own officers, and establish committees to deal with all aspects of their lives. In both groups the social worker's role is quite similar. Residents are helped to develop their abilities to effect change in their environment. When their physical and/or mental capacities impose limits, the social worker serves as an advocate.

One of the most important functions of the social worker is in developing facility services and programs to meet the changing needs of the resident community and to address particular problems as they arise. For example, the increase in the number of residents with Alzheimer's and related disorders has resulted in the development and implementation of a program designed to enhance communication involvement with and awareness of their surroundings and to decrease daily anxiety (Talerico et al., 2002).

IV. Potential for Role Development

After admission, social workers are involved in every aspect of resident care in retirement communities. The unique characteristics of the social work profession make it integral to client well-being and quality of life in this setting. Social work also has been essential in achieving the organizational mission described in the introduction. The role of the social worker is an evolving one that must respond to changes in individual residents and the resident community, the overall organizational context, and the larger community. The responsiveness and flexibility of practitioners in meeting a broad spectrum of needs and providing a comprehensive array of services have been noteworthy.

The potential for developing the social work role can be identified in several areas. First, the preadmission phase provides several opportunities for role development. As pointed out by Smallegan (1985), the decision to institutionalize is a decision of last resort, often leaving the family and client feeling trapped. Although retirement communities promote opportunities for independence and autonomy, admission signals a decrease in ability to control one's life and environment. Two possibilities for enhancement of the social work role at this point can be identified:

1. Provision of preadmission support groups for families and applicants
2. Involvement of applicants in activities provided by the facility prior to admission

These would support and, perhaps, prolong in-home care and make the transition to the long-term care environment easier when it becomes necessary.

Second, social workers possess a wealth of knowledge and skills that could be shared with other staff. For example, staff with the least amount of education and training provide much of the basic care and many services. This includes nurses aides, dietary employees, and maintenance staff, among others. Increasing their knowledge could result in an enhanced quality of care, early detection of problems, and more comprehensive assessments. Training initiatives should encompass organizational and system factors to be most effective (Alyward et al., 2003).

Third, the social worker's understanding of cultural diversity issues could be utilized to develop programming consistent and supportive of the aging lifestyles and patterns of ethnic and minority groups. This could broaden the composition of the retirement community and draw on the strengths found in a diverse population.

Finally, social workers should continue to expand their current role in increasing opportunities for making choices and taking control. Elders who feel they have control over their lives and environment experience better adjustment, higher morale, and satisfaction (Ryden, 1984).

Case Example

The following case exemplifies many of the issues addressed by social workers in a continuing care facility. The intervention strategy and associated social work activities are those often required in this type of setting.

Mr. and Mrs. S are a white, middle-class married couple, aged 65 and 63, respectively. They applied for admission to the life care community at the instigation of their two children. Mr. S is a native of Akron, Ohio.

He is the youngest of three children and the only surviving member of his family. His family medical history reveals a high incidence of cancer, diabetes, and stroke. He was diagnosed as having Alzheimer's disease at the age of 60. He has a master's degree and was employed as a high school teacher until the age of 61 when periods of irritability and disorientation resulted in his early retirement.

Mrs. S is from Cleveland. She has two brothers who live out of state. Even though she reported a family history of heart disease, she had no serious medical problems. After raising a family, she completed a bachelor's degree and worked full-time as a librarian. She retired at age 59 in order to care for her husband. They own their home and are financially stable despite early retirement. Their son, age 44, and daughter, aged 38, both have families and time-consuming careers. One lives in Columbus and the other in Cleveland.

After retirement, Mr. and Mrs. S became increasingly isolated from their community. As Mr. S experienced a greater degree of confusion and memory loss, Mrs. S became increasingly overburdened with his need for supervision and with household responsibilities. At this point their son and daughter urged admission to Rockynol. An intake interview with Mr. and Mrs. S and their children took place in their home. Since sudden changes upset Mr. S, a guest visit was not recommended. During intake, his family reported that Mr. S was still able to engage in all aspects of self-care and had no problems with mobility. The son and daughter felt he needed a protective environment, while she needed relief from her mounting responsibilities. Mr. S was cooperative and friendly during the interview, but was unable to respond to questions. The social worker discussed their different needs and abilities to engage in facility activities. All agreed that independent living was not appropriate. Mrs. S, however, expressed a desire to continue performing a number of household tasks.

It was the social worker's impression that currently Mr. S could be maintained in congregate living with supportive programming to provide structure and routine activities. This would allow Mr. and Mrs. S to remain together as long as possible and relieve her of some of her caregiving responsibilities.

Soon after admission, the staff team met to reassess their individualized care plans. Staff observations confirmed that the family had overestimated Mr. S's ability to care for himself. Furthermore, the stress of relocation seemed to accelerate Mr. S's deterioration. He began wandering the halls at night, experienced increasing problems with toileting, and began failing in other areas. Although Mrs. S was adapting well to the community, making new friends and finding activities she enjoyed, she was exhausted due to his increased need for supervision.

The social worker met with Mrs. S and the family and discussed the need for a level change to accommodate their differing needs. Mrs. S acknowledged that she could not provide the degree of care her husband required and would like some freedom. Initially, their son and daughter were reluctant to accept the fact that their father's condition was worsening. Finally, after much discussion with the social worker, they became supportive of his move into assisted living. With her encouragement, they made the move a family event to lessen the effects of relocation. They visit both parents frequently.

During the day Mr. S is in a community daycare program for Alzheimer's patients. He can converse in complete sentences and engages in more self-care. He also has adapted to assisted living. As his Alzheimer's disease progresses, skilled nursing will become necessary. The social worker has helped his family prepare and plan for this eventuality.

Mrs. S appears relieved and comfortable. After a period of hospitalization following a mild stroke, Mrs. S has returned to congregate living. The social worker continues to monitor their progress, referring them for services as needed, keeping their family aware and involved, and helping them build a lifestyle that affords them satisfaction.

V.   Concluding Remarks

The number of life care communities is growing. The exact number varies, based on the definition used. These facilities offer a quality of care that is inaccessible to many of the elderly. Those who choose this living arrangement are offered a range of long-term care services in addition to basic services.

The nature of the practice setting and client composition affects the roles and responsibilities of social workers in several ways. On the one hand the range of resources available, including financial, personnel, and environmental, offer the practitioner an unusual variety of options in planning interventions. By the same token, these factors tend to broaden the scope of duties performed.

In addition, clients vary from the well, active elderly to the frail, bedridden, and unresponsive. Developing treatment plans that are truly individualized requires innovation and creativity.

Another feature is the long-term nature of the setting. Although the specific practice roles and responsibilities performed are found in many other settings, social workers in continuing care communities come to know each resident and family very well. They observe them interact, identifying strengths and limitations, and noting changes as they occur.

Finally, the entire residential community may be termed a type of milieu intervention. Interventions and treatment are an integral part of daily community life. In addition to responding to problems, the facility staff is actively involved in promoting growth and achievement of potential among the residents. The social work practitioner is an integral part of making the community effective.

References

Abramovice, B. (1988). *Long-term care administration*. New York: Haworth.

Aylward, S., Stolee, P., Keat, N., & Johncox, V. (2003). Effectiveness of continuing education in long-term care: A literature review. *The Gerontologist, 43*, 259–271.

Beaver, M.L. (1983). *Human service practice with the elderly*. Englewood Cliffs: Prentice-Hall.

Evashwick, C.J. & Weiss, L.J. (eds.). (1987). Managing the continuum of care. There was nothing else to do: Needs for care before nursing home admission. *The Gerontologist, 25*, 364–369.

Gaugler, J. & Zarit, S. (2001). The effectiveness of adult day services for disabled older people. *Journal of Aging & Social Policy, 12*, 23–47.

Jenkins, C. (2001). Resource effects on access to long-term care for frail older people. *Journal of Aging & Social Policy, 13*, 35–52.

Keating, N., Otfinowsky, P., Wenger, C., Fast, J., & Derksen, L. (2003). Understanding the caring capacity of informal networks of frail seniors: A case for care networks. *Aging and Society, 23*, 115–127.

Myers, J.E. (1989). *Adult children and aging parents*. Alexandria: American Association for Counseling and Development.

Neugarten, B.L. (1981). Growing old in 2020. *National Forum, 61*, 28–30.

O'Shaughnessy, C. & Price, R. (1987). Financing and delivery of long-term care services for the elderly. In C.J. Evashwick & L.J. Weiss (eds.), *Managing the continuum of care*, pp. 191–224. Rockville: Aspen.

Ryden, M.B. (1984). Morale and perceived control in institutionalized elderly. *Nursing Research, 33*, 130–136.

Smallegan, M. (1985). There was nothing else to do: Needs for care before nursing home admission. *The Gerontologist*, 25(4), 364–369.

Talerico, K., Evans, L., & Strumpf, N. (2002). Mental health correlates of aggression in nursing home residents with dementia. *The Gerontologist*, 42, 169–177.

Internet Resources

AARP
  Research Centre for Health and Long-Term Care.
  http://research.aarp.org/health/
American Association of Homes and Services for the Aging
  Long-term care links.
  http://www.aahsa.org/public/links2.htm
The Assisted Living Federation of America
  Dedicated to the assisted living industry and the population it serves.
  http://www.alfa.org/
The Continuing Care Accreditation Commission
  http://www.ccaconline.org
Long-Term Care Link
  A comprehensive source of long-term care information.
  http://www.longtermcarelink.net/

Additional Readings

Castle, N. & Banaszak-Holl, J. (2003). The effect of administrative resources on care in nursing homes. *Journal of Applied Gerontology*, 22(3), 405–424.

Fox-Hill, E., Gibson, D., & Engle, V. (2002). Nursing home experiences of older African Americans with HIV/AIDS: Issues for future research. *Journal of Mental Health & Aging*, 8(4), 319–330.

Hubbard, G., Tester, S., & Downs, M. (2003). Meaningful social interactions between older people in institutional care settings. *Ageing & Society*, 23(1), 99–114.

Lichtenburg, P., MacNeill, S., Lysack, C., Bank, A., & Neufeld, S. (2003). Predicting discharge and long-term outcome patterns for frail elders. *Rehabilitation Psychology*, 48(1), 37–43.

Reid, R. & Chappell, N. (2003). Staff ratios and resident outcomes in special care units: Do activity aides make a difference? *Journal of Applied Gerontology*, 22(1).

CHAPTER 22

SOCIAL WORK PRACTICE WITH GERIATRIC PATIENTS IN A REHABILITATION HOSPITAL

VIRGINIA L. FITCH, LEE R. SLIVINSKE, JANICE GREEN, AND DEBRA HINKSON

Social workers have worked with geriatric patients in rehabilitation settings for many years. In the rehabilitation hospital, due to its medical focus, two primary social work contributions are formally recognized: liaison to the patient's family and discharge planning. However, they perform many additional tasks. These include assessment, education, networking, mediation, advocacy, linkage with community resources, team participation, consultation, counselling, case management, and discharge planning, among others. The entire array of responsibilities they assume allows elderly patients and their families maximum participation in rehabilitation, fosters adaptation to remaining handicapping conditions, and enables the disabled elderly to have maximum lifestyle choices.

I.   Introduction

Edwin Shaw Hospital is an accredited rehabilitation hospital servicing the needs of people disabled by head trauma, amputations, strokes, spinal cord injuries, degenerative joint and muscle diseases, and other disabling illnesses and accidents. It is located in the state of Ohio in southeast Summit County. Although no geographical catchment area is designated, in practice the hospital is viewed as a regional rehabilitation centre serving a 15-county area.

Edwin Shaw is considered a county hospital and receives a percentage of its funding from Summit County. Because of its location and the funding relationship, members of the board of trustees are appointed by the Summit County executive director. The appointees are bipartisan and represent different sectors of the community, including educators, corporate executives, and health care experts, among others.

The hospital's mission is to serve as the region's leading centre for comprehensive medical rehabilitation. Its purpose is to reduce the extent of disability and maximize the long-term functional independence of patients physically, emotionally, vocationally, and in every other way. The comprehensiveness of the services provided makes it unique. The services include a skilled nursing unit, day hospital for adolescents and adults, chemical dependency unit for adolescents and adults, out-patient services, and a 70-bed in-patient rehabilitation program. This chapter will describe the activities of social workers with geriatric patients in the in-patient rehabilitation program.

II.   The Clientele

Social work practice in rehabilitation involves both disabled persons and their families as clients. The first part of this section reviews the impact of disability on the elderly. In the second part, the geriatric patients receiving services at Edwin Shaw are described.

A.   The Effects of Disability

In general, the most salient factor in the quality of life expressed by the aged is physical health status (Elwell & Maltbie-Crannel, 1981; Markides & Martin, 1979; Furchtgott et al., 1985). Ward (1984) has even suggested that being old results not from arriving at a particular age but from a combination of experiences and situations that make elders "feel old." A subsequent reduction in quality of life is then experienced.

The incidence of chronic illness and disability among older adults is well documented. However, declines in physical capabilities do not uniformly lead to decreases in well-being. The degree of decline and its effects on activity level are important considerations. In addition, changes in social conditions, including role loss and loss of important reference groups, may ensue. These deprive the aged of feedback regarding their competencies (Holahan & Holahan, 1987). Certain factors such as having options from which to choose, positive sources of self-validation, and social supports serve as mediators between impairment and the impact of the loss (Decker & Schultz, 1985).

For the individual, impairment precipitates a crisis both socially and emotionally. Fear and uncertainty about prognosis and the life change that will be necessitated are aroused. Alterations have to be made in self-image and in social and family roles (Feibel & Springer, 1982). The individual also is likely to experience loss of control over self and environment. In turn, loss of control may lead to further deterioration in physical and psychological well-being (Langer & Rodin, 1976; Schultz, 1976; Fitch & Slivinske, 1987). When a patient comprehends the extent of loss, the grieving process will begin. This point may be reached days, weeks, or months after the precipitating crisis.

Most elderly maintain regular contact with their family. Thus, changes in the elder's health status affect the entire family system. Usually the family is the primary provider when an elder needs long-term care (Monk, 1983; Pezzin & Spillman, 2000). A disabling illness places new demands on the family and generally results in some degree of crisis. New stressors are added to those already affecting the family system. Their impact is influenced by family beliefs about disability and health and prior experiences with illness. Roles, approaches to decision-making, and other patterned behaviours may need to be modified. Families vary in their ability to make the changes needed in order to cope. Their ability to respond will determine whether the family in crisis is incapacitated. Often an early response to the crisis is denial. A belief in full recovery may be maintained by the family while the patient refuses to accept the degree of life change required (DePompei et al., 1988). Other families become overprotective and overinvolved, further decreasing the control and independence available to the patient.

The caretaking is financially, physically, and emotionally draining. The caretaking role for the geriatric patient is most often assumed by the spouse, secondly the daughter, followed by the son, female relative, and male relative. Where the spouse is caretaker, in addition to the assumption of unfamiliar tasks, loss of personal life, and often isolation, he or she may have one or more chronic health conditions that require special care. Children who become caretakers are often called the "sandwich generation." They find themselves caught between the needs of the parent at the top, their children at the bottom, and their spouse in the middle (Myers, 1989; Zarit & Zarit, 1984). These problems are exacerbated by the decreasing size of families, leaving fewer people to provide help, and the increasing tendency for both spouses to work outside the home.

Although a certain level of adjustment to disability may be achieved by the elder and the family, changes in treatment, prognosis, and functional capacity inevitably produce further stress. Long-term adjustment will require continuing effort (DePompei et al., 1988).

B. Geriatric Patients in In-patient Rehabilitation

With a few exceptions, all geriatric patients at Edwin Shaw are referred from acute-care hospitals. They are admitted based on the belief that: (1) they have the potential to improve their level of functioning, and (2) they are medically able to participate in an intensive, comprehensive rehabilitation program (Cunningham et al., 2000). Therapies are provided based on these criteria. This distinguishes the rehabilitation centre from a skilled nursing facility. The impairment must impact on several of the person's abilities, and rehabilitation must include a comprehensive array of therapies. A patient who can benefit from only one therapy, such as an individual with a hip fracture, is not a candidate for admission.

Clientele are admitted by admissions personnel who determine rehabilitation potential and medical status. The patient is assigned to a nursing unit and a social worker is assigned to the patient. Each social worker has a caseload of approximately 17 to 18 patients and is assigned patients on one or two specific units. When possible, patients are assigned to a social worker by diagnosis so that expertise may be developed in working with a particular impairment.

Length of stay is not predetermined. Some progress or improvement has to occur in order to justify continued hospitalization. Each case is subject to review prior to discharge. Quality of life, indicated by improvement in mobility, interpersonal behaviour, communication, and the like, is a good outcome measure of rehabilitation (Bauer et al., 2003). The average length of stay is 32 days, although this varies somewhat by diagnosis.

Geriatric patients comprise approximately 75 percent of individuals receiving inpatient rehabilitation at Edwin Shaw. Over 60 percent are female. Racial composition appears representative of the proportion of black and white residents in the region. No age limit is placed on rehabilitation potential.

Each client represents unique problems that challenge the skills of the social worker. However, two case scenarios typify often-encountered life situations of geriatric patients with disabilities. In the first scenario, the elder lives alone and has chronic health problems. The most recent illness or injury interferes significantly with the level of autonomy and control and precipitates a crisis. Generally, a daughter becomes involved, providing physical, financial, and emotional support. She represents the sandwich generation, trying to care for an aging parent while balancing other roles and responsibilities toward spouse, children, and work (Myers, 1989). In the other scenario, one member of an elderly couple experiences a debilitating impairment. They live alone and have few informal support systems. They may have some formal supports from community agencies. Often the spouse has health conditions that interfere with the ability to be caretaker.

III. Practice Roles and Responsibilities

The roles and tasks of the social worker in a rehabilitation centre may appear similar to those found in other settings. In practice, they are enacted in unique ways. Since physical rehabilitation is the main purpose of the centre, the social worker performs roles and takes responsibilities that support this purpose. The hospital formally assigns the social worker two responsibilities: (1) liaison to the patient's family and (2) discharge planning. In addition to these roles, the social worker informally takes on many others, including those of broker, advocate, educator, case manager, enabler, mediator, team participant, and consultant.

In the rehabilitation process, the social worker functions as part of a multidisciplinary treatment team. The team, led by a physician, is composed of representatives from each department, including a nurse, speech therapist, physical therapist, occupational therapist, social worker, psychologist, nutritionist, and recreational therapist. Each member works with a patient and conducts an assessment based on its disciplinary task. Each assesses whether the treatment provided can benefit the patient. However, throughout the treatment process, from the day of admission until the day of discharge, the social worker is involved with each patient and family. Limited contact may take place after discharge. In general, this involves making referrals to community resources.

The initial contact with patient and family usually is made on the day of admission. Many experience their first contact with a social worker at this point. They often have misconceptions about social work that must be addressed. In addition to role clarification and establishing a helping relationship with the clients, the social worker has several tasks to accomplish. First, a beginning assessment of the patient and the patient's family must be done. Both are interviewed at the same time. Several areas are covered in the assessment. For example, the patient's previous level of functioning, coping skills, formal and informal support systems, home setting, including obstacles to mobility, living situation, and expectations for recovery and willingness for rehabilitation (Ushikubo, 1998), are explored. This information will help identify obstacles to adjustment after discharge. If the patient is unable to respond, the family will be the primary source of information. The social worker will attempt to include the patient's participation by eye contact or other non-verbal gestures.

For the family assessment, information on each member's sense of the patient's likely degree of recovery, previous roles and interactions with the patient, experience with chronic illness, and ability to participate in aftercare is elicited. The spouse's physical health and cognitive level also are important. The social worker needs to determine whether the spouse can participate in rehabilitation and be the caretaker physically, mentally, and emotionally. Often the spouse also is impaired and unable to provide care.

A separate appointment with the family may be scheduled if cues indicating conflict or disagreement are noted in the joint interview. At other times the family may request a meeting immediately to discuss a possible nursing home placement after discharge. At this point the social worker will address the issues involved in discharge planning at a preliminary level. Further discussion will occur during the patient's stay.

A second task during the initial interview is to educate the family about rehabilitation. Families are often overly optimistic about recovery and vary in their understanding of rehabilitation. The social worker will attempt to help the family understand that the elderly patient rarely returns to the normal previous level of functioning and will need some degree of support after discharge. Greater knowledge of the disability and clear expectations of rehabilitations have been found to be associated with better outcomes at discharge (Clark & Smith, 1999).

In addition, general orientation to the treatment process and the hospital environment is given. Terms such as OT (occupational therapy), RT (recreational therapy), and PT (physical therapy), among others, are explained. The social worker demystifies the process and empowers the client and family to participate effectively and have input in the rehabilitation process.

The third and final task, at this point, is to make an informal contract with the family. The contract will indicate the person(s) to serve as primary contact, how to reach them, and their plans for participating in treatment.

After completing the assessment, the information is recorded on a form that is placed in the patient's chart. The assessment is presented at the next team meeting. At the meeting, all information on the patient and family is summarized and developed into a highly individualized rehabilitation program. A baseline of current status and initial goals is established and tentative plans for projected length of stay are discussed.

Weekly team meetings are held with a review of each patient scheduled every two weeks. The social worker represents the patient and family and advocates for them. For instance, plans for discharge may be postponed if the social worker feels the family is unprepared to provide aftercare. Content from each meeting including all therapy reports, prognosis, projected length of stay, ongoing assessments, aftercare needs, equipment requirements, and the like are discussed with the family and explained by the social worker. The family in turn is encouraged to provide feedback regarding how the patient is coping and behavioural changes noted since the treatment began. Initial team assessments are revised and updated as new information emerges.

Throughout hospitalization, the social worker is viewed as a liaison. The team expects families to attend therapy training once a week. There they receive education about the patient's activities, kinds of assistance needed, and training in continuing therapies after discharge. Through the social worker, the team approaches the family and obtains their cooperation. The family views the social worker as a means of having input into team decision-making.

The mediator role also is often needed. On the one hand, if the rate of physical progress is not consistent with the patient's expectations, anger may be directed toward self, the health care system, hospital personnel, or anyone perceived as being at fault. On the other hand, a conflict may arise between team members and the family. The social worker helps facilitate a resolution of the problem.

During hospitalization, a minimum of one formal appointment is made to meet with the family and patient after each team evaluation.

Consistent with the concepts of personal assumption of responsibility and self-determination that are basic to rehabilitation, families are encouraged and expected to initiate contacts with the social worker whenever a need arises. The degree to which they do so varies. Each contact is documented in the medical chart and includes comments on the family dynamics observed and the social worker's activities and interventions.

Interventions such as counselling occur informally and often focus on problem solving and provision of social support. The family typically is the focus of many social work interventions. Still in a state of crisis, members require reassurance and help in dealing with role change, establishing new patterns of interaction, and in managing stress levels.

Discharge planning begins with the initial social work interview. As the time of discharge approaches, plans are finalized and written in summary form. The discharge plan usually addresses the following: when the patient is leaving and where, the identified caretaker, referrals for services, and equipment recommended. The social worker identifies the range of long-term care services available, acts as their guide in choosing services, and helps them explore their personal resources. Although discharge planning may appear to be a simple task, it is based on multiple contacts with the patient and family and community resources for the purpose of linking them. At times, discharge planning presents the social worker with a dilemma. A geriatric patient, without a family to provide needed aftercare, may choose to return home to live alone against medical advice. The patient's right to self-determination is held paramount. Aftercare decisions must be consistent with the patient's wishes unless he or she is adjudicated incompetent. A conflict between this principle and the value systems of other professions within the hospital may arise. The social worker will likely make a referral to adult protective services for follow-up. Where indicated, a court referral requesting a guardian appointment may be initiated.

IV.   Potential for Role Development

Social work's importance to successful medical treatment has been recognized for many decades (Bartlett, 1975). The process of rehabilitation in a medical setting tends to be very fragmenting with many disciplines making contributions. The social worker performs an integrating function and makes rehabilitation a more cohesive experience for the family and patient. Rehabilitation is placed in context through the social worker's contributions, which include psychosocial assessment, counselling, team participation, linkage of clients with community resources, and consultation to the other disciplines involved. The list of contributions is both comprehensive and impressive.

Nevertheless, several areas for role development can be identified. Development of these areas would require the provision of additional resources. First, outreach services providing follow-up to discharged geriatric patients and families would help to ensure continuity of rehabilitation and support. Achievement of an optimal level of functioning would be more likely with the addition of such services. Also, problems could be addressed before developing into a crisis.

Second, patients and families would benefit from support groups during hospitalization and after discharge. Groups are used very effectively in many rehabilitation settings. However, Medicare requirements for a daily therapy regimen in inpatient rehabilitation have eliminated a time for group meetings in many hospitals, including Edwin Shaw.

Third, although social workers often provide case management informally, a formal designation as case manager could enhance patient care. As noted by Kane (1981), this would allow them to formally coordinate services and integrate care within the hospital setting and ensure the patient is viewed holistically.

Finally, social work involvement in preadmission screening and assessment or in marketing strategies could result in better-informed patients and families. Often patients are admitted with no understanding of what will be expected of them. They are ill prepared to act assertively on their own behalf in the hospital setting.

V. Concluding Remarks

Social workers in a rehabilitation centre work closely with clients beginning with assessment and through discharge. The roles and tasks are the same regardless of diagnosis. However, the patient's age makes a significant difference in the problems they encounter and the resources available. They apply the principle of self-determination to enable patients with impairments to reach their potential and have maximum life choices. They recognize that the patient is part of a system also affected by the impairment. Interventions are formulated with the entire client system in mind. Physical rehabilitation is meaningful only to the extent that it returns the client system to a functional state. Social workers accomplish this by helping the patient and family fit the rehabilitation process into their lives.

As non-medical personnel, their roles and responsibilities often go unrecognized by other disciplines. The social work knowledge and skills brought to the setting may be less visible than the therapy regimens of other disciplines. Nevertheless, the outcome of rehabilitation would be less than successful without social workers. Although often credited only as discharge planners, they do much more. They assess the psychosocial impact of the impairment on patients and families, provide direct services to facilitate adaptation and post hospitalization planning, monitor and evaluate the effectiveness of discharge planning, and identify gaps in service in the community. In sum, through effective discharge planning and coordination with formal and informal systems, they see that the progress achieved during hospitalization is maintained after discharge. Rehabilitation succeeds, in large part, through their efforts.

Case Example

The case described in this section illustrates the importance of the social worker's contribution to rehabilitation. The unique problems and life situations of the geriatric patient also are evident.

Mr. M is a 69-year-old white male referred to Edwin Shaw Hospital for rehabilitation following a cerebral vascular accident (stroke). He is a native of Youngstown, Ohio, and is the youngest and only surviving one of five siblings. As a result of the stroke, Mr. M was unable to speak during the initial interview with the social worker. He was alert, oriented to place and time, but easily distracted. He was accompanied by his daughter, Joanne, age 32, and his ex-wife, age 58. Assessment information was obtained from them in his presence.

Mr. M completed a high school degree and was employed in a steel mill for 45 years until his retirement. He retired at age 63 due to complications arising from diabetes. At that time circulatory problems resulted in amputation of the left leg above the knee. He walks with the aid of a prosthesis and a walker. His income is modest and adequate for his needs until the recent expenses incurred as a result of the stroke.

Mr. M has been divorced 28 years and has one daughter. He remains on good terms with his former wife and her second husband. He is a member of a Greek Orthodox church, but rarely attends services.

All social activities involve his family. Joanne described him as kind, generous, and family oriented with a dislike for change. His lifestyle following the amputation has become a sedentary one. She reported that he coped well following the amputation. She described him in very loving terms and stated that he would cope well with the stroke as long as he could go home.

The social worker found the daughter and ex-wife to be very supportive. Both reside in Youngstown, approximately one hour from the hospital. Joanne is married and has three children, ages 14, 13, and 8. The youngest is hyperactive. She works full-time, but plans to visit every other night. Both she and her mother intend to participate in therapy education once a week.

Their expectations for his recovery differed. His former wife expressed concern that he would need nursing home placement after discharge. The daughter refused to consider a nursing home and expected her father to live with her and her family until he could return to his apartment.

The social worker's impression was that although the daughter had a high level of involvement, she verbalized unrealistic expectations. In addition to her work and family responsibilities, she refused to acknowledge the physical barriers present in her small rural home. All bedrooms were on the second floor, entries had several steps, and the first floor had no bathroom facilities. These would limit the patient's movements and capacity for developing independence. Mr. M's need for 24-hour supervision, equipment for aftercare, and out-patient rehabilitation therapy were beyond her physical, emotional, and financial capacities. When the social worker talked with Joanne about these concerns, she insisted that she could manage.

Mr. M was hospitalized for two months. Through rehabilitation, his mobility improved, although he continued to require assistance getting in and out of bed, bathing, toileting, and in other self-care. He was able to formulate simple sentences regarding his basic needs, but could not engage in conversations.

Joanne visited each week, but rarely attended therapy training sessions. She had counted on her mother's assistance. However, her mother experienced a mild coronary and was unable to help. The focus of social work intervention was to help the daughter to explore her roles at home with her family and at work, the resources available to her in the community and from informal supports, and her father's needs. Her anxiety and agitation grew as it became more obvious that she could not provide in-home care for her father. Three weeks prior to his discharge she was able to acknowledge this after his first overnight home visit. With the social worker's support, Joanne told her father that she was unable to provide the care he needed and that a nursing home placement would be necessary. For the first time, Mr. M realized the extent of his impairment and began the process of grieving for his loss. Joanne expressed feelings of guilt. The social worker helped Joanne and her father begin to work through their feelings. Together they developed an aftercare plan and identified options.

Joanne chose a skilled nursing home in the Youngstown area. Staff there were contacted by the social worker and arrangements were made to provide for his special needs. Mr. M was discharged into the facility. Although initially he was very upset, he became accepting of the arrangement. His family visits him frequently.

References

Bartlett, H. (1975). Ida M. Cannon: Pioneer in medical social work. *The Social Service Review*, 49, 208–228.

Bauer, B., Eisemann, M., Richter, J., & Schwarz, M. (2003). Quality of life as an indicator for successful geriatric inpatient rehabilitation—a validation study of the "Vienna List." *Archives of Gerontology and Geriatrics*, 37(3), 265–276.

Clark, M. & Smith, D. (1999). Psychological correlates of outcome following rehabilitation from stroke. *Clinical Rehabilitation*, 13(2), 129–140.

Cunningham, C., Hogan, F., & O'Neil, D. (2000). Clinical assessment of rehabilitation potential of the older patient: A pilot study. *Clinical Rehabilitation*, 14(2), 205–207.

Decker, S.D. & Schultz, R. (1985). Correlates of life satisfaction and depression among middle-aged and elderly spinal cord injured persons. *American Journal of Occupational Therapy*, 39, 740–745.

DePompei, R., Hall, D.E., West, J.D., & Zarski, J.J. (1988). Chronic illness: Stressors, the adjustment process, and family-focused interventions. *Journal of Mental Health Counseling*, 10, 145–158.

Elwell, F. & Maltbie-Crannel, A. (1981). The impact of role loss upon coping resources and life satisfaction of the elderly. *Journal of Gerontology*, 36, 223–232.

Feibel, J.H. & Springer, C.J. (1982). Depression and failure to resume social activities after stroke. *Archives of Physical Medical Rehabilitation*, 63, 275–280.

Fitch, V.L. & Slivinske, L.R. (1987). The effect of control-enhancing intervention of the well-being of elderly individuals in retirement communities. *The Gerontologist*, 27, 176–181.

Furchtgott, E., Karley, C., Milligan, W., & Powell, D. (1985). Physical health correlates of attitudes toward aging in the elderly. *Experimental Aging Research*, 11, 75–81.

Holahan, C.K. & Holahan, C.J. (1987). Correlates of life stress, hassles and self-efficacy in aging: A replication and extension. *Journal of Applied Social Psychology*, 17, 574–592.

Kane, R.A. (1981). Education for teamwork revisited: Caveats and cautions. In J. Brown, B. Kirlin, & S. Watt (eds.), *Rehabilitation services and the social work role: Challenge for change*, pp. 304–315. Baltimore: Williams and Watkins.

Langer, E.J. & Rodin, J. (1976). The effects of choice and enhanced personal responsibility for the aged: A field experiment in an institutional setting. *Journal of Personality and Social Psychology*, 34, 191–198.

Markides, K. & Martin, H. (1979). A casual model of life satisfaction among the elderly. *Journal of Gerontology*, 34, 86–93.

Monk, A. (1983). *Resolving grievances in the nursing home: A study of the ombudsman program*. New York: Columbia University Press.

Myers, Jane E. (1989). *Adult children and aging parents*. Dubuque: Kendall/Hunt.

Pezzin, L. & Spillman, B. (2000). Potential and active family caregivers: Changing networks and the "sandwich generation." *The Milbank Quarterly*, 78(3), 347–374.

Schultz, R. (1976). Effects of control and predictability on the psychological well-being of the institutionalized aged. *Journal of Personality and Social Psychology*, 33, 553–573.

Ushikubo, M. (1998). A study of factors facilitating and inhibiting the willingness of the institutionalized disabled elderly for rehabilitation: A United States–Japanese comparison. *Journal of Cross-Cultural Gerontology*, 13(2), 127–157.

Ward, R.A. (1984). The marginality and salience of being old: When is age relevant? *The Gerontologist*, 24, 227–232.

Zarit, S.H. & Zarit, J.M. (1984). Psychological approaches to families of the elderly. In M.G. Eisenbert, L.C. Sutkin, & M.A. Jansen (eds.), *Chronic illness and disability through the lifespan: Effects on self and family*, pp. 269–288. New York: Springer.

Internet Resources

Elderly Health Promotion, Disease Prevention, and Rehabilitation
    http://www.bham.ac.uk/arif/elderlyhealth.htm
Injury Prevention Web
    http://www.injurypreventionweb.org/
National Alliance for Caregiving
    http://www.caregiving.org/
Universal Health Care Action Network
    A national resource and strategic centre supporting organizations
    and advocates working for comprehensive, affordable, and publicly
    accountable health care for all in the U.S.
    http://www.uhcan.org/
University of Maryland Medicine
    How Is Stroke Recovery Managed?
    http://www.umm.edu/patiented/articles/how_stroke_recovery_
    managed_000045_10.htm

Additional Readings

Arksey, H. (2002). Combining informal care and work: Supporting careers in
    the workplace. *Health & Social Care in the Community, 10*(3), 151–161.
Caplan, L. & Schooler, C. (2003). The roles of fatalism, self-confidence,
    and intellectual resources in the disablement process in older adults.
    Psychology and Aging, 18(3), 551–561.
Deeg, D., Pot, A., & Van Dyck, R. (2000). Psychological distress of caregivers:
    Moderator effects of caregiver resources? *Patient Education and
    Counseling, 41*(2), 235–240.
De Witte, L., Meyboom-de Jong, B., Sanderman, R., Schure, L., & Van den
    Heuvel, E. (2001). Risk factors for burn-out in caregivers of stroke
    patients, and possibilities for intervention. *Clinical Rehabilitation, 15*(6),
    669–677.
White-Means, S. (2000). Racial patterns in disabled elderly persons' use of
    medical services. *Journals of Gerontology Series B: Psychological Sciences &
    Social Sciences, 55B*(2), S76–S90.

CHAPTER 23

ASSISTED LIVING, SOCIAL WORK PRACTICE, AND THE ELDERLY

ELAINE T. JURKOWSKI, MARGERY KEMP, AND SUSAN PATTERSON

Technological and medical advances within the Western world have led to adults living longer with varying degrees of functional ability. This, coupled with the rise of expectations for community-based alternatives to institutional care, has led to the development of an assisted living option for older adults and people with chronic health care conditions. This chapter provides some insights into the concept of assisted living, describes the clientele, explores the roles and responsibilities for social workers working in assisted living facilities, and compares and contrasts how social workers will carry out these roles within the spectrum of long-term care options. The chapter concludes with challenges and recommendations for social workers working with people who are older adults in assisted-living care settings.

I. Assisted Living Defined

The independent living movement, born in the 1960s in North America (DeJong, 1979) made a concerted effort to ensure people could remain living in their homes and in the least restrictive environment. The group of people with disabilities, who had originally sought community-based living options that were not based on the medical model, are now aging and demanding community-based options for people who are aging and in need of supportive-living services. The increased demand for community living options for people as they age has led to an option known as "assisted living," which is a step between independent living within one's own independent home or a senior living complex and skilled-nursing care. The concept of assisted living is in its infancy in both the United States and Canada, but is a growing form of semi-independent living option.

The initial concept of assisted living (AL) emerged in the United States in the mid-1970s when community care options with varying forms of assistance were possible. However, the term was not recognized nationally until the Assisted Living Federation of America was officially incorporated in 1992. AL offers service delivery options, which developed between two opposing needs: 24-hour availability of custodial care staff and help in daily living activities as opposed to the need to have one's own place where as many decisions as possible are still made by an older individual with the option of assistance. AL and shared housing are options for seniors who may not be able to live alone, but who need 24-hour nursing home care (Illinois Department on Aging, 1999). Such options allow seniors to choose from a "package of services," typically only the ones they will require, including meals, housekeeping, laundry, and assistance with activities of daily living (ADL).

Atchley (2000) described the apartment or accommodation settings characterized as AL facilities as "independent apartments with full bath and toilet facilities, kitchen space, lock-able doors, temperature controls for heating and cooling the unit and the residents' own furniture. These buildings usually include dining rooms, group cooking facilities, laundry and living rooms" (p. 347). In addition to housing, assisted living facilities can offer several types of specific services, namely: (i) assistance with cooking; (ii) assistance with housekeeping, and (iii) assistance with personal care. These are designed to assist with activities of daily living (AOL) and fall predominantly within the following two areas: (i) hotel-type services such as housekeeping, meals, and laundry; and (ii) personal care services such as help with walking, bathing, dressing, or grooming. Routine nursing services, such as catheter maintenance or skin care, and special care, such as service coordination, monitoring, or behaviour management, are found within some facilities, but not consistently across all facilities.

AL encourages family and community involvement, while the organizational mission maximizes dignity, privacy, and independence. Unlike nursing homes, which often provide care in routinized and standardized ways using regulatory guidelines as the benchmark for progress, such facilities are organizationally designed to deliver a customized constellation of services negotiated with the consumers and their families. Residents are assumed to be autonomous and capable of developing individualized care plans to meet their needs. While it appears that there are no real alternatives to nursing homes for those who have acute illnesses and long-term severe health needs, those who are suffering relatively lesser decrements in AOL functioning find AL to be an attractive alternative to a traditional long-term care facility when they can no longer live safely at home. AL maximizes dignity, privacy, and independence and supports the needs and preferences of individual tenants in private residential services.

AL is, in most North American locales, a solely privately funded alternative not generally available to those with lower incomes. Naturally, the private assisted-living industry has marketed its product to those individuals who can afford these services, and most AL facilities are placed in communities where there is an opportunity to target more the more affluent, older consumer.

In some places, however, alternatives for AL options that can be accessed by those in lower income groups are being developed. Some of this impetus stems from the desire of those who manage public funds to find a less expensive alternative to traditional long-term care in nursing homes. This is particularly so when it is realized that some individuals enter long-term care facilities only because there are no lesser viable alternatives, and are being maintained at an inappropriately high (and expensive) level of care. Since government programs in both the United States and Canada pay for long-term care when an individual's resources are not sufficient, this issue of care provision becomes a public as well as a private matter of concern.

II.   The Clientele

The typical client suited for AL is someone who has a need for help in instrumental activities of daily living (IADL), such as cooking, shopping, or transportation, getting to medical appointments etc., or may also have need for help in more personal aspects of ADL functioning, e.g., bathing or other personal care needs. The range of people and their ability levels, when considering the target client type for assisted living, is broad. Some are almost independent, but not quite up to living alone comfortably. They will find AL to be the place where accommodations need to be made as they become less able to do things for themselves. Others will have moderate to fairly demanding IADL and ADL needs for AL facilities.

AL is less appropriate as persons evolve to a need for a nursing home level of care, either because they require specialized nursing care on a long-term basis, or because they are almost totally dependent on staff for almost all ADLs. Similarly, individuals who have been diagnosed as having mild or beginning dementia may find AL fits their needs perfectly for a while. With meals, cleaning, scheduling reminders, and activities provided, this type of client can have support without an overly restrictive institutional level of care. However, once dementia becomes severe, another placement will probably be necessary.

Barrow and Hiller (1999) described those who utilized AL services as engaged in a conscious "hands-off" approach to care. They received whatever services were necessary in order to maximize their independence. The clientele within this context can be contrasted with those in nursing homes or board and room care, where a "hands-on" approach to providing assistance with all one's needs is a necessity.

III. Practice Roles and Responsibilities

In light of the description of the concept of AL, one may ask the question: Is it effective and should social workers promote this as a viable option for care? Some researchers have begun to examine the efficacy of the model, but the empirical evidence to answer these questions is still in its infancy. For instance, Sikorska (1999) examined the relationship between organizational factions and resident satisfaction with AL. In this study, 13 facilities were sampled to create a population cohort of 156 residents. The findings revealed that the more satisfied residents were happier, more functionally independent, more involved in housing decisions, and less educated. The highest satisfied group of residents was in smaller facilities, had moderate levels of physical amenities, greater availability of personal space, fewer socio-recreational activities, and non-profit ownership. Similarly, Capitman, Leutz, Sceigaj, and Yee (1999) surveyed administrators, staff, and residents in 20 AL facilities. Residents suggested that they led independent lives; however, health and long-term care needs were unmet, and they reported limited participation in community-based activities. These researchers concluded that AL settings offered elders a safe and independent living opportunity; however, AL facilities did not necessarily promote choice, community building, and care.

Turning to the issue of practice roles, Hill et al. (1999) identified several roles for social workers as components in generalist practice.

These include counsellor, educator, broker, case manager, mobilizer, mediator, facilitator, and advocate.

As indicated in Figure 23.1, the *counsellor* provides support, encouragement, and suggestions, while the *educator* conveys information to the client, provides group participants with new information, structures presentations, and uses modelling to help members within the group setting adopt new skills/behaviours. Within AL settings, the role of counsellor provides supportive counselling services to include problem-solving, empowerment, and psychosocial issues of adjustment. These issues generally relate to loss, change, and transitions and adaptation. Counselling may also be directed at encouraging functional activity on the part of the individual. Counselling may also include dealing with depression. Hence the role is somewhat different in AL settings (see Figure 23.1), when compared to community and skilled-nursing care, because the focus of intervention in AL facilities is to maximize the individuals' capacity for independence (Wilson, 1996).

The *broker* links clients with needed services, and helps clients obtain needed resources by connecting them with community agencies. Within AL settings, clients are offered information about connections they can choose to make. Since such facilities are not regulated for a standard level of care, social workers are not mandated to actually carry out the necessary connections to "broker" for services per se, as would be required in board and care, or nursing home settings. Hence, the *case manager/mobilizer* seeks out resources, plans service delivery, and monitors progress. In AL settings, a customized yet flexible individualized care plan is developed for the individual and negotiated between the facility, individuals, and their family, with a vision of maximizing independence. In contrast, the nursing home or continuing care options provide specific, medically based care delivered as a result of standardized care plans based upon levels of nursing care/service needed.

The *mediator* helps conflicting parties settle disputes and agree on compromises. In AL settings, this role may include mediating the perception of resident needs and maximizing options for independence. The focus of mediation usually takes place between family members and the individual resident, or between residents. The *facilitator* guides or expedites the way for others, while the advocate champions the rights of others. The focus of *advocacy* efforts within AL settings are designed

Figure 23.1: Practice Roles Compared and Contrasted across Three Settings: Assisted Living, Long-Term Care or Skilled Nursing, and Community-Based Home Settings

Roles	Activities within Assisted-Living Setting	Long-Term Care or Skilled Nursing	Community-Based Home Setting
Counsellor	• Support to client as needed • Issues related to maintaining independence, adjustment to setting	• Daily support may not include any level of intense counselling issues	• Referral to mental health agency
Educator	• Training on health promotion and prevention issues • Individual and group settings • Support groups for families	• Arrangements often made with external resources for programs/ services/ presentations	• Individualized based upon individual need • Can include community-based support groups
Broker	• Assist with application for services, funding mechanisms, etc. • Level of services to be input is fairly independent • Goal is to maximize independence	• Assist with application for services directed as medically necessary, custodial, or to the medical needs of individual • Focus is medical model in orientation	
Case manager/ mobilizer	• Oversees and arranges for services • Networking and advocacy services		
Mediator	• Often includes families and consumer and focus of mediation directed between expectations of independence	• Between clients, service providers/owner of facility • Focus is on best strategies for care, quality of care, etc.	• Between family members only • Focus is directed on bridging family supports to meet needs of individual

con't

Figure 23.1 (continued)

Facilitator	• Similar to other roles in accessing services		
Advocate	• Advocate for client rights • Advocacy on a systems level • Advocacy for improved resources	• Advocacy for the development of new resources/ additional care facilities	• Advocacy for increased level of community-based services

to maximize independence, while normally the advocacy efforts in nursing home or continuing care settings focus on improved medical, nursing, or custodial care.

McMahon (1996) and Hill et al. (1999) identified several stages within generalist practice framework. Inherent within the problem-solving model are several steps within which social work practice is exercised. These include engagement, assessment, data collection, planning, intervention, evaluation, termination, and follow-up. While these steps are transferable across various practice settings [as indicated in numerous chapters in Section II of this text], it is important to understand how they may be similar or different, depending upon the setting in which the social worker is working.

In Figure 23.2, in the *engagement* phase, the social worker aims to develop rapport, build relationships that will lead to problem-solving, and introduce the service components available to the client. In AL settings, social workers strive to develop a relationship in the engagement phase, which will [typically] lead toward a long-term working relationship with the client. This is in direct contrast to the process of engagement, which occurs in a long-term care or skilled-nursing care settings, whereby cognitive impairments on the part of the individual may interfere with establishing this relationship.

In the *assessment* phase, AL options seek opportunities that maximize rehabilitation plans, with a focus on functional ADLs and IADLs. The focus here is rooted in a rehabilitation and social/independent living paradigm in contrast to a medical model, which guides the assessment process in a long-term care or skilled-nursing care facility.

The AL social worker's role in the next *planning phase* will be similar across all settings in the sense that the social worker works with the individual, regardless of ability level or impairment. The

Figure 23.2: Steps in the Social Work Process Compared and Contrasted across Three Settings: Assisted Living, Long-Term Care or Skilled Nursing, and Community-Based Home Settings

Steps in the Generalist Intervention Model		Community-Based Home Settings	Assisted-Living Options	Long-Term Care or Skilled-Nursing Care
Engagement	Similarities	• Families as well as clients		
	Differences	• Short-term relationship	• Working in a long-term relationship	• Impairments may interfere with relationship
Assessment	Similarities	• Social model		• Medical model
	Differences	• Consider person-in-environment model and strengths-based approach	• Opportunities to maximize rehabilitation plans • Examine functional status in activities of daily living and instrumental activities of daily living	• Assessment tools focus on care needs • Regulatory paperwork
Planning	Similarities	• Working with individual, needs based upon abilities despite impairment		
	Differences	• Focus on care plan based upon medical need	• Focus on a customized individualized plan negotiated with consumer	• Staff members as well as consultants are part of the planning process
Intervention	Similarities	• All levels include client consent and active participation in intervention		• In the real world, less likely at this level
	Differences	• Uses a variety of community resources	• Blend between community and in-house	• In-house interventions

con't

Figure 23.2 (continued)

Evaluation	Similarities	• Need to better document outcomes and practice interventions across all settings		
	Differences	• Focus is on maintaining stability	• Study is in infancy • Focus is on maximizing independence	• Focus is on medical and health outcomes
Termination	Differences	• Results in move to nursing home facility	• Usually results in move to facility with higher level of care	• Usually results due to death of resident
Follow-up	Differences	• Monitor the level of service and individual need	• Monitor of efficacy of services	• Client satisfaction with facility

main difference in AL settings is that the focus of the care plan is on a customized, flexible, individualized plan negotiated with the consumers, which is designed to maximize their strengths, while in nursing care or community care settings, the focus is to maximize the safety needs of the individual through a medical model's auspices. In addition, such AL plans are designed to be revisited and amended with consumers as their needs and situations change in the future.

Social workers design *interventions* with their clients in order to assist in achieving the clients' goals. Interventions generally are designed between in-home and community-based resources within an AL facility. In contrast, community-based care offering home health services use a variety of intact community resources. Social workers working in skilled-nursing care settings typically design interventions for their clients based upon resources and services offered solely "in-house."

Social workers also have a responsibility to *evaluate* the impact of their care plans and interventions, document outcomes, and identify areas for further intervention or recommend termination. The practice of evaluation is standard across all three settings; however, the focus differs. The outcome desired in AL settings will is to maximize independence, while the outcome [dependent variable] in a long-term care/skilled-nursing care setting is to focus on medical and health outcomes. Hence, while evaluation of practice occurs across all settings, the outcome or focus [dependent variable] differs.

Social workers do not engage in competent social work practice without considering the final stage of the process, termination. *Termination* of residency in an AL facility usually occurs due to a need for a higher level of care or need for skilled-nursing care. Termination from long-term care or skilled-nursing care usually results due to the eventual passing on of residents. Finally, as indicated in Figure 23.2, the role of *follow-up* includes an evaluation of the efficacy of services, the need to monitor the levels of service and individual needs, as well as client satisfaction with services and the facility. While all three can occur within all settings, the emphasis in AL settings is on monitoring the efficacy of services as related directly to client satisfaction (as they are the "paying customers").

In summary, the roles of social workers, working within AL settings, will be somewhat different from working with the elderly in long-term care or skilled-nursing facilities. This is largely due to the difference in focus (independence), and in the overriding philosophy (social/rehabilitation model versus a medical model).

III.   Potential for Role Development

Foremost, in general social workers, employed in settings focused on for-profit motives, need to develop their identity and standards around ethical social work practice. Dilemmas may ensue between social workers co-ordinating services (fee-for-service basis) offered on-site (e.g., meal preparation, dining, laundry) and negating the potential of the individuals and their actual ability, or maximizing their own potential for independent action.

As well, social workers will need to develop a comfort level with making public presentations both in group and community settings. Group presentations for individuals, family members, and members will be required both on issues related to the aging process, and the alternatives to long-term care that will include AL. Within the macro-practice arena, one may need to challenge the community of prejudices related to aging and potential disability (Gilson, 2000). In addition, an educational process may need to be developed to challenge the medical model perspective of social work, and adapt features of a community-living model. Understanding medical aspects of aging will inevitably be important within the vision of a community-living perspective.

Another area for role development will include the need for counselling related to psychosocial issues of adjustment. These will usually relate to loss, change, and transitions. The adaptation process will involve stages of disbelief, developing awareness, reorganization, resolution, and identity change (Mackelsprang & Salsgiver, 1999).

More frequent contacts, especially for social workers who work on-site, will mean an increase in demand for case management. There will be a need to work at empowering individuals, but the level of contact will differ because the focus will be on maintaining the consumer/clients' independence.

Social workers will also need to develop skills in advocacy for changes in funding mechanisms, Medicaid or Medicare coverage, and Blue Cross coverages. In addition, it will be necessary to take legal action when necessary, and to provide evidence when appropriate. The role of advocacy will also require that documentation, quality assurance, and monitoring be maintained, so that records can support advocacy claims. As AL facilities become increasingly in vogue, there will be an increased demand for advocacy and documentation.

The evaluation of practice, outcomes, and impact of these congregate-living settings is limited because of the dearth of empirical evidence available. AL social workers will need to examine the role facilities play, impact on functional status, maintenance of specific ADL, and impact of social support. Social workers can also contribute to our understanding of these facilities and their impact for their consumers in areas such as physical health status, functional abilities, psychosocial well-being, consumer satisfaction, autonomy, utilization and cost of hospitals, physicians, and other services.

Another role for future development in the area of AL social work is marketing. As AL becomes less the exclusive province of the profit-driven industry, and its potential for diverting individuals from unnecessarily expensive and restrictive nursing home care are recognized entities such as state governments or not-for-profit agencies, there will be efforts to reach out to moderate- to lower-income individuals. Social workers may find that their traditional roles as brokers, educators, or providers of linkages need to be expanded to take on the focus of marketing for an AL facility. For instance, they may have to present to interested community groups or groups of potential consumers and their families about the concept of AL and about the characteristics of the particular facility that they represent. They may also have to meet with interested consumers and/or families at the AL residence, and provide a tour and informational material on the services available, as well as answer questions in person or by phone. This is both an appropriate and meaningful role as long as there is no effort to sell that which is inappropriate for client needs. Thus, the focus is on providing needed information and helping the consumers and their families begin the assessment process of identifying what their needs are, and whether AL fits those needs. While the role of marketing is important and seems "on the horizon," in this record, most social workers are uncomfortable with this role, and there is definitely a need for more role development in this area.

Social workers will also need to become familiar with financial-assistance programs as well as more complex issues such as insurance, wills, trusts, property, etc. Many social workers may have familiarity with the financial profiles and needs of the poor elderly, but may not be as familiar with or versed in financial strategies involving trusts or stocks/investment portfolios of healthier elderly. Thus, they may need to expand their knowledge base in order to help potential residents determine their ability to private pay for AL options.

When considering the role of brokerage with finances and macro practice settings, it is necessary to utilize creative funding options, to include waivers, tax incentives, etc., in efforts to reach clients who may be low income but interested in AL opportunities. In the United States, for example, there are some funding options available for housing to accommodate the low-income elderly with incomes of $15,000 or less. Section 42 of the *Internal Revenue Tax Code* provides a low-income housing tax credit to corporations investing in low-income elder housing. Medicaid offers a home and community-based waiver that allows for the financing of health care services in an AL setting. The challenge here [for social workers] will be to design programs that can utilize these options and reach those elderly who have limited incomes. In Canada, AL options have been primarily limited to people who have the means to privately pay for such services. An area for role development will include skills to effectively negotiate program and policy options to similarly accommodate the low-income and moderate-income elderly to also benefit from AL options.

In summary, social workers interested in working in AL settings and people who are growing older may be confronted with a wide range of areas for role development. These can include brokerage with finances, marketing, facility management, evaluation and research, ethical practice, documentation and case management, education, advocacy, and counselling. They also include [in the current financial reality] keeping the consumers happy with the services they provide—a role that may involve some interesting challenges for social workers unaccustomed to working in upper-income fee-for-service facilities.

IV. Concluding Remarks

Certainly, as the literature has documented, a majority of older people prefer to live within the comforts of their own home. For older people [as for most of society] home represents comfort, security, and control over one's immediate environment. By extension, control of the immediate environment means control over one's life as well, and the issues of control and independent decision making become even more important when an individual begins to fear that s/he might not be able to retain such control because of the physical or mental decrements that can accompany aging. This preference for "aging in place" even as one becomes more frail and more dependent is one of the primary factors that has led to development of some in-home services, either privately or publicly paid, which can enable people to live more comfortably and safely at home, even as they are experiencing health concerns, physical debilitation, or impairment of mental functioning, such as the onset of Alzheimer's disease.

The institutional bias within our society prevails, however, and public monies for long-term care services are still diverted overwhelmingly to institutional care. Publicly funded in-home services typically have delimited criteria and are in short duration (e.g., Medicare-funded Home Health care), or if provided for the long term, are still only intermittent, and often do not provide the number of hours that may be needed to fulfill funding dispersement allocations.

Even families of individuals who can afford to hire care for themselves often encounter significant problems. These may include:

- advertising, interviewing, and checking references for applicants: This is a difficult process for many families, and can be even harder for the older individuals who must do it on their own;
- hiring someone who has the knowledge, skills, and personality suited to a caregiving situation, and who will be reliable (and, if 24-hour care is needed, this usually means

finding at least two or three people who meet that criteria);
and finally
• private pay care is usually quite expensive and will often
  present a financial burden that cannot be sustained over a
  long period of time.

Institutional care, such as that offered in many nursing homes (or
long-term care facilities), may often be the only viable alternative an
older person has. Long-term care facilities accept public funds, are
staffed 24 hours a day, they offer health care for the person who has
ongoing health care needs, they provide assistance with ADL for those
who can no longer pay for their care.

What most long-term care facilities do not offer (and perhaps for the
most part cannot offer because of their existing structure and purpose)
are some of the very elements that people value the most: the comfort
and security of their own home, and the feeling of independence that
comes from being in control of one's own surroundings. As this chapter
has demonstrated, AL provides these opportunities in a unique case
management that has profound implications for the future of both the
elderly and the social work profession. As indicated, social workers in
the future can anticipate a growth in opportunities to working in AL
settings with unique roles, responsibilities, and challenges that will be
important for the actualization of these settings to provide competent,
respectful, and efficacious care.

Case example

Joan was a 65-year-old African American female with a sixth grade
education, who had not worked for several years due to a chronic
disability. She had been living with a daughter and son-in law for
several months following the death of her husband. The family
homestead where Joan lived for her entire life had been sold, and her
possessions put in storage in one of the storage units within the storage
company owned by her daughter and son-in-law. Joan had done the
cooking for her husband and the cadre of farmhands who worked on
the family farm for several years prior to her husband's death. She
had also taken care of the day-to-day laundry regularly, while items
for pressing went to the local dry cleaners. Joan had a driver's licence,
but chose not to drive regularly since her late husband enjoyed the
role of chauffeur.

Despite the loving and doting nature of Joan's daughter, Joan often felt intimidated by her as she took over all decision-making for her widowed mother, and insisted on letting the housekeeper do all of the cooking, laundry, and other household chores for the entire family.

Medically, Joan had recently undergone bypass surgery and was a diabetic. She also had developed some mental health issues. The conditions required her to take several medications on a daily basis, but due to the nature of her illnesses, her medications changed every several months.

Joan's situation came to the attention of Shawnee Alliance's Abuse, Neglect, and Exploitation (ANE) program when the housekeeper reported the family situation. Joan had repeatedly shared with the housekeeper her feelings of intimidation resulting from her relationship with [her] daughter. The housekeeper also noticed on several occasions that Joan's daughter refused to allow the mother to go to the bank and shopping mall on family outings with the family, left her mother at home alone, and suggested the family would "buy her some treats."

Consistently, the housekeeper noticed on such occasions that Joan would break down into tears for hours upon the exodus of the family.

The case manager explored the circumstances that led Joan to the point of referral to the ANE program. After interviewing Joan, the case manager understood Joan's viewpoint. Joan felt that her daughter had been intimidating, but also taken many of the things that Joan enjoyed doing from her repertoire of activities. In addition, Joan felt that she did not have an opportunity to thrive socially and meet other people who had been recently widowed or who could understand the experience.

The case manager proceeded to conduct an overall assessment of needs through using an assessment scale known as the "Determination of Need" (DON) index. The DON is a tool with a series of questions that are used to measure a person's physical and cognitive ability to function independently, and is focused specifically on Assisted Daily Living (ADL) tasks such as bathing, getting out of bed, dressing, housecleaning, feeding, and doing laundry. In addition, a second segment examines the Instrumental Activities of Daily Living (IADLs) to include shopping, banking, cooking, getting to medical appointments, and using the telephone.

Overall, Joan was capable of living in her own domicile and conducting ADLs; however, [she] felt that she would like to have some assistance with ironing her clothes. Although she needed someone to drive her to the local shopping mall and help her with loading and unloading groceries, she was capable of taking care of some her IADLs.

Following a tour of the Big Muddy Assisted Living Facility, and several meetings with Joan, her daughter, son-in-law, and case manager, it was decided that Joan would consider an Assisted Living Option at the Big Muddy Assisted Living Facility, which was located about 25 miles from where her daughter and daughter's family lived. Joan would have a one-bedroom unit with a living room/sitting area, kitchen, and bathroom. Home-care services would provide housecleaning and assistance with laundry (especially ironing) on a weekly basis. The van and transportation service, coupled with the local "Ride Share" program, would provide transportation to medical appointments and to the local mall for groceries or other shopping needs. The driver and their assistant would be responsible for loading and unloading groceries from the store, into the van, and from the van to the domicile unit. Lastly, the case worker encouraged Joan to attend the social programs offered within Big Muddy daily, where she could meet other residents. A referral was also forwarded to the on-site case manager to enable Joan's participation in the weekly bereavement and coping support group and women's health group, facilitated by the on-site case manager.

Three months following Joan's arrival, she reported to the case manager that she felt alive again, but still experienced feelings of intimidation when her daughter and family came to visit. The case manager worked with Joan to role play scenarios with Joan, so that she could feel a sense of independence and strength when communicating with her daughter. The case manager also offered to assist in mediation between the two when situations of conflict would arise.

References

Atchley, R. (2000). *The social forces of aging: An introduction to social gerontology.* Belmont: Wadsworth.

Barrow, G. & Hiller, S. (1999). *Aging, the individual and society.* Belmont: Wadsworth.

Capitman, J., Leutz, W., Sceigaj, M., & Yee, D. (1999). Resident-centered care in assisted living. *Journal of Aging & Social Policy,* 10(3), 7–9.

DeJong, G. (1979). Independent living: From social movement to analytic paradigm. *Archives of Physical Medicine and Rehabilitation,* 60, 435–446.

Gilson, S.F. (2000). Disability and aging. In R. Schneider & N. Kroph (eds.), *Gerontological social work: Knowledge service settings and special populations*, 2nd ed., pp. 368–395. Belmont: Brooks Cole.

Hill, G., Kurst-Asshman, K., & Vogel, V. (1999). *Understanding generalist practice*, 2nd ed. Chicago: Nelson Hall Publishers.

Illinois Department on Aging. (1999). Fact sheet on assisted living and shared housing. Springfield: Illinois Department on Aging.

Kane, R. & Wilson, K.B. (1993). *Assisted living in the United States: A new paradigm for residential care for frail older persons*. Washington: American Association of Retired Persons.

Litwin, H. (1998). The provision of informal support by elderly people residing in assisted living facilities. *The Gerontologist*, 38(2), 239–247.

Mackelprang, R. & Salsgiver, R. (1999). *Disability: A diversity model approach to human service practice*. Belmont: Brooks Cole.

McMahon, M. (1996). *The generalist method of social work practice*. Toronto: Allyn & Bacon.

Regnier, V. (1996). Factors affecting the growth of assisted living. *The supportive housing connection*. San Francisco: National Resources and Policy Center on Housing and Long-Term Care.

Seifert, A. (1999). Thoughts from the front line. *Assisted Living Today*, 6(7). Assisted Living Federation of America.

Sikorska, E. (1999). Organizational determinants of resident satisfaction with assisted living. *The Gerontologist*, 39(4), 450–457.

Welton, E.P. (1999). How to choose a residence: Making the right choice easier. *Assisted Living Today*, 6(8).

Wilson, K.B. (1996). *Assisted living: Reconceptualizing regulations to meet consumers' needs and preferences*. Washington: American Association for Retired Persons.

Internet Resources

The Assisted Living Federation
> Provides a perspective from assisted living providers.
> http://www.alfa.org

The Assisted Living Workgroup
> An advocacy group that assures quality in assisted living and offers guidelines for federal and state policy, state regulations, and operations.
> http://www.aahsa.org/alw.htm

Canada's Care Guide
> Everything under the sun related to seniors' housing and care in Canada. It provides tools and information to help one make informed

decisions about housing, care services, and other related issues.
http://www.thecareguide.com
The Consumer Consortium on Assisted Living
   This site provides information to consumers and their loved ones on
   issues about assisted living.
   http://www.ccal.org
FIRSTGOV for Seniors
   An overview of key concepts and issues related to Assisted Living
   developed by the United States government.
   http://www.seniors.gov/retirementplanner/housing/assisted_living.html
The National Centre for Assisted Living
   A collection of broad-based groups that have coalesced to create an
   advocacy and educational collective for the benefit of assisted living.
   http://www.ncal.org/

Additional Readings

Cummings, S.M. (2002). Predictors of psychological well-being among
   assisted-living residents. *Health and Social Work,* 27(4), 293–302.
Feinberg, R.K. (2002). The increasing need for social workers in assisted
   living. *Journal of Social Work in Long-Term Care,* 1(3), 9–12.
Franks, J. (2002). Social workers need to know more about assisted living
   and vice versa. *Journal of Social Work in Long-Term Care,* 1(3), 13–16.
Weiner, A.S. (2002). Social work practice—clinical, programmatic and
   training dimensions: The role of social work in assisted living. *Journal of
   Social Work in Long-Term Care* (entire-issue), 1(3), 1–2.
Williams, H.M. (2002). Social work skills in assisted living. *Journal of Social
   Work in Long-Term Care,* 1(3), 5–8.

CHAPTER 24

SOCIAL WORK PRACTICE IN COMMUNITY PSYCHOGERIATRIC PROGRAMS

DARLENE H. KINDIAK, JANE L. GRIEVE, GLEN E. RANDALL, AND VICTORIA A. MADSEN

This chapter discusses psychogeriatric practice and describes the clinical and administrative roles that have emerged for social workers on community psychogeriatric teams. An overview of both the macro system (the health care reforms in Ontario) and micro system (the specialized areas of knowledge) provide a context to understanding the roles, responsibilities, and challenges facing social workers in providing specialized community-based psychogeriatric services. Within these roles, the variety of responsibilities, along with the complexities involved, is outlined. Discussion is oriented toward future trends and the importance of education and training for social workers working in this field.

I. Introduction

Community psychogeriatric services are regarded as a valuable and growing area of specialty within the mental health field. One of the first full-time Canadian psychogeriatric programs was established at Ottawa General Hospital in 1976, under the direction of Dr. David Harris, with the support of Dr. Gerald Sarwer-Foner (Harris personal communication, August 18, 1993). Due to an ever-increasing number and proportion of the elderly in Canada, along with an emphasis on maintaining individuals in the community, a growing number of outreach psychogeriatric services have been established across the country.

Within the province of Ontario, there are currently more than 50 community psychogeriatric programs whose mandate is to service the mental health needs of elderly persons. While there is no standard age to be eligible for services (they can range from 50 to 70 years of age), most psychogeriatric programs are targeted to those 65 years of age and older. These programs are primarily based on three types of models: assessment/consultation; assessment/consultation and treatment; and assessment/consultation, treatment, and teaching. These programs tend to differ according to their sponsorship (teaching hospital, non-teaching hospital, community mental health clinic, etc.); location (urban or mixed); composition of team members (social workers, nurses, occupational therapists, psychologists, psychiatrists, etc.); and team size (ranging from one to ten clinical staff). In the past, there had been no established norm of service delivery, with programs typically operating idiosyncratically. However, more recently, through the ongoing cooperative efforts of Ontario's psychogeriatric teams, there has been progress toward an established service delivery approach.

Due to the multifaceted biological, psychological, and social problems frequently presented by elderly clients, the social worker is challenged to broaden his or her clinical knowledge and skills in order to work effectively with this population. There is also a need for social workers to be able to articulate and delineate their roles within the context of the multidisciplinary team. The specific mandate of the program, the parameters that define each program model, the blend of disciplines, the history of inter/multidisciplinary functioning within the organization, plus the amount of flexibility that each social worker is comfortable maintaining, inevitably determines the role that the social worker formulates within each setting.

The role of the social worker in community psychogeriatric programs has typically had three different components: clinical, administrative, and a dual one (both clinical and administrative). While each of these may be clearly outlined in job descriptions specific to each work environment, the overlapping of functions and the degree of support received within the sponsoring organization ultimately affects the range of responsibilities that are translated into practice. Regardless of the specific position the social worker fills within a psychogeriatric program, it is essential that s/he has a clear understanding of the broader macro-system environment within which the program must function. This includes gaining knowledge of ongoing health care reforms and their impact on the psychogeriatric field.

A. Health Care Reform: The Ontario Context

At the beginning of the 21st century, health care continues to be at the centre of much of the political and economic debate in Canada. In 2002, two major federal government-sponsored reports on health care were released. The first was the *Kirby Report*, produced by the Standing Senate Committee on Social Affairs, Science, and Technology under the chairmanship of Senator Kirby (Kirby, 2002). The second was a report from the Commission on the Future of Health Care in Canada, led by Roy Romanow (Romanow, 2002). Both reports concluded that there remains strong public support for medicare and the *Canada Health Act*, as well as a need for health care reform.

Despite this general public support for Canada's health care system, all governments in Canada are grappling with growing health care costs and public demands for services in the face of seemingly conflicting public pressure to limit government spending and to bring government debt under control. In Ontario, the result has been cuts to the budgets of most health care provider organizations and a sustained period of confusion, frustration, and anxiety as health care reforms are implemented. It is within this broader context of health care reform, fiscal restraint, and growing public demand for services that psychogeriatric programs in Ontario have been struggling to provide adequate community-based mental health services for seniors.

Throughout most of the 1970s and 1980s, both institutional and community-based health care services in Ontario expanded dramatically. However, the lack of a grand vision of how the system should evolve, combined with the "piecemeal" addition of services, has contributed to an increasingly fragmented and inefficient health care system. This was especially true of community-based services. Many of these, including psychogeriatric programs, were offered through different sponsoring agencies, had different levels of funding, and their ability to meet community needs varied widely throughout the province.

Most importantly, the complex system of provider agencies has made it difficult for the public to access these specialized community-based services (Mechanic, 1991). Those individuals who did access such services could expect to find an alarming absence of coordination between their various health care providers and a lack of continuity of care across their various health care needs. In addition, health care costs were growing at an alarming rate and it was clear that an aging population and the use of increasingly expensive technologies, along with a reduction in the federal government's contribution to health care costs, would make the Ontario government's task of controlling costs even more challenging.

Ontario took aggressive steps toward reforming the health care system in the mid-1990s. However, mental health services did not appear to be a government priority. In 1996, the Ontario government began reforming the acute care system with the formation of the Health Services Restructuring Commission (HSRC). Through the course of its four-year mandate, the HSRC called for the consolidation of specific hospital services within regions, an overall reduction in hospital beds, and the closure or merger of entire hospitals (Health Services Restructuring Commission, 2000). While these changes were intended to create efficiencies and shift emphasis from acute to preventive and primary health care services, funding to community-based programs to support this shift was slow in coming. Hospital restructuring also resulted in an overall reduction in institutional beds available. This had a significant impact on psychogeriatric programs. As beds are eliminated, greater pressure is placed on community-based services to meet client needs. Not only are there more clients requiring services, but the services are increasingly resource intensive and specialized.

History has shown that mental health services have traditionally been the "poor cousin" in Ontario's health care system. While hospital and long-term care restructuring have been a government priority during the past decade, community-based mental health services in general, and psychogeriatric programs in particular, have not always received the amount of attention and government funding they deserve. This is not to say that the issue of mental health reform has been totally ignored. The Ontario government has looked at the issue of mental health reform in the past and continues to do so. Back in 1993, the Ontario government released two reports, *Partnerships in Long-Term Care* and *Putting People First: The Reform of Mental Health Services in Ontario*. These reports left many people with a feeling of optimism since they acknowledged that the mental health system was underfunded, fragmented, and needing reform. However, progress has been slow.

On a more positive note, additional funding has begun to flow to some specialized community-based programs, in particular, Assertive Community Treatment Teams (ACTTs). In order to bring decision making closer to the local communities, the Ontario Ministry of

Health and Long-Term Care (MOHLTC) implemented regional offices around the province. In addition, through its divestment of mental health facilities, which were primarily placed under the governance of hospitals, the Ontario government's hospital reforms have resulted in greater integration of institutionally based mental health and other health services. This shift in governance to community hospitals may help to motivate hospitals to work more closely with other community-based mental health services in forming a more integrated mental health system.

In the late 1990s, the Ontario government reinvigorated its mental health reform initiative. Specifically, in 1999 the Ministry completed its work on a comprehensive strategy to address challenges related to Alzheimer disease and released the paper entitled *Ontario's Strategy for Alzheimer Disease and Related Dementias: Preparing for Our Future* (Ministry of Health and Long-Term Care, 1999c). In the same year, the Ministry also released the *Making It Happen* policy papers. These were intended to provide the operational framework and direction for implementation of mental health reform (Ministry of Health and Long-Term Care, 1999a, 1999b). This reform initiative recognizes first-line, intensive, and specialized services as the three levels of need within the continuum of mental health services. Psychogeriatric programs fall under the category of "specialized" services, which the reports defines as a "… highly specialized mental health programs provided in community or hospital settings and which focus on serving people with serious mental illness who have complex, rare, and unstable mental disorders" (Ministry of Health and Long-Term Care, 1999b, p. 16).

In 2000, the MOHLTC announced the funding of nine regional Mental Health Implementation Task Forces assigned to determine how best to implement mental health reform. Over a two-year period, these Task Forces have been looking at ways of making the system more accountable; supporting the shift from institutional care to community-based care; standardizing the services and the funding for those services across the province; and enhancing the integration of mental health services into the broader health care system so that client care may become seamless. The final reports from these Task Forces were completed in Fall 2002 and are expected to be available for public circulation in 2004. With a brief overview of the macro-system environment, specifically the broader health care context, one can now shift to focusing on the micro-system components, beginning with the characteristics of this unique area of specialty.

B. Psychogeriatrics Defined

The psychiatry of old age, otherwise known as psychogeriatrics, has evolved from a movement originating in the U.K. during the 1960s. Up until that time, interest in the mental health of old age had been largely confined to clinical research. Arie (1990) identified the following five factors as the basis for the development of this emerging specialty:

- pressure from the increase in the numbers of the aged and particularly the very aged;
- the growth in psychiatry's capacity to treat conditions previously regarded as hopeless (Post, 1978);
- the movement of psychiatry from mental hospitals into people's homes and into the general hospital;
- the effectiveness of geriatrics in British medicine; and
- the writings and teachings in the 1960s of a small group of figures ... on the epidemiology, clinical features, prognosis, and pathology of the mental disorders of old age. (p. 70)

Canadian interest in this area was initially sparked at McGill University in Montreal during the late 1940s, with the establishment of the first gerontological group within a department of psychiatry (Reichenfeld & Tourigny-Rivard, 1989). This original group included Drs. Stenn, Prados, Grad, and Kral. The 1970s served as a turning point, with the development of geriatric psychiatry extending beyond the borders of Montreal (Reichenfeld & Tourigny-Rivard, 1989). Specifically, in 1974 the first multidisciplinary psychogeriatric association in Canada—the Ontario Psychogeriatric Association (OPGA) was formed and contributed to the establishment of services, education, and research for various health-related disciplines. Furthermore, during the late 1970s the Canadian Psychiatric Association formed a section on geriatric psychiatry and the University of Toronto established the first division of geriatric psychiatry.

Over the years, the term psychogeriatrics has been used interchangeably with *geriatric psychiatry* and *geropsychiatry* to identify the psychiatric subspecialty that addresses the care of the mentally impaired elderly (Health and Welfare Canada, 1988). At the same time, there has been wide variation in the meaning, with some confining the word to the care of the confused and demented elderly and others applying it where mental and physical disease occurred simultaneously (Pitt, 1982).

While the term psychogeriatrics has often been criticized for being an "ugly word" (i.e., cumbersome, overtly clinical) as well as denigrating to the individual who is identified as a psychogeriatric patient (Pitt, 1982), its use reflects the broad specialty area that concerns itself with all aspects of care and functioning of older persons. In 1988, Health and Welfare Canada defined psychogeriatrics as follows:

> It comprises a body of knowledge on the psychodynamics and psychopathology of old age, special expertise in the pharmacological and psychosocial treatment and management of the mentally ill elderly, and a unique organization of services. It represents an innovative use of existent resources rather than a new specialty, for it has had contributions from many fields and disciplines. (p. 14)

More recently, the Ministry of Health (1995) has defined the target population for "psychogeriatrics" as including individuals with dementia and behavioural problems, late-onset psychogeriatric disorders, medical psychiatric disorders associated with medical illness, functional difficulties, individuals with psychiatric and co-morbid substance abuse. In essence, in response to the combination of psychosocial, physical, and social needs as experienced by older people with serious mental health problems, there has developed a need for psychogeriatrics/specialized geriatric mental health services. The complexity of their multiple needs has resulted in the need for ongoing support, more structures, and intensive treatment and a higher level of coordination, security, and support.

C. Community Psychogeriatric Services

The provision of community psychogeriatric services is quite distinct in that it is premised upon a community-based approach to care. This need to assess and treat the elderly in the community as much as possible has been expressed by Gutkin (1985) to include the following:

> ... I believe that the vast majority of patients are best managed in their own environment. This is not to say that in-patient units are not necessary or important, but that well-balanced and relevant services for the elderly must include both facilities. (p. 179)

Several reasons for a community orientation have been outlined by Hemsi (1982). First, due to the nature of mental disorders, there is often little to be gained by admitting an elderly person to the hospital. Since older people are integral members of social networks, it is essential to have a good working knowledge of that network as observed in the community. Further, in order to provide the necessary support that may be required, it is important to understand the individual's situation and the psychosocial processes that are having an impact on them. Although one would not expect there to be a shift toward institutional care, the reality has been that an expansion of the long-term care capacity in the province has placed pressures on the system to fill these surplus beds despite contradictions to the philosophy of mental health reform.

The majority of psychogeriatric teams provide assessment and treatment in an elderly person's own home or long-term care facility. Such views have also been reinforced by Health and Welfare Canada (1988), whereby the home is considered the "optimal setting" for assessment of persons with psychiatric disorders. While this allows greater comfort and privacy for the client, working in the home setting may induce increased stress for the professional. In this regard, the loss of control experienced by the professional needs to be acknowledged and understood.

The approach taken by health care professionals in the assessment and treatment of the psychogeriatric population has evolved over time. Initially, as programs became established, team functioning often focused upon a multidisciplinary approach to care, whereby each team member takes responsibility for activities related to his or her own particular discipline (Halper, 1993).

As team building became an important component in the delivery of service, and there was a greater need to interact among the disciplines, teams often experienced a shift from multidisciplinary to interdisciplinary functioning. Compounding the responsibility of team members working toward a common goal, the interdisciplinary approach also incorporates group effort and outcomes along with active family involvement (Halper, 1993).

A further change has also emerged in light of current economic constraints, staffing cuts, limited resources, and professional staff obtaining higher levels of education. The so-called transdisciplinary approach is based upon the premise that:

> ... one person can perform several professionals' roles by providing services to the patient under the supervision of the individuals from the other disciplines involved. Representatives of various disciplines

work together in the initial evaluation and care plan, but only one or two team members actually provide the services. (Halper, 1993, p. 35)

This type of approach is becoming more common and is particularly prevalent with programs operating in rural settings where staffing and/ or community resources are frequently limited. In essence, the type of approach used within each community psychogeriatric program is dependent upon flexibility and such factors as the number of team members, the types of disciplines, the sponsoring organization's philosophy of care, and the degree of psychiatric input, among other things.

Despite the orientation taken, the community approach to care requires cohesive teams. Since optional team functioning often means a blurring of roles, each team member must be able to transcend the role of a specific discipline while maintaining professional uniqueness in terms of specific knowledge and skills. Obviously, such collaborative processes also involve the learning and incorporation into one's clinical practice of a variety of knowledge and skills from the other disciplines. Thus, the ultimate goal for the team is to enable its members not only to retain the expertise of their specific disciplines, but also to develop a commonality of skills as applied gerontologists (Knight, 1989).

While team functioning and the operations of practice vary from one program to another, it has become recognized that the expertise needed to conduct home assessments is commonly associated with the professions of nursing and social work (Jackson et al., 1989). However, regardless of which practitioners participate in the actual home visit, the basic premise of a team approach is that all the team members have an equal opportunity to contribute to the diagnosis and treatment plan (Health and Welfare Canada, 1988).

II.   The Clientele

As we enter the twenty-first century, projections of the Canadian population 65 years of age and older are expected to increase dramatically [see Chapter 1]. According to the Ontario Ministry of Finance (2002),

The population age 65 and over will more than double, from 1.5 million or 12.6 percent of the population in 2001 to 3.2 million or 20.3 percent in 2028. The population age 75 and over will also more than

double, increasing from 0.7 million or 5.6 percent of the population
in 2001 to 1.4 million or 8.9 percent in 2028. (p. 13)

As further noted by the Clarke Consulting Group (1996), the oldest
age group, i.e., individuals more than 80 years, are expected to increase
by 80 percent between 1986 and 2001 to 557,700 individuals (p. 2).

Given such projections, the need for psychogeriatric services will
also escalate. According to the Ministry of Health (1993), "by 2010, the
actual number of moderate and severe cases of dementia will increase
by 85 percent and by 2021 the increase will be 150 percent. The number
of people with Alzheimer's Disease and related dementias in Ontario
in 1999 is estimated to be 117,000" (p. 18).

Dementia is a particularly severe problem because there is presently
no cure. Furthermore, the course of the disease is one of progressive
deterioration, compounded by the onset of difficult behaviours as a
result of the cognitive impairment. Consequently, caregivers for persons
suffering from dementia are at risk themselves for the development of
mental health problems, i.e., mood and anxiety disorders.

Aside from dementia, depression is the most pervasive and
possibly the most frequently underdiagnosed mental health problem
experienced by the elderly (Health and Welfare Canada, 1988). To date,
epidemiological information about depression has been contradictory,
with early studies identifying higher rates of prevalence (Butler, 1975;
Myers & Weissman, 1979), yet more recent evidence has challenged
this once prevailing view. It has more currently been identified that
the proportion of elderly who suffer from "clinical depression" is not
higher than among their younger counterparts (Aboraya & Anthony,
1992; Feinson, 1989; Newman, 1989).

Despite these conflicting findings, almost all epidemiologic data
demonstrate that depression among older adults is too prevalent
a problem to be ignored (Aboraya & Anthony, 1992). In addition,
depression in elderly persons is often "masked" by major symptoms
in other areas. For instance, somatic complaints, especially pains of
unknown origin, are common along with such presenting complaints
as tiredness, fatigue, and lack of energy. Depression may also hide
behind any alteration in usual behaviour, i.e., impulsive sexual
behaviour, outbursts of rage, and drug/alcohol abuse (Wasylenki, 1987).
Furthermore, the suicide rates among the elderly are higher than among
other age groups, with elderly white males having the highest rate for
suicides (Butler, 1975; D'Arcy, 1987; Wasylenki, 1987).

Although it is not within the scope of this chapter to detail the problems associated with the diagnoses and treatment of depression in later life, the fact that depression is a common and treatable problem for elderly persons needs to be emphasized. Frequently, depression remains undetected in this age group due to the misperception that depression is a normal reaction to the losses associated with aging.

Other psychiatric disorders that are common among the elderly include anxiety, somatoform disorders, personality disorders, psychosis, and substance abuse. In addition, there are individuals who developed psychiatric disorders earlier in life, which they carry to their senior years. This subgroup is often not represented statistically in the data, but rather subsumed under "other diagnoses." Various disturbances of mental functioning or behaviour in later life, notably confusion or delirium, may also be associated with systemic infections, adverse drug reaction, trauma, or surgery (Health and Welfare Canada, 1988).

The identified mental health problems of elderly persons as described in the literature reflect the types of referrals currently received in community psychogeriatric programs. In particular, two of the more prevalent reasons for referrals to these programs are depression and dementia/memory loss, with the additional complication of behavioural management problems. Other common presenting problems include complicated and non-complicated grief reactions, and suspicious/paranoid behaviours. In addition, problems related to retirement, marital conflict, and elder abuse are increasingly being identified among the reasons for referral.

Psychogeriatric services are not only targeted to the identified elderly client but also to their spouses and adult children. In particular, family members who are caring for someone who is cognitively impaired are at risk for the development of a range of emotional difficulties such as depression, anxiety, guilt, social isolation, marital/family/interpersonal conflicts, and ultimately physical health breakdown (Mace & Rabins, 1991).

In addition to the unique presentation of mental health problems of elderly persons, there are also specific difficulties related to the delivery of service. Traditionally, elderly persons have constituted a disproportionately small percentage of the population receiving mental health services. Barriers to the provision of mental health services are evident not only among this clientele but also with service providers. For example, elderly persons do not tend to perceive of their problems in psychological terms and are inclined to be wary about involvement with mental health services (Carner et al., 1984). Likewise, service

providers may be pessimistic and question the value of the provision
of mental health services for elderly persons or feel inadequate in their
ability to provide these services (Knight, 1989).

In essence, given the broad range of clinical presentation of
mental health problems of elderly persons and the reluctance among
this age group to accept help, the approach to treatment requires
knowledgeable, skilled, sensitive, and creative practitioners. A review
of the roles and responsibilities of the social worker will demonstrate
the wide versatility required of this discipline in working in community
psychogeriatric programs.

III. Practice Roles and Responsibilities

Social workers are represented on almost every community
psychogeriatric team currently functioning in Ontario. As indicated
earlier in this chapter, three types of roles characterize social work
practice on these teams: clinical, administrative, and the dual clinical/
administrative. The following provides a description of these clinical
and administrative roles, with a caveat that these descriptions are
neither inclusive nor definitive.

A. The Clinical Role

The clinical roles include a composite of both direct and indirect
practice skills. Subsumed under direct practice skills are the following
competencies: to conduct a comprehensive biopsychosocial assessment;
to provide supportive counselling and psychotherapy with individuals,
families, and groups; to locate and coordinate linkage with appropriate
resources; and to offer case management services (i.e., coordination,
monitoring, and advocacy).

Within the context of these various clinical responsibilities, the
process of assessment demands the acquisition of important skills. The
significance of the assessment process has been stated emphatically by
Health and Welfare Canada (1988).

> Assessment is the cornerstone of good psychogeriatric care. Careful,
> broad-based, systematic examination of the patient is essential for
> accurate diagnosis and appropriate treatment decisions. Assessment
> is necessary for determining priority of needs, for establishing

competency or incompetency, for patient monitoring, for outcome or program evaluation, and hence for resource allocation. (p. 8)

The clinical psychogeriatric assessment extends beyond the psychosocial assessment to include the following components: physical and mental health, behaviour and self-care abilities, and the individual's physical environment (Ontario Psychogeriatric Association, 1990). In assessing the mental status component, there needs to be an examination of the individual's psychological/emotional state and cognitive functioning. Martin (1987) offered a breakdown of mental status categories, which need to be observed and recorded as follows: (1) *Appearance and Behaviour*—manner of relating to the interviewer, appropriateness to the interview, gross neglect of hygiene and grooming, inanition and dehydration, mobility, and bizarre behaviour; (2) *Speech*—rate and articulation and vocabulary; (3) *Affect*—subjective and objective mood, self-esteem, future orientation, and suicidal ideation; (4) *Thought Form and Content*—coherence and logic, themes with which the patient is preoccupied, obsessional thoughts, and delusions; (5) *Perception*—illusions, hallucinations, and depersonalization/derealization; (6) *Cognitive Function*—level of consciousness, orientation, memory, attention and concentration, language, visual-spatial organization, abstract thinking, judgment, and insight (p. 121).

To assist in the assessment of mental status and cognitive functioning, standardized assessment tools are also commonly utilized. There are numerous instruments used in geriatric psychiatry, including delirium screens, functional status assessments, and caregiver stress/burden scales. For example, one of the more commonly used instruments for screening cognitive function is *The Mini-Mental Status Examination* (MMSE) (Folstein et al., 1975). Another popular instrument used in assessing the level of depression in the elderly is *The Self-Rating Geriatric Depression Scale* (GDS) (Yesavage, 1986) and the *Cornell Depression Scale* (CDS) (Alexopoulous et al., 1998). A comprehensive listing of the numerous structured instruments that are available and useful in working with the psychogeriatric population is offered by the Ontario Psychogeriatric Association (1990) and the *Putting the PIECES Together* reference manual (Ministry of Health, 2002).

In 1988, Ontario's community psychogeriatric teams had the opportunity to become involved in a training initiative for the staff of long-term care facilities with the goal of increasing their skills in caring for residents who were presenting with increasingly complex physical and mental health problems. The manual, *A Psychogeriatric Guide and Training Program for Professionals in Long-Term Care Facilities in Ontario* (Ministry of Health, 2002), incorporates a systematic approach to assessment and management involving a variety of techniques and strategies. A core concept in this training approach was PIECES (an acronym developed by Dr. Ken LeClair), a holistic framework for understanding the various factors that may be contributing to the behaviour of elderly persons.

> PIECES is an acronym that attempts to convey the individuality and importance of the various factors in the well-being, self-determination, and quality of life of seniors.
>
> It provides a framework for the understanding why we behave the way we do and what resources we have to build on.
>
> - The first three letters *P-I-E* represent an individual's *P*hysical, *I*ntellectual, and *E*motional Health.
> - The *C* can be seen as the centre-piece or focus in care, i.e., maximizing *C*apabilities which promotes the achievement of the highest quality of life as possible for an individual.
> - The *E-S* represents the environment that an individual interacts with—physical as well as the emotional environment. *E*nvironment (physical) *S*ocial environment. (Ministry of Health, 2002)

Attention to all of these six factors in the PIECES template is important in thinking through complex problems in a systematic way. It is also integral to conducting a comprehensive assessment and implementing appropriate interventions whether or not the elderly individual resides in an institution or in the community.

It is clearly apparent that specialized knowledge and skills are required for direct practice with this clientele. The social worker must be able to understand such features as: the unique presentation of mental health problems among elderly persons; the progression of dementia and the utilization of behaviour management strategies to deal with difficult behaviours; the necessary adaptations required in communicating with sensory and cognitively impaired older adults; and the issues involved with the provision of multigenerational family intervention.

Furthermore, psychotherapy with older adults also requires subtle changes in one's practice. For example, reminiscence is effective therapy for elderly clients, although this process can be misconstrued as being repetitive storytelling rather than "real therapy." The location, frequency, timing of sessions, use of self-disclosure, and physical touching are also subject to variation in working with the elderly person. However, other therapeutic conditions such as the provision of an atmosphere of safety and trust, skilled listening, awareness, and use of transference and counter-transference issues remain constant.

As is evident from the previous overview about the evolution of psychogeriatrics, psychiatry has strongly influenced the development of mental health services for the elderly. Consequently, there has been a reliance on descriptive nomenclature such as the *Diagnostic and Statistical Manual of Mental Disorders*, 4th edition (DSM IV) and its bias toward the medical model of diagnosis and treatment. Within the context of the "person-in-environment" perspective, the social worker can serve to broaden the domain of mental health services for elderly persons beyond the realm of psychiatric pathology and medical management. In the process of assessment, for example, consideration needs to be given to the political, social, cultural, gender, and economic realities and their impact on elderly persons. The current emphasis on pharmacological dispensation, as the primary mental health intervention with older persons, needs to be addressed while alternate forms of treatment are considered. Thus, the varying theoretical orientations common to social work practice (i.e., psychodynamic, family systems theory, cognitive behavioural) can serve to broaden the understanding of symptomatic behaviour and the scope of intervention strategies. In addition, the focus to relationship and differential use of self can be helpful for other team members in understanding their work with this clientele. Another reason for the medical emphasis in psychogeriatric practice is due to the prevalence of physical illness coexisting with mental health concerns. Consequently, social workers on psychogeriatric teams may find themselves in a similar position as their colleagues working in hospital settings, in that they lack the medical knowledge and skills that are common to the other team members. In addition, as the other team members become more proficient in dealing with psychosocial issues, the social worker may feel threatened and become defensive or succumb to the pressure of the prevailing model. It is important [that] social workers functioning on community psychogeriatric teams be able to articulate for themselves and the team their unique knowledge that can contribute to understanding elderly persons and their specialized skills in working with this age group.

Nevertheless, social workers on community psychogeriatric teams are required to expand their knowledge and skills beyond traditional social work practice to include a familiarization with related areas in pharmacology, psychology, and medicine. Teams need social workers who have an understanding and working knowledge of the diagnostic model of medical illness in elderly persons. In addition, social workers need to develop comfort with the use of standardized screening and assessment tools such as mental status tests and depression inventories. In order to incorporate such new knowledge and skills within the social work perspective and to function effectively as a member of the team, one must have a strong professional identity and self-awareness about both one's own collaborative style and interpersonal biases (Lowe & Herranen, 1981). Failure to do so may unduly restrict and even jeopardize the role of the social worker on psychogeriatric teams.

In addition to the numerous direct practice skills required of social workers in community psychogeriatric programs, there are also indirect practice skills. These include such competencies as consultation to long-term care institutions; collaboration with other community agencies; education to professionals and laypersons; supervision of students; and program and community development (to identify unmet needs and to promote the development of new resources).

In working with this clientele, there is a need for the provision of education regarding aging and related problems for professional and personal caregivers. Social workers are skilled in understanding the issues regarding the impact of illness on individuals and family functioning, along with the resulting difficulties that can ensue. Also, social workers have an appreciation of some of the dynamics involved regarding the provision and acceptance of help. The interpretation of these dynamics can be useful for other caregivers who are frequently frustrated with the tendency among elderly persons to resist or refuse assistance. In practice, there is considerable variation among each psychogeriatric program regarding the focus given to education. For those teams that operate on the assessment and consultation model, a greater emphasis may be given to education. Whereas, for those teams that operate within the assessment and treatment models, there may be less opportunity to provide this service.

Overall, it is evident that the clinical role for social workers on psychogeriatric teams is broad in scope, encompassing both the direct and indirect practice skills. The balance of the emphasis that is given to either direct or indirect practice will depend to a large degree on the nature of the individual team in combination with education, specialized skills, and interests of the social worker.

B. The Administrative Role

The other major role for the social worker functioning on a psychogeriatric team is administrative. Currently in Ontario, only a small number of the operational community psychogeriatric teams have social workers designated in management positions. The job titles of these "administrators" can vary anywhere from manager to coordinator to team leader.

Similar to the clinical component, the division of administrative responsibilities for these administrators varies with the functioning of each team as well as the structure of the sponsoring organization. While the administrative role is essentially comparable to any middle management position, there are some unique administrative functions common to psychogeriatric programs.

The first identifiable feature is the budgetary responsibility. In Ontario, the majority of psychogeriatric programs are funded by the Ministry of Health and Long-Term Care (MOHLTC). Each program receives separate dedicated funding that is funneled through a sponsoring organization. Hence, the social work "administrator" is often accountable both to the Ministry and the sponsoring organization.

This dual reporting relationship also comes to the forefront in relation to other administrative expectations. For example, the program may be required to submit separate statistical data reporting requirements—one directly to the Ministry and another to the sponsor organization. In addition, in the recently released document *Mental Health Accountability Framework* (Ministry of Health and Long-Term Care, 2003), the Ministry requires all government-funded organizations that provide mental health services to have operating plans, legal agreements with the government regarding the use of funds, and measurable performance indicators.

Another dual reporting relationship occurs in regard to the evaluation process. Both the MOHLTC and the sponsoring organization have specific program guidelines, standards, and expectations that must be adhered to. Thus, it is very common for community psychogeriatric programs to participate in two types of evaluations. For example, one of the author's experiences in a newly funded program during their three-year probationary period was to undergo three separate evaluations by the MOHLTC and participate in two accreditations processes by the sponsoring hospital.

A final dual reporting relationship occurs in relation to the program advisory committee (if one exists). The MOHLTC recommends that specialty programs establish an advisory body comprised of consumers/family members, service providers, etc., to serve in assessing, developing, guiding, and promoting its community psychogeriatric service. The design of these advisory committees may vary in accordance with the sponsoring organization's structure.

In essence, the social work administrator has two sources of responsibility—to his or her supervisor within the sponsoring organization and to the regional consultant at the Ministry. While some managers are permitted full access and communication with their Ministry representative by their sponsoring organization, in other cases the responsibility for contact is redirected to other management personnel. Whichever system is practised, the social work manager is always in the delicate position of having to balance all of the responsibilities and maintain open communication from all avenues. In addition to the normally expected administrative responsibilities that a social work manager would have to fulfill within the organization's expectations, this individual also needs to focus a large amount of energy in the local community. Since community psychogeriatric programs are mandated to maintain a community outreach focus, the manager is often actively involved in local community services, (i.e., Alzheimer societies, adult day programs, CCACs, VON., etc.) as well as planning bodies (i.e., district health councils, long-term care committees, mental health committees, etc.) that are relevant to psychogeriatric issues.

Overall, the administrative role in psychogeriatric programs is both complex and challenging. The social work manager must be able to balance internal obligations with external community endeavours along with Ministry expectations. While the social worker is well equipped to utilize the principles of social work practice at the macro level in managing the tasks, ongoing administrative upgrading and education is required for the individual to meet all these demands.

IV.   Potential for Role Development

There are numerous opportunities for role development of social work practice within community psychogeriatric programs. From a clinical perspective, ethical dilemmas are common to social workers working with elderly persons. For example, issues regarding euthanasia, competency, autonomy, and the right to refuse treatment are an integral part of psychogeriatric practice. In particular, referrals to psychogeriatric teams frequently include the request for a recommendation regarding the safety of an individual to remain living in his or her own home. It is important for social workers to gain expertise and comfort with the process of assessing competency and to develop a framework for working through ethical dilemmas.

The ability for social workers to work effectively on multidisciplinary teams is key to the provision of comprehensive care. Expanding one's professional role, as noted by one author, is critical to functioning in the work environment.

> In assessing the importance and usefulness of social work practice in gerontology, we must note that working with the aged and responding to their many complicated needs requires a multidisciplinary and multitheoretical approach. Professionals (including social workers) who work with the elderly are still far from reaching a consensus on their respective domains, but they are more and more aware that the knowledge explosion is not the property of any one discipline. (Guttmann & Lowenstein, 1992, p. 495)

There is also a need for ongoing research into both the effectiveness of community psychogeriatric teams as well as client problems commonly encountered by social work practitioners, e.g., social isolation, poverty, and substance abuse. Traditionally, social workers have tended to focus more on the immediate clinical demands of practice rather than participating in research activities. However, greater involvement in research will inevitably serve to enhance the credibility of the role of social work in the overall provision of community psychogeriatric services.

The potential for role development also exists in the role of program and client advocacy. Within the past few years, the Ontario provincial government released documents that are intended to serve as a guide for service provision in the areas of long-term care and mental health reform. Both of these reports—*Making It Happen: Implementation Plan for Mental Health Reform* (Ministry of Health and Long-Term Care, 1999a) and *Making It Happen: Operational Framework for the Delivery of Mental Health Services and Supports* (Ministry of Health and Long-Term Care, 1999b)—offer recognition of the problems and needed services for the psychogeriatric population. At the same time, social workers in administrative positions need to become actively involved in bringing these concerns to the forefront. Advocacy, at the provincial level, is definitely a role that must be developed if psychogeriatric programs are to have a chance for future survival.

V.   Concluding Remarks

In light of the positive developments in mental health reform noted above, we anticipate some increased funding being made available to community psychogeriatric programs that will support the expansion of existing programs and the creation of new ones. Given that social work practice in community psychogeriatric programs has emerged as an important area of specialty within the social work profession, one can expect further room for expansion of professional positions.

In order to adequately prepare new social workers for psychogeriatric practice, educational issues need to be addressed. At the present time, graduates from baccalaureate and masters level social work programs are not always adequately prepared to provide knowledgeable and skilled service in working with an elderly population. As a result, social workers in this area tend to have obtained on-the-job training and search out additional courses to gain the required knowledge and skills. Whether it is possible for the inclusion of an adequate number of courses on mental health care for the elderly within the current curriculum offered by the existing facilities of social work is no longer an issue for debate but rather a necessity if the profession is going to seize this opportunity. Mellor and Solomon (1992) described an innovative post-graduate social work interdisciplinary geriatric education model offered at Hunter/Mount Sinai Geriatric Education Center in New York City. These authors stated: "... interdisciplinary geriatric education for social workers is best approached after graduation, in the workplace and as a continuing education process" (p. 184). Further exploration of the utilization of this education model would seem advisable in order to adequately prepare social workers for practice with this rapidly growing segment of the population.

Finally, the social work profession has been an integral player in the development of community psychogeriatric teams. This specific field of practice has required practitioners to move beyond the traditional social work into an area of specialty where one must work intensely with other disciplines. The demands of team functioning, the blurring of roles between disciplines, the difficulties involved with the shift to conducting home rather than office visits, along with the need to expand one's knowledge base and assessment skills, can all contribute in making this type of position very strenuous. At the same time, the challenges and continued growth opportunities offered in community psychogeriatric programs can also serve to provide the social worker with an extremely rewarding work experience.

Case Example

Mr. G, aged 72, was admitted to hospital as a result of a heart attack. Following the stabilization of his medical condition, Mr. G appeared to be quite depressed and a referral was made to the medical social worker. At the time of discharge, the medical social worker recommended follow-up by the psychogeriatric clinic. When the social worker from the clinic was introduced to Mr. G, he responded to her in a brusque manner, stating that he was quite capable of managing on his own. However, he did accept her card with the name and phone number of the clinic. The family physician prescribed an anti-depressant medication and Mr. G was discharged home having refused any referrals for community support.

Two days following his discharge home, Mr. G contacted the clinic by phone. He appeared to be in a state of acute anxiety and he agreed to having the social worker make a home visit later that afternoon. A biopsychosocial assessment was completed by the social worker and presented at the team conference. The following problems were identified: (1) reactive depression to cardiac illness, (2) unresolved grief reaction following the death of his wife six years ago, (3) suspected alcohol abuse, and (4) refusal of community supports. A concurrent mental status examination revealed mild confusion attributed to his depression rather than the early onset of dementia.

When the social worker met with Mr. G, he was somewhat formal but cordial and he reported that he did not recall meeting her at the hospital. Mr. G stated that he was agreeable to seeing her on a weekly basis only on the condition that she was not to discuss emotional issues. The social worker respected Mr. G's strong need for control in these early sessions and concentrated on establishing a trusting relationship with the client. Mr. G proved to be an intelligent and articulate man and he enjoyed sharing with the social worker aspects of his former career. He also talked about his only child, a son, with whom he appeared to have had a close relationship. Initially, when

Mr. G appeared to be overwhelmed with emotion, he would leave the room. However, in time, he was able to disclose and weep openly with this worker regarding some of the painful losses that had occurred during his life.

One day, the social worker was notified that Mr. G had suffered a coronary attack and had been admitted to hospital. When the social worker went to see Mr. G, he introduced her to the nurses as his friend. He died the following day.

Case Comments

Due to the multiple natures of problems presented by the elderly, the likelihood that adaptive interventions are required and the lack of other services, social workers can rarely confine themselves to playing a single preferred role, such as therapist. Rather, they will often be required to display a high degree of flexibility geared to the specific needs of the client (Edinberg, 1985). This brief case example has attempted to illustrate this feature of the clinical role.

When the social worker first met with Mr. G, he seemed to be a contentious and somewhat confused elderly man. Frequently, elderly people present very differently in hospital and a return to the familiarity of their own home can effect a remarkable improvement in their physical, emotional, and cognitive functioning. While in hospital, Mr. G seemed to have perceived of the offer of support as an intrusion into his personal life. His rejection of community resources upon discharge may be interpreted as [a] defence reaction and a need to regain a sense of himself through his refusal to allow others into the privacy of his own home. Nevertheless, Mr. G was able to accept the worker's invitation and did contact the clinic two days later.

Building a relationship—the cornerstone of the social work practice—is crucial to therapeutic involvement with older adults. The core conditions (respect, non-judgmental attitude, genuineness, empathy) are frequently absent in the interpersonal relationships experienced by elderly persons. Their experience, more often, is of being ignored or treated in a paternalistic manner. The social worker allowed Mr. G to set the terms of her involvement and focused on the development of a trusting rapport. It took considerable time for a therapeutic relationship to develop with Mr. G, and initially the social worker experienced concern that she was more like a friendly visitor than a professional. These feelings were intensified by seeing Mr. G at his home where they would meet in the kitchen over coffee.

Frequently, older people do not differentiate among professionals or may, as Mr. G did, prefer to perceive the social worker as a friend. This attempt to minimize the status of the social worker may be interpreted as another illustration of the tendency of elderly persons to resist help. Indeed, by perceiving the social worker as a friend may have enabled Mr. G to accept her help. As long as the professional boundaries are maintained, for the worker to dispel the notion of friendship (at least with this particular client) might have been counterproductive. During the course of involvement with the social worker, Mr. G eventually was able to engage in a meaningful and purposeful helping relationship. It was the impression of the social worker that Mr. G had made considerable progress toward the integration of his formerly disavowed painful emotional states.

Death is a reality in working with elderly clients. However, Mr. G's death was unexpected as he had been managing quite well. The death of a client (expected or unexpected) with whom one has had a significant relationship is a loss and the feelings of grief need to be acknowledged and validated. To be able to experience the intensity of the feelings of loss and grief that are frequently the crux of the problems presented by elderly persons, without the worker becoming overwhelmed, is one of the challenges of working with this population.

As illustrated by this case example, elderly people tend to have several issues and problems impacting them at the same time. Clients and caregivers have different values, beliefs, attitudes, and interaction patterns. All of these factors influence the care of the elderly person. To provide the best care and service strategies for the client, all of these factors must be considered together.

References

Aboraya, A. & Anthony, J.C. (1992). The epidemiology of selected mental disorders in later life. In J.E. Birren, R.B. Sloane, & G.D. Cohen (eds.), *Handbook of mental health and aging*, 2nd ed. New York: Academic Press.

Arie, T. (1990). Psychogeriatrics. *British Journal of Hospital Medicine*, 44, 70–71.

Baranek, P., Barnsley, J., Deber, R.B., Leggat, S., & Williams, A.P. (1999). Long-term care goes to market: Managed competition and Ontario's reform of community-based services. *Canadian Journal on Aging*, 18, 125–153.

Blazer, D.G. (1980). The epidemiology of mental illness in later life. In E.W. Buss & D.G. Blazer (eds.), *Handbook of geriatric psychiatry*, pp. 249–271. New York: Van Nostrand Reinhold.

Butler, R.N. (1975). Psychiatry and the elderly: An overview. *The American Journal of Psychiatry*, 9, 132.

Carner, E., Klein, M., & Waxman, H. (1984). Underutilization of mental health professionals by community elderly. *The Gerontologist*, 24, 23–30.

Clarke Consulting Group. (1996). *Establishing benchmarks for psychogeriatric outreach programs*. [On-line]. Available at: www.health.gov.on.ca/english/providers/pub/mhitf/central_east_whitby/app_i.pdf

Cohen, G.D. (1976). Mental health services and the elderly: Needs and options. *The American Journal of Psychiatry*, 1, 133.

D'Arcy, C. (1987). Aging and mental health. In V.W. Marshall, ed., *Aging in Canada: Social perspectives*, 2nd ed., pp. 424–450. Toronto: Fitzhenry & Whiteside.

Desjardins, B. (1993). *Population, aging and the elderly: Current demographic analysis*. Ottawa: Statistics Canada.

Edinberg, M.A. (1985). General considerations in mental health practice with the elderly. In *Mental health practice with the elderly*, pp. 140–156. Englewood Cliffs: Prentice-Hall.

Feinson, M.C. (1989). Are psychological disorders most prevalent among older adults? Examining the evidence. *Social Science and Medicine*, 29, 1175–1181.

Folstein, M.R., Folstein, S., & McHugh, P.R. (1975). Mini-mental state: A practical method for grading the cognitive state of patients for the clinician. *Journal of Psychiatry Research*, 12, 189–198.

Gutkin, B. (1985). Psychogeriatrics. *The Medical Journal of Australia*, 143, 178–179.

Guttmann, D. & Lowenstein, A. (1992). Psychosocial problems and the needs of the elderly in mental health. In F.J. Turner (ed.), *Mental health and the elderly: A social work perspective*, pp. 478–502. Toronto: Maxwell Macmillan Canada.

Halper, A.S. (1993). Teams and team work: Health care settings. *American Speech-Language Hearing Association*, 35(617), 34–35.

Harris, D.J. (1993, August 18). Director, Psychogeriatric Community Clinic, Victoria Hospital, London, Ontario, personal interview.

Health and Welfare Canada. (1988). *Guidelines for comprehensive services to elderly persons with psychiatric disorders*. Ottawa: Department of National Health and Welfare.

Health and Welfare Canada. (1991). *Mental health problems among Canada's seniors: Demographic and epidemiologic considerations*. Ottawa: Department of National Health and Welfare.

Health Services Restructuring Commission (HSRC). (2000). *A legacy report*. Toronto: Health Services Restructuring Commission.

Hemsi, L. (1982). Psychogeriatric care in the community. In R. Levy & F. Post (eds.), *The psychiatry of later life,* pp. 252–287. Oxford: Blackwell Scientific Publications.

Herranen, M. & Lowe, J. (1981). Understanding teamwork: Another look at the concepts. *Social Work in Health Care, 7,* 1–11.

Hopkins, R.W. (1990). Dementia projections for the counties regional municipalities and districts for Ontario. Unpublished manuscript, Kingston Psychiatric Hospital, Geriatric Unit, Kingston, Ontario.

Kirby, M.L.J. (2002). The health of Canadians—the federal role, volume six: Recommendations for reform. The Standing Senate Committee on Social Affairs, Science and Technology. Retrieved from http://www.parl.gc.ca/37/2/parlbus/commbus/senate/Com-e/SOCI-E/rep-e/repoct02vol6-e.htm

Knight, B. (1989). *Outreach with the elderly.* New York: University Press.

Mace, N.L. & Rabins, P.V. (1991). *The 36 hour day,* rev. ed. Baltimore: The Johns Hopkins University Press.

Martin, B.A. (1987). Clinical assessment. In D.M. Clarke, M.K. Harrison, E.L. Lennox, B.A. Martin, L.A. Perry, & D.A. Wasylenki (eds.), *Psychogeriatrics: A practical handbook,* pp. 115–137. Toronto: Gage Educational Publishing Company.

Mechanic, D. (1991). Strategies for integrating public mental health services. *Hospital and Community Psychiatry, 42*(8), 797–801.

Mellor, M. & Solomon, R. (1992). Interdisciplinary geriatric education: The new kid on the block. *Journal of Gerontological Social Work, 18,* 175–186.

Ministry of Finance. (2002). Update to Ontario population projections, 2001–2028. Toronto: Queen's Printer for Ontario. Retrieved from http://www.gov.on.ca/FIN/english/demographics/demog02e.pdf

Ministry of Health. (1993). *Putting people first: The reform of mental health issues in Ontario.* Toronto: Queen's Printer for Ontario.

Ministry of Health. (1995). *Policy framework and implementation guidelines for mental health and long-term care interface for older people with mental health needs.* Toronto: Queen's Printer for Ontario.

Ministry of Health. (2002). *Putting the PIECES together: A psychogeriatric guide and training program for professionals in long-term care facilities in Ontario.* Toronto: Queen's Printer for Ontario.

Ministry of Health, Ministry of Community and Social Services and Ministry of Citizenship. (1993). *Partnership in long-term care: A new way to plan, manage and deliver services and community support.* Toronto: Queen's Printer for Ontario.

Ministry of Health and Long-Term Care. (1999a). *Making it happen: Implementation plan for mental health reform.* Toronto: Queen's Printer for

Ontario. Retrieved from: http://www.health.gov.on.ca/english/public/pub/mental/MOH-imp.pdf

Ministry of Health and Long-Term Care. (1999b). *Making it happen: Operational framework for the delivery of mental health services and supports.* Toronto: Queen's Printer for Ontario. Retrieved from: http://www.health.gov.on.ca/english/public/pub/mental/MOH-op.pdf

Ministry of Health and Long-Term Care. (1999c). *Ontario's strategy for Alzheimer disease and related dementias: Preparing for our future.* Toronto: Queen's Printer for Ontario.

Ministry of Health and Long-Term Care. (2003). *Mental health accountability framework.* Toronto: Queen's Printer for Ontario.

Myers, J.K. & Weissman, M.M. (1979). Depression in the elderly: Research directions in psychopathology, epidemiology and treatment. *Journal of Geriatric Psychiatry, 12,* 187–201.

Newman, J.P. (1989). Aging and depression. *Psychology and Aging, 4,* 150–165.

Ontario Psychogeriatric Association. (1990). *Creating links: Review of assessment for persons with dementia.* Toronto: Ontario Psychogeriatric Association.

Pitt, B. (1982). *Psychogeriatrics: An introduction to the psychiatry of old age,* 2nd ed. New York: Churchill Livingstone.

Post, F. (1978). Then and now. *British Journal of Psychiatry, 133,* 83–86.

Ramsdell, J.W., Swart, J., Jackson, J.E., & Renvall, M. (1989). The yield of a home visit in the assessment of geriatric patients. *Journal of the American Geriatrics Society, 37,* 17–24.

Reichenfeld, H.F. & Tourigny-Rivard, M.F. (1989). Teaching the psychiatry of old age: A Canadian perspective. In B. von Hahn (ed.), *Interdisciplinary topics in gerontology,* Chapter 6. Basle: S. Karger.

Romanow, R.J. (2002). *Final report: Building on values: The future of health care in Canada.* Commission on the Future of Health Care in Canada. Retrieved from http://www.hc-sc.gc.ca/english/care/romanow/index1.html

Wasylenki, D.A. (1980). Depression in the elderly. *Canadian Medical Association Journal, 122,* 525–532.

Wasylenki, D.A. (1987). Depression. In D.A. Wasylenki, B.A. Martin, D.M. Clark, E.A. Lennox, L.A. Perry, & M.K. Harrison (eds.), *Psychogeriatrics: A practical handbook,* pp. 41–58. Toronto: Gage Educational Publishing Company.

Yesavage, J.A. (1986). The use of self-rating depression scales in the elderly. In L. Pivon (ed.), *Clinical memory assessment for older adults.* Washington: American Psychological Association.

Internet Resources

Health Canada Online
  http://www.hc-sc.gc.ca/english
Ministry of Health and Long-Term Care (Ontario)
  http://www.health.gov.on.ca
Ontario Association of Community Care Access Centres
  The CCACs provide a simplified service access point and are
  responsible for several aspects of the health of their community.
  http://www.oaccac.on.ca/index.php
Ontario Psychogeriatric Association
  An interdisciplinary association dedicated to enhancing the quality of
  life of the elderly.
  http://www.opga.on.ca/opga_home.html
PIECES
  Advocates for the individuality and importance of the various factors in
  the well-being, self-determination, and quality of life of seniors.
  http://www.pieces.cabhru.com

Additional Readings

Bloom, H. & Carswell, M. (1996). *A practical guide to mental health, capacity and consent law of Ontario*. Toronto: Professional Publishing.

Conn, D. (ed.). (2001). *Practical psychiatry in the long-term care facility*. Toronto: Hogrefe and Huber Publishers.

Dawson, P., Kline, K., & Wells, D. (1993). *Enhancing the abilities of persons with Alzheimer's and related dementias: A nursing perspective*. New York: Springer.

Kane, R.L. & Kane, R.A. (2000). *Assessing older persons*. Toronto: Oxford University Press.

Kaplan, H. & Saddock, B. (1998). *Synopsis of psychiatry*. New York: Lipinkott Williams and Wilkins.

SECTION III

FUTURE CONSIDERATIONS

CHAPTER 25

GERONTOLOGICAL SOCIAL WORK PRACTICE IN 2005 AND BEYOND

MICHAEL J. HOLOSKO, LINDA J. WHITE, AND MARVIN D. FEIT

I.   Introduction

Gazing into a crystal ball and projecting what the future will hold for social workers practising in the field of gerontology is less risky if one examines what is currently known about such practice and then extrapolates from that knowledge. This textbook is rife with topical and rich illustrations of social workers practising with the elderly in both unique and creative ways. It reminds us that to do so they must utilize knowledge and practice, which transcends conventional social work curricula. We are also reminded that this often requires being effective at "doing more with less." Indeed, all of the chapters in this text serve as testimony to the fact that social work practitioners have important roles to play in helping the elderly in health and human service organizations (HSOs), and they are operationalizing these roles in most efficacious ways.

Three main themes, which require some elaboration at this point, underpin each of the chapters of this text. They are: (1) the social work profession has a decidedly important role to play in practising in this field; (2) in order to be more effective in the future, the profession will have to adapt accordingly to the many demands, resources, and needs of this client group; (3) changes will have to be made in our policy responses to the elderly; and (4) the future is now.

No statistician, epidemiologist, or Malthusian [demographer] need remind us that the numbers of elderly both with the general population and also in need of services are increasing at an alarming rate all over the world. The many practitioners who have diligently described their practice activities in this text have successfully fulfilled their roles within the frameworks of their respective health and HSOs in most adroit ways. Indeed, the various psychosocial, familial, social support, and unique service needs of the elderly described in these various settings require both comprehensive and creative social work intervention. Thus social work, more so than any other profession that helps the elderly (e.g., medicine, nursing, and/or any other specialty field), has such a diverse range to its practice repertoire that its service potential is apparent to all clients in need of help. It is also typically complementarily [to some other one] tied to the multiple needs of the vast majority of elderly clients in care. In other words, regardless of what other services elderly persons require, they seem to also require social work services, if not immediately, then at some point in the near future.

This reality certainly shifts the importance of many social workers practising in this field from offering tangential or supportive services to providing cornerstone service delivery. In this regard, the impassioned accounts of the current and future practice roles of gerontological social workers in this text consistently reiterate the point that social workers often hold leadership roles and key roles in serving the needs of the elderly. There is also no doubt that this trend will continue in the future.

In regard to the second theme expressed in this text, that is, social work's adaptation to the changing needs and resources of the elderly, the hallmark of social work's evolution has been characterized by its flexibility (Holosko, 2003). Historically, clients' needs have determined how the profession has evolved, and the only troubling notion in this equation is whether there will be adequate resources to "do the job" in the future. To date, policy-makers at both the macro (governmental) and meso (organizational, agency) levels have made sporadic attempts in providing meaningful programs and services for the elderly, and any consideration of whether the profession can adapt accordingly must be framed contextually in whether resources will be made available. Certainly, not only resources, but also policies that promote such services and administrative supports, are equally important factors to consider in this regard. Thus, our ability to adapt is based less on our malleability [which is a "given"] and more on other variables in our external environment, which loom as potential impediments to our ability to "do our job."

The final point about timeliness speaks to the fact that social work practitioners (as was noted throughout this manuscript) have already filled many cracks in various health and human service delivery systems and are the primary caretakers for many elderly persons. We are never more certain about the fact that the future is *now* for the profession in this very exciting and challenging field. Thus, we need to evolve and share our practice knowledge and wisdom through practising, researching, educating, and promoting ourselves if we are to be effective in serving this client group in the future.

Future practice directions are many and varied and involve us moving forward in both indirect and direct practice. However, since frontline direct practitioners have been on the leading edge of working with the elderly, the impetus for understanding where the profession is emerging in gerontological social work practice will be discussed from this perspective. Four areas that are projected as areas for emerging practice include: (1) prevention, (2) community-based initiatives and policy responses, (3) practice considerations and challenges, and (4) education and training. Rather than present a prescription for what the profession should do in each of these areas, our intent here is to create some awareness about how we may envision or think about such inevitable practice realities the loom on the horizon of 2005.

II.   Prevention

Prevention is a notion that we [the profession] have embraced and have difficulty defining (Bloom, 1981). Not unlike other helping professions, funding agencies that define their fiduciary parameters in quantitative terms, based on "body count" data, has supported social work practice in North America. In other words, how many you see, how many you treat, and how many return for service are the basis for how much money HSOs and health care organizations receive (Canadian HSOs do not differ significantly from American ones in this regard). Not surprisingly, therefore, prevention programs or strategies currently provide a disincentive for HSOs as they "keep the monthly statistics down" of clients who form the units of service for funding purposes. This is referred to as the "rhetoric of prevention" (Holosko et al., 1998).

Herein lies the rub. As evidenced in this text, when one examines the various settings of care for the elderly, they are being inundated with demands for service. Waiting for health and social services today is the norm, not the exception. Indeed, existing structures, institutions, or programs are being "stretched to the limits" to provide minimal services basic to their organizational mandates. Such programs and their personnel are already working within their full capability, and guess what—*there is no relief in sight*. No large chunks of federal, provincial (Canada), or state monies are being earmarked to meet these disproportionately increased demands for service, and guess what—*there are more elderly in sight*. This means only one thing—that sooner or later prevention must emerge as a reality for future service provision in this area and because social work, *more so than any other helping profession*, can be "had on the cheap," we may find ourselves right "smack dab" in the middle of this issue!

In this regard, we hope that the profession doesn't entrap itself in the long-standing public health and health care dilemma of getting hung up defining elaborate models of prevention and funding unique, sporadic primary, secondary, or tertiary prevention programs. Certainly, one of social work's strengths has been its theoretical orientation and getting to the heart of practice by letting their clients determine their prevention needs. What is required, therefore, is for the profession to sense and act accordingly to these needs and develop low-cost strategies to infuse them into their existing programs and services. What is also required is for a different mindset to emerge (on behalf of funding agencies) about prevention activities and coherent agency policies and procedures to support these activities (Holosko et al., 1998). For example, it really doesn't cost that much for a social worker who is conducting a psychosocial assessment (in-home or in the office) to call a public health nurse to assist a client with something that we (the under-60 cohort who can touch their toes, or have someone else touch our toes) consider as mundane as podiatric care, which can slowly evolve (if not treated) into a chronic debilitating problem for many elderly persons.

III. Community-Based Initiatives

Another area on the horizon for gerontological social work practice involves practitioners taking more community-based initiatives for either providing direct care for elderly persons or supporting service provision in a complementary fashion. As we know, institutional and residential care facilities are costly and needed; however, data about this issue clearly point out that much can be done to support community-based care for the elderly.

At one level, better integration of services using technology information systems, referral networks, resource sharing, and interorganizational models is necessary. This involves a regional conceptualization of health and social services as defined by a community's needs, and implies that communities can provide minimal of comprehensive community care. To date, policy-makers have touted the importance of community-based care, but have not adequately resourced the issue. In short, the infrastructure to embrace the concept has lagged far behind the concept and policy-makers can no longer continue to exercise "conscious avoidance behaviour" about developing their communities of care. Service models that promote a sensitivity of the changing demographics of the elderly, e.g., more women, more foreign born, the escalating 85-plus cohort, etc.; integrated approaches to service delivery; improved strategies to access care; adequate funding levels; more models of community care; more evaluation of community-based initiatives; approaches that respond to morbidity trends; and services that have a prevention, education, and health promotion emphasis definitely need to be on the next agenda of North American policy-makers (Holosko & Dunlop, 1989; Jurkowski & Tracy, 2000). At another level, social supports and social networks for helping the elderly need to be defined and utilized more effectively by communities, helping professionals, and laypersons. Our current knowledge of social supports and their integral role in service delivery cannot be overstated and the potential for practice in this area is both exciting and promising. The trend from family supports to community supports, for instance, for the elderly needs to be incorporated into service delivery models. In sum, it will be a challenge for the profession to evolve in this area in meeting the multifaceted and various needs of the elderly and practice that routinely incorporates social support can only lead to better community-based service provision.

IV. Practice Considerations and Challenges

A creative shift in how we look at this stage of life flies in the face of our ageist and death-defying culture. The vision of old age as a viable, dignified, and hopeful stage of life is met with societal denial, which is intense, pervasive, and often unconscious. It follows, then, that the foremost qualification for any practitioner dealing with this age group is a belief in the importance of seeing and understanding the real problems of old age. The stigmatizing, minimizing, and general discounting of older individuals often exacerbates the obvious issues of disease and frailties. Life-giving and life-promoting practice in a context that sometimes denies these realities is a formidable challenge for the field.

Not only do practitioners need to be realistic about the problems they assess, they will have to be prepared to highlight issues that our institutions and service agencies have not considered and are not yet ready to consider. Because most of our existing health and social services are based on stereotypical and euphemistic thinking about old age, they are currently often inadequate at best.

The paradigmatic shift that needs to take place is a "hard sell." Other professionals, particularly those who have been the "experts" in the field and our own colleagues who have practised in the "old" system, will ironically present the most resistance. A practitioner needs to be prepared to teach, persuade, cajole, and force a different way of "seeing" the problems on administrators, existing service agencies, and funders. We will need to develop and use our expertise in advocacy, research, writing, proselytizing, and public speaking as well as our full range of clinical skills in order to prove a point such as prevention saves money.

Practitioners who take up these challenges will be unpopular and misunderstood at times by the families of their own clients. What they have to offer is not a neat package with no loose ends. Rather, it is a philosophy and a style that is open-ended and uncertain as yet. It involves a capacity to deal with messy, half-baked situations with an open mind and intelligent curiosity. It involves resisting the status quo when things get tough and holding out for recognizing the uniqueness of each new client and situation. It entails a willingness to learn from clients and their families, as all good social work practice does. However, add to that the absolute necessity of being willing to experiment, take risks, and make mistakes and to document what works when it works.

The challenge is obvious. The questions yet to be answered are: Who will meet it and how?

V.   Education and Training

Despite the rather convincing evidence presented throughout this text that social work has a decidedly important role to play in serving the elderly, the profession has had a reticent educational orientation toward moving in this direction. This probably has more to do with its reluctance to provide specialization and training than anything else. The empirical data on this subject are fairly clear; that is, professional social work education in North America is oriented toward generalist practice at both the BSW and MSW levels; however, graduate programs are more likely to provide any specialized education and training (if it occurs at all) (Holosko, 1995).

As noted by legions of social work authors who have debated *ad infinitum* the generalist-specialist issue, the question of what specifically constitutes a generalist versus specialist curriculum is germane to it. Certainly, one course, a practicum, and perhaps a term paper in gerontology does not make anyone a "specialist" (Erickson & Erickson, 1989). Also, one must be mindful that specialty courses or specialty fields of practice do not constitute specialized education and training (Brengarth, 1981). Without sinking too deep into the nuances of this issue, the chapters in this text remind us that we have much to learn about how to practise effectively with the elderly and much of this learning is not being offered in most North American schools of social work.

However one perceives this issue, it appears that education and training must go beyond traditional learning objectives in a curriculum that enhances a student's knowledge, values, and skills and moves toward developing self-awareness, compassion, and a sense of more humanism among social work students. Thus, issues such as death and dying, intergenerational families, intrapsychic awareness assessing capacity, dealing with complex ethical issues, communication skills, tolerance, cultural awareness, attitude shaping, and teaching social workers how to become competent in two to three practice interventive repertoires that are used with the elderly need to be addressed. The extent to which current formal or continuing professional education and training can provide such learning seems uncertain at this point in time. Within the future, however, we (the profession) must take the responsibility for such educational initiatives if we are serious about our commitment to providing minimally competent care for elderly persons.

VI.   Concluding Remarks

Gerontological social work practice holds a promising future for our profession. The future directions noted in this chapter are but a few of many challenges we will face in the next decade and beyond. We believe that social work has much to offer. However, it needs to better orient itself to the needs of the elderly, educate and train its entry-level professionals in more comprehensive and unique ways, and promote and market its skills and competencies in more dynamic ways. Both indirect and direct practitioners will face very real challenges of working effectively in another era of belt-tightening and economic constraint. The time is now for the profession to meet these and future challenges and the sooner we throw ourselves into the mix, the better. We [the authors and editors] feel that we have something special and important to offer this field. Let's not get bogged down by conceptualizing it but by proactively going out and doing it, and to beat the drum one final time (at the expense of overkill) ... the *future is now*!

References

Bloom, M. (1981). *Primary prevention, the possible science*. Englewood Cliffs: Prentice-Hall.

Brengarth, J. (1981). What is "special" about specialization? *Health and Social Work*, 5(2), 91–94.

Erickson, G.D. & Erickson, R. (1989). An overview of social work practice in health care settings. In M. Holosko & P. Taylor (eds.), *Social work practice in health care settings*, pp. 3–19. Toronto: Canadian Scholars' Press.

Holosko, M.J. (1995). The inclusion of gerontology content into undergraduate social work curricula in Australia and New Zealand. *Gerontology and Geriatrics Education*, 15(4), 5–20.

Holosko, M.J. (2003). The history of the working definition of practice. *Research on Social Work Practice*, 13(2), 400–408.

Holosko, M.J. & Dunlop, J. (1989). *A program evaluation of the interorganizational family violence project*. Chatham: The Chatham-Kent Women's Centre.

Holosko, M.J., Feit, M.D., & Bulcke, G. (1998). Health care prevention: Real or rhetoric? *Journal of Health and Social Policy*, 10(1), 101–104.

Jurkowski, E. & Tracy, M. (2000). Social policy and the aged: Implications for health planning, health education, and health promotion. *The Health Education Monograph Series 2000*, 18(2), 20–26.

ABOUT THE EDITORS

Michael J. Holosko is Professor of Social Work at the University of Windsor. He has taught in schools of social work (primarily), nursing, public administration, and applied social science in Canada, the United States, Hong Kong, Australia, and the U.S. Virgin Islands. For the past 24 years, he has been a consultant to a variety of large and small health and human service organization in the areas of: program evaluation, outcomes, organizational development, communication, leadership, conflict resolution, and stress management. He has published numerous monographs, chapters, articles, and texts in the areas of evaluation, health care, gerontology, social policy, and music intervention. He is on the editorial boards of: *Research of Social Work Practice, Journal of Health and Social Policy, Journal of Human Behaviour and Social Environment, the Hong Kong Journal of Social Work,* and the *Journal of Evidence-Based Social Work Practice.* He has served on numerous boards of directors for a variety of local, provincial, federal, and international human service agencies, including Health and Welfare Canada's Research Advisory Committee. In the past years he has taken his concerns for advocacy and social justice to the airwaves where he is billed as "The Community Doctor" on AM800 CKLW and The New WI out of Windsor, Ontario, Canada.

Marvin D. Feit is Professor and Dean of the Ethelyn R. Strong School of Social Work at Norfolk State University. He has taught social work graduate and undergraduate courses in administration and treatment and served as a consultant to a variety of health and human service organizations for over 30 years. His areas of expertise are financial management, administration, group work, substance abuse, and health care. He has published many chapters, articles, monographs, and books over the years, including: *The Management and Administration of Drug and Alcohol Programs, Evaluation of Employee Assistance Programs,*

Adolescent Substance Abuse, Capturing the Power of Diversity, Health and Social Policy, and *Financial Management in Human Services.* He is also a founding editor of the *Journal of Health and Social Policy,* the *Journal of Human Behaviour in the Social Environment,* and the *Journal of Evidence-Based Social Work Practice,* all published through the Haworth Press.

LIST OF CONTRIBUTORS

Austin, Carol D., PhD, University of Calgary, Calgary, AB
Birnie-Marino, Susan, MSW, RSW, Regional Mental Health Care, London, ON
Bobyk-Krumins, Jacqueline, MSW, Children's Aid Society, Windsor, ON
Cuevas-Feit, Nuria, PhD, Norfolk State University, Norfolk, VA
Dicks, Barbara, PhD, University of Connecticut, West Hartford, CT
Fabino, Len, FCS, RN, Port Perry, ON
Feit, Marvin D., PhD, Norfolk State University, Norfolk, VA
Fitch, Virginia, PhD, University of Akron, Akron, OH
Gallant, Melanie, MA, doctoral candidate, University of Windsor, Windsor, ON
Giannetti, Vincent J., PhD, Duquesne University, Pittsburgh, PA
Green, Janice, MSSA, deceased, OH
Greive, Jane L., MSW, RSW, Saskatoon Health Region, Lanigan, SK
Hinkson, Debra, MSW, retired, OH
Holosko, D. Ann, MSW, MEd, St. John's Senior Community Center, Detroit, MI
Holosko, Michael J., PhD, University of Windsor, Windsor, ON
Jurkowski, Elaine T., PhD, Southern Illinois University, Carbondale, IL
Kemp, Margery, MSW, Shawnee Alliance for Seniors, Carterville, IL
Kindiak, Darlene H., MSW, RSW, Clinical Legal Coordinator, St. Joseph's Healthcare, Hamilton, ON
Kleiner, Fran, MSW, RSW, Baycrest Centre for Geriatric Care, Toronto, ON
Kopstein, Rhoda, MSW, retired, Toronto, ON
Lagunoff, Joyce, MSW, RSW, Baycrest Centre for Geriatric Care, Toronto, ON

Leslie, Donald R., PhD, University of Windsor, Windsor, ON
Leslie, Kaye, Scotia Bank Group, Toronto, ON
MacKenzie, Patricia, PhD, University of Victoria, Victoria, BC
Madsen, Victoria A., MA, St. Joseph's Centre for Mountain Health
    Services, Hamilton, ON
Martyn, Ron, PhD candidate, Silver Meridian Consulting and Training
    in LTC, Courtice, ON
McClelland, Robert W., PhD, University of Calgary, Calgary, AB
Nichols, Sally, LSW, retired, OH
Patchner, Lisa S., PhD, Ball State University, Muncie, IN
Patchner, Michael A., PhD, Indiana University-Purdue University,
    Indianapolis, IN
Patterson, Susan, BSW, Egyptian Area Agency on Aging, Carterville,
    IL
Randall, Glen E., MBA, PhD candidate, McMaster University, Hamilton,
    ON
Slivinske, Lee, PhD, Youngstown State University, Youngstown, OH
Smith, Tamara L., PhD candidate, Institute of Gerontology, SUNY,
    Albany, NY
Soifer, Ahuva, MSW, CSW, retired, Hamilton, ON
St. John, Natalie, MSW, RSW, Youth Court Program, Newmarket, ON
Taylor, Laura, PhD, University of Windsor, Windsor, ON
Toseland, Ronald W., PhD, Institute of Gerontology, SUNY, Albany,
    NY
Urman, Sorele, MSW, RSW, private practice, Toronto, ON
Venturini, Vincent, MSW, Mississippi Valley State, Itta Bena, MS
Watt, Susan, DSW, CSW, McMaster University, Hamilton, ON
Wheeler, Judith, MSW, In-Touch Consulting, Essex, ON
White, Linda J., MSW, RSW, Canada Customs and Revenue Agency,
    Windsor, ON
Zinoman, Michele, MSW, Institute of Gerontology, SUNY, Albany,
    NY